Care of the mentally disordered offender in the community

Edited by

Dr Alec Buchanan

Senior lecturer
Department of Forensic Psychiatry
Institute of Psychiatry
London, UK

D0770733

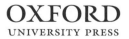
OXFORD
UNIVERSITY PRESS

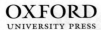
OXFORD
UNIVERSITY PRESS

Great Clarendon Street, Oxford OX2 6DP

Oxford University Press is a department of the University of Oxford.
It furthers the University's objective of excellence in research, scholarship,
and education by publishing worldwide in

Oxford New York

Auckland Bangkok Buenos Aires Cape Town
Chennai Dar es Salaam Delhi Hong Kong Istanbul Karachi
Kolkata Kuala Lumpur Madrid Melbourne Mexico City Mumbai Nairobi
São Paulo Shanghai Singapore Taipei Tokyo Toronto

with an associated company in Berlin

Oxford is a registered trade mark of Oxford University Press
in the UK and in certain other countries

Published in the United States
by Oxford University Press Inc., New York

© Oxford University Press, 2002

The moral rights of the author have been asserted

Database right Oxford University Press (maker)

First published 2002

A catalogue record for this title is available from the British Library

Library of Congress Cataloging in Publication Data
Care of the mentally disordered offender in the community / edited by Alec Buchanan.
(Oxford medical publications)
Includes bibliographical references and index.
1. Mentally ill offenders—Mental health services. 2. Community mental health
services. I. Buchanan, Alec. II. Series.
[DNLM: 1. Community Mental Health Services—Risk Management. 2. Ambulatory
Care–legislation & jurisprudence–Risk Management. 3. Mental Disorders–Risk
Management. 4. Public Policy–Risk Management. 5. Sex Offenses–legislation &
jurisprudence–Risk Management. WA 305 C271 2001]
RC451.4.P68 C374 2001 362.2'2'086927–dc21 2001036221

ISBN 0 19 263058 X (Pbk. : alk. paper)

10 9 8 7 6 5 4 3 2 1

Typeset in Minion
by Footnote Graphics, Warminster, Wiltshire
Printed in Great Britain
on acid-free paper by
T.J. International Ltd., Padstow, Cornwall

OXFORD MEDICAL PUBLICATIONS

Care of the mentally disordered offender in the community

Whilst every effort has been made to ensure that the contents of this book are as complete, accurate and up to date as possible at the date of writing, Oxford Univeristy Press is not able to give any guarantee or assurance that such is the case. Readers are urged to take appropriately qualified medical advice in all cases. The information in this book is intended to be useful to the general reader, but should not be used as a means of self-diagnosis or for the prescription of medication.

To Calum and Anna

Editor's preface and acknowledgements

I have been surprised by the degree to which the contributors have noted the same things and interpreted them differently. I have chosen not to intervene, not out of dedication to editorial catholicism or parsimony, but because I think that, both within disciplines and across them, this is a subject where a range of ideas have currency. I am indebted to Adrian Grounds, Paul Bowden and Graham Robertson, who discussed with me the outline for the book, and to Philip Joseph and David James, who helped me to assemble the present company.

Contents

Part 3 **The relationship between psychiatric services for mentally disordered offenders and other agencies**

List of contributors

Dr Alec Buchanan,
Senior lecturer,
Department of Forensic Psychiatry,
Institute of Psychiatry,
London, UK

Professor Joan Busfield,
Department of Sociology,
University of Essex,
Colchester, UK

Dr Philip Fennell,
Reader in law,
Cardiff Law School,
Cardiff, UK

Dr Claire Henderson,
Medical Research Council training fellow,
Health Service Research Department,
Institute of Psychiatry,
London, UK

Dr Frank Holloway,
Consultant psychiatrist and
clinical director,
South London and Maudsley NHS Trust,
London, UK

Ian Jewesbury,
Formerly assistant secretary,
Department of Health,
London, UK

Dr Andrew McCulloch,
Director of Policy,
Sainsbury Centre for Mental Health,
London, UK

Dr James McGuire,
Senior lecturer in clinical psychology
Department of Psychology,
University of Liverpool,
Liverpool, UK

Professor Paul Mullen,
Clinical director,
Victorian Institute of Forensic
Mental Health,
Victoria, Australia

Dr Edward Mulvey,
Professor of psychology,
Western Psychiatric Institute and Clinic,
University of Pittsburgh School of
Medicine,
Pittsburgh PA, USA

Dr Kingsley Norton,
Director,
Henderson Hospital,
Sutton, UK

Professor Nikolas Rose,
Department of Sociology,
Goldsmiths College,
University of London,
London, UK

Dr Jennifer Skeem,
Assistant professor of psychology,
University of Nevada,
Las Vegas NV, USA

Dr Jeffrey Swanson,
Associate professor of psychiatry,
Department of Psychiatry and
Behavioral Sciences,
Duke University,
Durham NC, USA

Dr Marvin Swartz,
Professor of psychiatry,
Department of Psychiatry and
Behavioral Sciences,
Duke University,
Durham NC, USA

Professor Graham Thornicroft,
Head,
Health Service Research Department,
Institute of Psychiatry,
London, UK

Dr David Tidmarsh,
Formerly consultant psychiatrist,
Broadmoor Hospital,
Crowthorne, UK

James Tighe,
Clinical research fellow,
Oxleas NHS Trust,
Bexley, UK

Dr Michael Travis,
Lecturer,
Section of Clinical Neuropharmacology,
Institute of Psychiatry,
London, UK

Dr Jonathan Vince,
Consultant forensic psychiatrist,
Springfield University Hospital,
London, UK

Victoria Yeates,
Senior lecturer,
School of Law,
University of Glamorgan,
Pontypridd, UK

Introduction

Paul E. Mullen

Risk assessment and risk management now occupy the centre of the mental health stage. This is impacting on community mental health services who, in practice, manage the majority of mentally abnormal offenders, and to whom falls the responsibility of predicting and preventing further violent and criminal acts. This new imperative has emerged at a time when community care is not infrequently blamed by the media and by politicians for a supposed increase in the rate of acts of violence by mentally disturbed individuals (see Chapter 4). As this book's contributions amply illustrate, the emerging emphasis on managing mentally disordered people who have an increased probability of acting violently with the aim of minimising such aggression is neither a cause for innocent rejoicing nor is it an unmitigated disaster. This book is about how this new emphasis has come about, how it affects clinical practice and, most importantly, how to respond to this new reality in a manner which extracts benefits for patients. Equally it is in part about the dangers inherent in an over-enthusiastic and uncritical assumption of the technologies and ideologies imminent in the new culture of risk and blame.

The debates which used to rage over whether the mentally ill were dangerous, and if so how to recognise that unfortunate quality, were gradually replaced in the 1990s by discussion of risk assessment and risk management (Monahan 1988, Snowden 1997, Mullen in press; also see chapters 2, 5 and 6). This shift in terminology is often presented as a product of the progress of knowledge. In the past, dangerousness was all too often regarded as the property of an individual, as uncertain in manifestation as it was unchangeable in practice. Employing the notion of risk, rather than dangerousness, should move attention from qualities to probabilities, and from the immutable to the inherently variable. The language of dangerousness has been transmuted into the language of risk which has the comforting resonance of the actuarial, the calculable and the avoidable. Risk management is about applying the knowledge generated from risk assessment to minimising the actual occurrence of violent and criminal behaviour.

The language of risk came relatively late to the field of mental health. The notion of risk and risk management first surfaced in the 1970s in the context of concerns amongst large corporations or governmental agencies about being blamed for the damage their activities inflicted on individuals and on the environment. Soon, it was not only governments and big business which were held responsible for increasing the risks to the individual citizen's health, it was also professions, most particularly the health professions. Mary Douglas (1992) wrote of the new culture of blame "we are ..

almost ready to treat every death as chargeable to someone's account, every accident as caused by someone's criminal negligence, every sickness a threatened prosecution. Whose fault? is the first question … then what damages? What compensation? What restitution?" (pg 15-16). The response of corporations, governments and professionals who are being increasingly blamed for the impact of their actions on others was to resort to risk assessment and risk management strategies. Risk assessment aimed at estimating the exposure of the individual, or corporation, to future claims. Risk management attempted to obliterate, or mitigate, the chances of damage occurring or, alternatively, of being held responsible for such ills and misfortunes.

Frank Holloway (see Chapter 10) notes that the culture of blame is influencing mental health policy in the UK which has, in his words, "become peculiarly and increasingly dominated by a preoccupation with the risks that people with a mental illness present to themselves and others". Any damage or distress which occurs to someone who is, or has been, a client of a mental health service is at risk of being transformed into a preventable tragedy for which professionals are to be held responsible. Rose (1996) has suggested that mental health professionals are increasingly controlled through standards, audits and inquiries which not only regulate their professional conduct, but hold them personally responsible for unwanted outcomes. Blame is all too easily shifted from politicians and administrators, responsible for poorly financed and inadequately managed services, to individual clinicians, who are judged to have failed to follow procedures. In response, professionals are increasingly pushed into a situation where they regard their patients first and foremost as the embodiments of varying degrees of risk which it is their duty to control. In the area of the risk of violence to others the mental health patient is in danger of being metamorphosed from an individual who evokes our professional concern into someone who presents a greater, or lesser, risk of inflicting harm on others. The mental health professional becomes not the mediator of science and skill to the benefit of the patient but the protector and rescuer of unknown others from the potential threat presented by their patient. Risk management one might have hoped would have been primarily about improving the patient's situation but all too often it seems driven by the desire to reduce the organization's and the professional's future liability. Time honoured ethical imperatives, like confidentiality and the avoidance of harm, tend to wilt in the face of the supposed new duties to warn and to rescue (for further discussion see Chapter 10).

There was a time, not so long ago, when issues of dangerousness rarely impinged on mental health professionals in general psychiatry. The assessment and management of dangerousness used to be a piece of arcane clinical alchemy to be performed by specialist forensic psychiatrists or psychologists. Today, in it's new guise, risk assessment and management has established a central role in much of mental health practice. Risk assessments are no longer the exclusive domain of the forensic specialist but are rapidly becoming one of the skills defining clinical competence for all mental health professionals. The rise to prominence of risk assessment and risk management, as Fennell &

Yeates (Chapter 13) point out, has occurred at a time when the mental health field is also coming under increasing influence from ideologies around populist retributivism and the protection of the rights of victims, or potential victims. To the fear of blame are added increasingly coercive and punitive attitudes towards deviance of all types. There is also a black and white approach favoured by the popular media which sees perpetrators and victims as inhabiting entirely different worlds, not just at the moment of victimisation but for all time. The mentally disordered all too easily are placed into the role of potential perpetrator in need of containment with the mental health professional being held responsible for ensuring such control. Understanding the cultural and ideological roots of the increasing hegemony exerted by this rhetoric of risk in no way frees the individual mental health professional from the need to function in the new environment.

It seems so obvious as to be self evident that mental health professionals should consider the possibility that their patients may not only harm themselves but harm others. It is not just coroners and litigation lawyers but the media and many fellow professionals who discern a duty for the clinician to prevent their patients attacking, or otherwise incommoding, their fellow citizens. Surely it is obvious that the chances of a mentally disordered person acting violently should be carefully evaluated and every step taken to prevent such a consequence. It is, perhaps, not quite as obvious that a central, if not the primary, responsibility of a mental health professional is to the wider community rather than their patient. It is not entirely obvious how a responsibility to predict risk is to be discharged. It is certainly not obvious how a clinician should act if they do suspect their patient is more probable to act violently. And finally, it is far from obvious that we should allow concerns about the risk which some of our patients may present to others to become a major determinant of our approach to all our patients.

Assessing and managing the risk of future violence is often bracketed with assessing and managing the risk of suicide. I have to plead guilty to being one of those who has in the past glibly asserted such a correspondence. Though there are similarities in the proper approach to assessing and managing the probability of both suicidal behaviour and violent behaviour the differences are at least as important. If we take for example a young person with schizophrenia. The chances of their killing themselves may be as high as 1 in 10 but the chances of them killing someone else is far less than 1 in 1000 (Hafner and Böker 1982, Wallace et al. 1998). This difference in level of risk, quite apart from its obvious relevance to likely future harm, also profoundly effects the chances of predicting such future behaviour with any degree of precision. (For further discussion Chapters 2 & 5). One by-product of this new 'age of risk' is that professionals need to become more mathematically literate if they are to understand and effectively employ probability estimates. One contributor to this book writes that when patients make threats to kill the outcome is surprisingly benign as only 1% carry out their threat. The chances of an individual committing a homicide varies from country to country but in most industrialised nations it is between 2 & 5 per 100,000 (i.e. 0.0002% to 0.0005%). One percent represents, therefore, an astronomical inflation in risk. The usual errors tend, however, to be in the opposite direction: assuming, because, for example, homicide rates in schizophrenia are 4 to 10 times higher than expected (Taylor & Gunn 1984, Eronen *et al.* 1997, Wallace *et al.* 1998), that identifying in advance those individuals at high risk is practical. Such predictions would require unrealisable precision in evaluating future probabilities. Risk assessment and management to be a practical method of crime reduction has either to focus, as Joan Busfield (see Chapter 4) indicates, less on individuals and more on populations, or on behaviours which occur with sufficient frequency in the target population (e.g. threatening behaviours or pushing and shoving).

The implications for the patient of being placed in a high risk category for suicidal or violent behaviour, though in theory not necessarily diverging are, in practice, quite different. Suicide risk evokes primarily greater care and concern and usually only secondarily coercive responses. Risks of violence are prone to evoke withdrawal more often than greater engagement, and various forms of coerced containment tend to come high on the list of responses. Mental health professionals assume, perhaps too readily, that self destructive intentions are the product of mental disorder. Conversely they often assume, with even more ill considered alacrity, that violent intentions are the product not of illness but of personality or moral failings. Given these different constructions, one tending to illness and one to wickedness, different professional responses are likely to be engendered. One might expect in these risk averse times that patients judged to present a high probability of acting aggressively would attract particular and intensive clinical interest. Sadly this is often far from the case. Frank Holloway (Chapter 10) and Alec Buchanan (Chapter 11) both discuss how mentally disordered offenders find themselves regarded by mental health services not as priorities for treatment but as distinctly undesirable. When they present, such patients may simply be denied services or deflected towards alternative providers (on a good day social services, on a bad, the criminal justice system). As Alec Buchanan notes, no one has found a way of making a doctor, or indeed a service, look after a patient who they in their wisdom have deemed "inappropriate" or "in need of services which we are unable to provide". Perhaps the greatest task facing academics and educators who aim to make risk management work for patients is to change the culture amongst mental health professionals. Currently this culture is prone to resort to de-legitimising the mentally abnormal offender by labelling them offender not patient, or as personality disordered with no 'formal' mental illness (irrespective of how many psychotic experiences they report). All too often the favoured option is to banish them from our services. In practice adequate care for such patients will only be provided through the development of forensic mental health services staffed by professionals whose pride is in caring for those whose disorder causes, or is accompanied by, potentially serious antisocial behaviours.

The Pandora's box of assessing and managing the probability of future violence in our patients is well and truly open. However misbegotten we may believe it to be, it is no longer an option to distance ourselves from the process. The clinician's liability based on failures to predict and manage future violence in their patients is now established.

In many states in the US the Tarasoff decision, and its progeny, have been approved by civil courts awarding damages against clinicians for failure to predict, failure to prevent and failure to warn (Carstensen 1994). Though the Tarasoff decision carries little, if any, legal weight outside of the US, it's ghost haunts clinicians throughout the English speaking world where intense, if largely specious, arguments are advanced over duties to warn and to rescue. In the UK homicide enquiries have cut a swathe through forensic psychiatric clinicians, and not a few of their generalist colleagues, as they are publicly pilloried for their failures to prevent the murderous acts of their patients. (e.g. Ritchie *et al.* 1994). Media and coroners often combine to similar effect. Such developments should elevate risk management to near the top of the agendas of both clinicians and risk averse administrators.

Traditionally, predicting dangerousness was an activity in which clinical experience was paramount. Risk assessment in contrast is often regarded as an essentially actuarial endeavour (Monahan 1999). A risk factor is simply an empirically established association with the unwanted outcome. To be a risk factor does not require a causal connection but merely a significant association to the predicted future event. Risk management in contrast necessitates identifying factors which can be influenced so as to alter outcomes. At least for health professionals this should be the implication. For courts and parole boards risk management may amount to simply incapacitating the risky person by incarceration but this can never be an ethically justified approach for a health professional. Risk factors are ideally events, or states of affairs, which can be established by observation and inquiry and the recognition of which requires little or no processing by the evaluater. Actuarial approaches aspire to a reduction to the administration of standardised questionnaires (instruments) which, based on the scores, divide the target population into high, low and medium categories of risk. In theory the actuarial approach should provide valid, reproducible, value free predictions.

There is a substantial literature on the use of actuarial methods in the prediction of recidivism among convicted offenders (Quinsey *et al.* 1998). It is asserted that the risk factors established among offender populations as predictive of future violence are directly applicable to psychiatric patients (Bonta *et al.* 1998). This has smoothed the way for an uncritical transfer of instruments developed on offender populations into the mental health field. Among such instruments in current use are the Psychopathy Check List and the Violence Risk Appraisal Guide (Hare *et al.* 1990, Hare 1998, Harris & Rice 1997). The advocates for these instrumentalities are not overly troubled by doubt or reservation about effectiveness and appropriateness. Hare (1998) asserts psychopathy as measured by the Psychopathy Check List is the single most important clinical construct in the criminal justice system. In its modified form it is claimed to be useable in both civil and forensic mental health patients (Hart *et al.* 1994). Quinsey and colleagues (1998), though less sanguine about the Psychopathy Check List, are absolutely certain about the value of their Violence Risk Appraisal Guide. This they write it is a "guarantee (of) both reliability and validity" (p165) and "further weakens any remaining support for the idea that clinical intuition (or indeed any variables relying on unstructured clinical judgement) can yield accurate predictions of violent recidivism" (pg 164-165).

Most existing attempts to advance risk assessment instruments depend on what are presumed to be abiding characteristics, like psychopathy or a history of antisocial behaviours. These constants contribute to a once and for all estimate of the probability of future violent, or criminal, activities. Skeem and Mulvey (Chapter 6) characterise such approaches as static and their predictions as estimates of ongoing risk status. But they emphasise that the potential to act violently is the product of complex reciprocal interactions between an individual and current situational variables. Skeem and Mulvey regard violence as primarily a transactional process involving interactions between an individual and their environment. The individual's current risk status may be influenced by static and abiding characteristics of the individual but will be best predicted by understanding the dynamics of the ever changing interactions between the individuals vulnerabilities and the environment. This process seems to require at least a partial rehabilitation of the derived clinical approach.

The problems associated with static risk factors are not confined to their failure to appropriately encompass the ever-changing nature of the probability of violent behaviour. The static factors advocated as predictors of risk may be historical and therefore essentially unchangeable (i.e. they are the abiding stigmata of violence risk). Further, once ascertained, the "high risk" patient, or prisoner, is in danger of carrying this label with them for the rest of their lives. The MacArthur Violence Risk Assessment Study, which involves many of the leading researchers in this area, have advanced an actuarial tool for assessing violence risk (Monahan *et al.* 2000). The risk factors on which their assessments were based included historical, and therefore immutable, elements, such as, seriousness of prior arrests, father used drugs, legal status, and "parents engaged in physical fights with one another when the patient was growing up" (pg 317). Fathers recreational choices and the quality of parental relationships are not only beyond change, and therefore in principle unmanageable, but they are also related to the behaviour of others of which the subject may have been a victim. The direct use of histories of abuse and neglect in the subject's childhood as risk factors would be even more egregious, amounting potentially to a true re-victimisation.

If risk management is to emerge out of risk assessments; if risk management is to amount to more than coercion and incapacitation; if risk management is to be a legitimate activity for health professionals, then, assessments must focus on establishing those vulnerabilities contributing to offending which are open to modification through appropriate health related treatments. Health professionals have to approach risk management as an exercise in therapeutics in which decreased symptoms and improved function are the primary aims, with risk minimisation being a by-product. Ultimately, mental health professionals can best contribute to the overall safety and peace of their communities by acting as therapists, not as jailers.

References

Bonta J, Law M, Hanson K. (1998) The prediction of criminal and violent recidivism among mentally disordered offenders: A meta analysis. *Psychological Bulletin* 122: 123–142

Carstensen P C. (1994) The evolving duty of mental health professionals to third parties: a doctrinal and institutional examination. *International Journal of Law and Psychiatry* 17: 1–42

Douglas M. (1992) *Risk and Blame: Essays in Cultural Theory.* London, Routledge

Eronen M, Tiilhonen J, Hakola P. (1997) Psychiatric disorders and violent behaviour. *International Journal of Psychiatry in Clinical Practice* 1: 179–188

Hafner H, Böker W. (1982) *Crimes of Violence by Mentally Abnormal Offenders* (Trans. H. Marshall). Cambridge: Cambridge University Press

Hare R D, Harpar T J, Hakstian A R, Forth A E, Hart S D, Newman J. (1990) The revised psychopathy checklist: Reliability and factor structure. Psychological Assessment: *A Journal of Consulting and Clinical Psychology* 2: 338–341

Hare R D. (1998) The Hare PCL-R: Some issues concerning its use and misuse. *Legal and Criminological Psychology* 3: 99–112

Hart S D, Hare R D, Forth A E. (1994) Psychopathy as a risk marker for violence: Development and variation of a screening version of the revised psychopathy check list. In: Monahan J, Steadman HJ, eds *Violence and Mental Disorder*. University of Chicago Press, Chicago, 81–98

Harris G, Rice M. (1997) Risk Appraisal and Management of Violent Behavior. *Psychiatric Services* 48: 1168–1176

Monahan J. (1988) Risk Assessment of Violence Among the Mentally Disordered: Generating Useful Knowledge. *International Journal of Law and Psychiatry* 11: 249–257

Monahan J. (1999) Clinical and Actuarial Predictions of Violence. In: Faigman D, Kaye D, Saks M, Sanders J, eds. *Modern Scientific Evidence: The Law and Science of Expert Testimony*. St Paul, Minnesota: West Publishing Company, 41–49

Monahan J, Steadman, HJ, Applebaum PS, Robbins PC, Mulvey EP, Silver E, Roth LH, Grisso T. (2000) Developing a clinically useful actuarial tool for assessing violence risk. *British Journal of Psychiatry* 176: 312–319

Mullen P.E (in press) Dangerousness, Risk and the Prediction of Probability. In: Oxford Textbook of Psychiatry. Eds. M G Gelder, J J López-Ibor, N C Andreasen. Oxford: Oxford University Press

Quinsey V L, Harris G T, Rice M E, Cormier C A. (1998) *Violent Offenders: Appraising and Managing Risk*. Washington D.C.: American Psychological Association

Ritchie JH, Dick D, Lingham R. (1994) *The report of the inquiry into the care and treatment of Christopher Clunis*. HMSO, London

Rose N. (1996) Psychiatry as a political science: advanced liberalism and the administration of risk. *History of the Human Sciences* 9: 1–23

Snowden P. (1997) Practical aspects of clinical risk assessment and management. *British Journal of Psychiatry* 170 (suppl. 32): 32–34

Taylor P T, Gunn J. (1984) Violence and Psychosis: I. Risk of violence among psychotic men. *British Medical Journal* 288: 1945–1949

Wallace C, Mullen P E, Burgess P, Palmer S, Ruschena D, Browne C. (1998) Serious criminal offending and mental disorder: Case linkage study. *British Journal of Psychiatry* 172: 477–484

Part 1

The social, administrative and clinical context in which mentally disordered offenders are cared for in the community

Chapter 1

Society, madness and control

Nikolas Rose

Introduction

What role does psychiatry play in contemporary strategies of control? How do psychiatrists and their institutions operate within all those ways of thinking and acting that aim to eliminate, minimize, manage or contain types of conduct that authorities consider to be undesirable? Since the middle of the nineteenth century, two great assemblages for the control of pathological conduct have taken shape in western societies. On the one hand stands the criminal justice system with its laws, codes and jurisprudential arguments, its constables, judges, lawyers and warders, its judgements of guilt and innocence, its prisons and reformatories. On the other stands the psychiatric system, with its diagnostic systems and its theories of aetiology and prognosis, its psychiatrists, psychologists, nurses and therapists, its diagnoses and treatments, its hospitals and clinics. Most accounts suggest some kind of basic contradiction between the rationales of these two 'complexes'. Within the domain of law and penality, the subject of regulation, the criminal, is apparently deemed a rational actor to be controlled, capable of being incarcerated, punished—and possibly reformed—for his or her criminal actions. Within the domain of psychiatry, the subject of regulation is apparently considered to be a sick person to be cured, requiring care, treatment and rehabilitation. Within the one, then, the questions posed to the problematic individual are 'what law have you broken?' and 'what do you deserve?'. Within the other, the questions posed are 'what kind of a person are you?' and 'how can we help you?'. For a hundred and fifty years, lawyers, psychiatrists and philosophers have explored and tried to clarify or even resolve this apparent philosophical, constitutional and juridical contradiction.

This image of a fundamental opposition between the subject of law and the subject of psychiatry—legalism versus welfarism, punishment versus treatment, the austerity of the rule of law versus the expansive obligations of care—is not altogether misleading. Its emblematic moments—the famous trials of the first half of the nineteenth century—Hadfield, Bellingham, M'Naghten—where lawyers and doctors contested their respective powers and capacities to understand, judge and respond to 'dangerous individuals'—have cast a long shadow. In different ways some of these foundational controversies over the attribution of responsibility and culpability are still being played out (on the nineteenth century trials, see Smith 1981). But, in practice, these two domains were never so distinct—they intersected, interacted and supported one another at a multitude of cross-over points. At the level of their actual operation, one does not find a conflict between two 'systems'—historically or today—so much as an array of heterogeneous and internally contradictory practices and policies pursued in different locales with different kinds of relations and conflicts running across them (cf. Johnstone 1996). Since at least the middle of the nineteenth century, judicial and penal procedures have become caught up with the diagnostic question—the criminal is no longer merely the judicial subject of the crime, but must be *understood* if the verdict is to be fully legitimate and sentencing is to be appropriate (Pasquino 1991). And since that time too, psychiatric judgement has had to concern itself with a problem that is penal in its implications—what might this person do, and how can that propensity be controlled: how, that is to say, can this person be *managed* in the interests of social defence or public safety (Foucault 1978). For about a hundred and fifty years, those who some now term 'forensic' psychiatrists have claimed, or been given, the task of managing a multiplicity of points of tension, friction and conflict within this dual logic of control. Thus one way to begin an exploration of the contemporary place of psychiatry in strategies of control is to consider the role of 'forensic psychiatry'.

Forensic psychiatry unlocked

Across the English-speaking world, and perhaps elsewhere, the last decades of the twentieth century saw a considerable expansion of forensic psychiatry: increasing numbers of those who used this term to describe themselves, the growth of professional organizations, government reports calling for improvement and expansion in forensic psychiatric services, conferences, textbooks, journals, training courses, the multiplication of the sites in which forensic psychiatric activities take place and so forth. In the process, forensic psychiatry was transformed. It is no longer, if it ever was, focused exclusively on a small and exceptional group of 'mentally disordered offenders'. It embraces all those offenders or suspects who are suspected of being or thought to be acutely, chronically or even mildly 'mentally ill' including those who may be suffering from neuroses, have behavioural disorders, be personality disordered, be abusing alcohol or drugs, or who have committed certain types of offences believed to involve a component of psychiatric disturbance—sex offences, anti-social or aggressive conduct, child abuse and more. And it includes all those in touch with psychiatric services thought to actually present a threat to others, or to have the potential to present such a threat. Indeed, the very idea of 'forensic psychiatry' is thrown into question, for it now seems to be accepted that every practising psychiatrist inescapably deals with 'forensic' issues, not just assessing individuals referred from police, courts, prisons or special hospitals, not just being prepared to make reports to, or give evidence in court, not just dealing with individuals who have broken the law but are receiving psychiatric treatment in the community, but also evaluating almost every patient according to criteria of 'risk' that are explicitly or implicitly 'forensic', with an eye to their potential for ending up in the criminal justice system. What is the problem—or are the problems—to which forensic psychiatry now appears to be, claims to be, or is required to be a solution?

In one respect, the recent expansion of forensic psychiatry is surprising. It would be difficult to attribute it to some remarkable advance in either the knowledge base of the profession, or in the practical efficacy of forensic psychiatrists in the various tasks with which they are charged. Are they more effective or convincing in their judgements as to whether an accused person was 'responsible' for the offence which they are alleged to have committed? Are they more accurate in ascertaining whether an individual is competent to stand trial? Is their evidence in the courtroom less marked by controversy and less criticized and disputed by lawyers, the mass media and 'public opinion'? Are they better at making judgements of dangerousness—and hence of the necessity for individuals to be detained in secure provision under the various provisions of the Mental Health Acts and other legislation that requires such an assessment? Have they made advances in determining or providing appropriate regimes for prisoners who are mentally disordered? Have they agreed upon ways of defining, diagnosing or treating those who the law—and the mass media —term 'psychopaths': those today that psychiatrists prefer to consider under the category of 'anti-social personality disorder'? Have the accusations of ethnic bias in forensic psychiatric judgements and gender bias in treatment recommendations finally been answered? Have forensic psychiatrists achieved what some attempted in the first half of this century—a fully psychological theory of offending and a therapeutic practice for treating offenders, whether juvenile or adult, female or male? Even a sympathetic observer would be reluctant to answer all, perhaps any, of these questions in the affirmative. Of course, introductory textbooks for trainee doctors, general psychiatrists, psychiatric nurses, social workers, solicitors, probation officers and the like often present an account of forensic psychiatry in terms of a number of settled and routinized practices underpinned by accumulated professional wisdom. But, even being generous, the most a dispassionate observer could report was that, in each of these areas, research is under way, conflicting theories and hypotheses abound, competing programmes are suggested and occasionally implemented, and failure rather than success is the norm.

Yet, in another respect, the expansion of forensic psychiatry as a set of activities, a profession, a variety of claims and demands, is not in the least surprising. Professional ambitions and the like have undoubtedly played their part. But the conditions which made this growth possible are to be found in the changes that have taken place more generally within regimes of control. For the activities that we know as forensic psychiatry—or retrospectively unify and seek to codify under this name—do not manifest the unity of an academic discipline or sub-discipline. Forensic psychiatrists operate at all those disparate points where the coercive powers of law and its regimes of punishment seem insufficient to constrain troublesome individuals on the basis of what they have done, and must be supplemented or supplanted by psychiatric determination of who they are (cf. Owen 1991). And when the crime control complex and the psychiatric complex each mutate as radically as they have in the last decades of the twentieth century, it is inevitable that problems that seem to call for forensic psychiatry will also be reconfigured. Thus if we are to understand the expansion of contemporary forensic psychiatry, and its problems and dilemmas, we must try to map the nature of these transformations, and their implications for these transactional spaces that shape the problems of forensic psychiatry.

Many critics are tempted to make a rather simple evaluation of these developments: that forensic psychiatry is a new instance of power. They suggest that forensic psychiatry takes the strategy of the medicalization of deviance from general psychiatry; it uses this strategy to legitimate coercive treatment under the guise of therapy; it pathologises subjects who are merely different and who breach the assumptions about class, race and gender built into the prevailing norms of a society; it individualizes problems that actually arise as a result of the damage wrought upon individuals by an unjust and oppressive social system; it panders to the processes of stigmatization, scapegoating and moral panic that beset those with mental health problems in contemporary western societies. There is much truth in these simple slogans. But I do not think one can understand the role of forensic psychiatry today in isolation—it needs to be assessed in relation to the changing social obligations of psychiatry itself. Perhaps most significant has been the rise, within both crime control and psychiatry, of strategies for the assessment, management and control of *risk*.

Risk thinking and crime control

Risk thinking has certainly infused many recent changes in the rationalities and technologies of crime control. On the basis of detailed empirical investigation, Ericson and Haggerty (1997) claim that the role of the public police has been fundamentally restructured in terms of risk. They argue that policing is no longer principally focused upon investigating and solving crimes and apprehending criminals *ex post facto*. Rather, police are risk managers. Their principal aim is preventive—reducing the chances of criminal behaviour occurring. Police now work as advisors on risk management in public and private spaces, managing public order and disorder prospectively rather than reactively, mapping crime neighbourhood by neighbourhood and seeking to minimize it by targeted interventions aiming to increase the community's own risk management capacities. Police are involved in licensing and certifying security technology. Police advise on all aspects of environmental design—from the location of automatic cash machines to the provision of street lighting—from the perspective of reducing the risks of offending behaviour. More generally, Ericson and Haggerty suggest that almost all major institutions—education, welfare and social security, insurance, the retail industry, employers, the credit and banking sector etc.—have become organized around 'risk knowledge'—that is to say, attempts to assess, predict, minimize, control or manage in order to avoid undesirable events in the future.

The police are thus an institution organized around risk knowledge. They both shape and are shaped by the kinds of risk knowledge required by many others. Police have become 'risk knowledge workers'—'categories and classifications of risk communication and ... the technologies for communicating knowledge [about risk] internally and externally' prospectively structure the actions and deliberations of police and other professionals (Ericson and Haggerty 1997). Such risk classifications 'format' the gaze of the professional in a specific manner: they are more or less formalized rules which also shape the ways in which information is organized and presented into certain 'communication formats'. Risk, that is to say, is not just a language of communication. Risk becomes the means by which professionals think, act and justify their actions. These rationalities of risk 'format' the thought and practice of many other professionals. Like police, psychiatrists too have become knowledge workers. But, in many ways, the knowledge work of the psychiatrist is formatted by the criteria and demands made by others:

> Even in medicine the doctor on the ground is a subordinate of expert systems and those who manage them. He or she is one of many contributors to the expert system of risk management that creates the patient's dossier, and therefore loses control over particular outcomes as well as over the progress of cases (Ericson and Haggerty 1997)

And the 'risk-formatted knowledge' generated by psychiatrists is extracted, organized, packaged and communicated with consequences far removed from those of professional practice.

Macrosociologists, notably Ulrich Beck, have gone so far as to argue that we now live in a 'risk society' (Beck 1992). Risk society is no longer structured by the distribution of 'goods'—resources, wealth, class—but by the distribution of 'bads'—exposure to potential harms whether environmental, medical or psychological. It is a society whose anxieties are pervasively structured by fears of future dangers and attempts to avert them. This idea seems attractive when one considers the proliferation of the language of risk in the mass media, policy debates and advice about everything from diet to procreation. But the notion of 'risk society' obscures as much as it reveals. We need only to recall rates of infant mortality, changes in life expectancy, or waves of epidemic disease to doubt that our society is objectively 'more risky' than societies in the past. Nor is it useful to think of risk as a 'spirit of our age', structuring everything from public policy to personal experience. I think it is more useful to think of risk as a more modest and localized phenomenon—a *style of thought* that has come to characterize a variety of practices of regulation and management (Hacking 1991). It is a style of thought that seeks to bring the future into the present and make it calculable. It obliges authorities and individuals to take actions in the present in the light of beliefs and predictions about that future. It renders them potentially accountable at some future time for the success or failure of those actions in achieving their objectives or averting the unwanted. Risk thinking has proliferated, in part, because it can be deployed within very different rationalities. The nature, conceptualization and calculation of epidemiological risk, for example, differs from that of environmental risk, which differs from assessments of the risk of engineering failure, which differs again from the assessments of clinical risk, in particular medical procedures. And each of these forms of risk assessment, and these obligations of risk management, operates in a different problem space, and in relation to different kinds of strategies and objectives.

The rise of risk thinking in the crime control complex is an element in a wide ranging reshaping of control (Rose 2000). In the 1970s and early 1980s, some sociologists suggested that a general process of 'decarceration' was taking place, with the reduction of the populations of both prisons and asylums in the face of social, political and economic changes that rendered incarceration expensive, inefficient and unnecessary (notably Scull 1984). More detailed examination and international comparisons failed to show any relation between such developments and any supposed 'fiscal crisis'. More fundamentally, it soon became clear that these new strategies were no simple 'reduction' of control. Rather, a new configuration of control was taking shape that was no longer captured in the stark image of the carceral institution with its closed walls. As Cohen (1985) pointed out, the rise of provisions for the management, regulation and control of offenders—and psychiatric patients—outside the institutional enclosure of prison and hospital actually expanded the scope of control. It blurred the boundaries between the 'inside' and the 'outside' of the system of social control. It widened the net of control, bringing individuals into the field of formalized control mechanisms who would previously have been dealt with informally. It thinned the mesh, so that the 'net' of control caught smaller and smaller fish— individuals were brought into the new elements of the system, such as intensive community programmes, for violations which would previously have resulted in a one-off fine, non-invasive probation or a conditional discharge. The development of a whole range of community provisions, alternatives to incarceration and so forth did not reduce the prison population. In fact, it brought many more individuals into the web of control, which now encompassed smaller and smaller violations of the normative order. The spread of control mechanisms and techniques into the territory of everyday life also led to an intensification of the level of detail in which conduct is scrutinized and acted upon. For the first time, an individual's participation in the world of work was formally connected up with the discharging of penal obligations. And the minutiae of the behaviour of offenders, juveniles and even ex-offenders, their demeanour, time keeping and daily activities, were now monitored and tracked in 'the community'. Despite the rapid rise of the prison population in the UK and the USA, such trends have continued, for example in the use of electronic tagging techniques and curfews. At the close of the twentieth century, such programmes were further augmented by alternatives to custody such as reparation schemes, where the conduct of the offender is targeted by techniques designed to produce shame and remorse.

Cohen argued that, despite the shift he discerned, the pathological individual was still seen as distinct from the normal individual. The delinquent was still seen as someone with a deficit to be diagnosed and corrected. But this deficit was no longer understood as a deep internal flaw, a damaged psyche, that set the delinquent fundamentally apart from the law abiding citizen. Instead, pathological conduct was coming to be understood as arising from a lack of some acquired features of behaviour and capacities of personhood—the capacities necessary to manage existence in the external world: an absence of social skills, a failure of role competence, the lack of an appropriate moral code, an inability to obtain and hold down a job and the like.

More recently, Feely and Simon have claimed a new type of justice is taking shape on this open territory: a 'new penology' whose principle is that of 'actuarial justice', in which even the residual concern with responsibility, fault, moral sensibility, diagnosis or intervention and treatment of the individual offender is on the wane (Feely and Simon 1992, 1994). The new penology, they argue, concerns itself primarily with crime rates and probabilities, its principal techniques are those that seek to identify, classify and manage groupings, sub-populations or territories that manifest higher than average levels of crime. This is not a strategy that seeks to respond to particular deviants. It does not seek to normalize pathological individuals, to diagnose and treat the factors that lie internal to the criminal subject. It is a managerial attempt to regulate levels of deviance. It is actuarial in that it is concerned with the overall levels of undesirable events in a population at large. Rather than targeting and removing offenders from the social body, it seeks to manage potential offenders in place by shaping or reshaping the physical and social structures within which offending behaviour may or may not occur. Situational crime control, designing out crime through environmental measures, surveillance though closed circuit television cameras, security checks on credit and debit cards and the like all seek to reduce the overall probability of undesirable conduct. The new penology, then, does not aim to identify, apprehend, incarcerate, rehabilitate, reintegrate, retrain or provide employment for particular individuals. It seeks only to reduce rates of crime in populations, or risks posed by groups or sub-populations, by acting upon whatever factors seem to be correlated with increases or decreases in the risk of the acts in question taking place.

There is much of value in this analysis. But it is misleading in one respect. This has particular significance for the work of psychiatrists in relation to actual or potential subjects of the criminal law. Risk thinking certainly contains an actuarial dimension, directing attention to probabilities in populations. But this does not eliminate the demand for identification and management of particular risky individuals. In the practical deployment of risk management within contemporary control strategies, the reverse is true. In the complex territory of control that took shape in the closing decades of the twentieth century, individuals have to be assigned to, and administered across, a diversity of sites. Hence the decision points, and the demands for individual risk assessments and risk management, are multiplied. Professionals are increasingly obliged to assess the riskiness of individuals in order to make the decisions about their disposal in the present, with the aim of minimizing unwanted occurrences in the future. One source of the new demands on psychiatrists in relation to criminal justice arises from within this new dispersed and open field of corrections—or rather, from that grey area where the boundaries blur between criminal and psychiatric juris-dictions. Most significant here are all those points where the question is raised of 'diversion' from the apparatus of criminal justice to that of psychiatry: diversions to psychiatric services from the police station, remands to hospitals by the courts for psychiatric assessment, court-based schemes for psychiatric assessments of offenders to assess whether they should be diverted to psychiatric treatment before trial, or after trial and conviction, or given a psychiatric probation order. Peay and others have pointed to the potential 'net-widening' effects of all these provisions—that is to say, their tendency to lead to formal measures being taken for trivial offences, which might otherwise never have come before the courts, in the name of enhanced control and public safety (Peay 1994). Central to such net-widening potential is the assessment of risk. I will return to this later in this chapter.

If risk thinking reshapes responses to those at the lowest end of the risk continuum, it also reshapes ways of defining and responding to a set of problems that appear to be at the other end—those exceptions to normality and the constraints and obligations of its moral order that have long incited and frustrated psychiatrists. I refer here to those who one might term 'monstrous' individuals. Contemporary societies seem to be swept by waves of 'moral panics' that focus upon certain figures that seem to symbol-ize something in excess of the particular horror of their offences: psychopaths, sex offenders, paedophiles and child pornographers, calculating murderers, evil serial killers, intractably anti-social individuals. The imperative to act in relation to such individuals has a significance that is as much symbolic as instrumental. It forms part of what many perceive as a 'new punitiveness' in the politics of crime control (Garland in press; Pratt 2000). There are a number of elements to this new punitiveness. There is the widespread political use of harsh penal sanctions as a public display of political resolve in the face of the apparent intractability of the 'crime problem'. There is the inexorable rise of the prison populations in many western countries, notably in the USA, together with the abandonment of long-cherished beliefs about the reformative role of imprisonment. In the USA, and elsewhere, sentencing measures such as 'three strikes' clauses come into play to mandate life imprisonment for those who have proved unable or unwilling to manage themselves in the open territory of the commun-ity. At the same time, in the UK, the USA, New Zealand, Australia and elsewhere, preventive detention has been introduced, or is being contemplated , for certain 'risky individuals' who are considered to present an incorrigible or unacceptable threat to 'public safety'—whatever the actual statistical data may show of the relative levels of this 'threat' compared to others that are more mundane. And in the USA, the death penalty is increasingly used in many states—the list of those for whom execution is considered appropriate includes all those monstrous individuals listed above, notably for those whose mental state suggests that they are liable to be intractable to reform and to retain their dangerous propensities despite imprisonment.

The focus of such punitiveness is thus not crime as such. It is the conduct of those who are thought to be intractable, anti-social, amoral: in other words, those who refuse to conform their behaviour to the moral demands for responsible self-government in a free society. The measures introduced in the USA, Australia and other jurisdictions are not justified in the abstract terms of justice and the rule of law, but in the name of protection of the general public. Whatever the expert evidence may suggest, it appears that political authorities must be seen to be responding to the fears of public as shaped, organized and amplified by a mass media (cf. Pratt 2000; Brown and Pratt 2000). 'Risk to the public', as Pratt points out, is the recurrent factor that runs through these new measures of 'punitive' crime control: curfews for youth; preventive detention for 'sexual predators'; preventive detention for 'risky' psychiatric patients; public shaming of offenders in some states in Australia and the USA; castration as a condition for parole for sex offenders in some states of the USA. Similarly, Simon (1998) argues that sex offenders are emblematic of the public focus of punitiveness upon the new 'monsters'. They are not to be reformed—indeed they are emblematic of a penal philosophy which abandons hope of reform with the despairing sigh of 'nothing works'. They are merely 'predators' to be incapacitated in the name of public protection.

Psychiatrists are increasingly called upon to guard the entry and exit points to a new range of quasi-psychiatric institutions that seem to offer a solution to the problems thrown up by such public fears and political responses. There may, of course, be scope for limited therapeutic experiments within such institutions. But their socio-political role is that of incapacitating those potential offenders who may have committed no crime or have completed their sentence, but who seem to present a risk in the light of what has become the overriding political priority. They answer to the political—and professional—need to be seen to be acting to preserve the security of 'the public'. Bluglass (1990) was anticipating such developments when he wrote that 'Forensic psychiatrists will ... be anxious to resist being regarded as psychiatry's jailers in a re-organized health service; a risk which they may face as mental hospitals close down'. In the second half of the nineteenth century and the first half of the twentieth century there was an apparently limitless increase in the population of the asylums, as they came to be used as receptacles for all manner of failed or anti-citizens unable or unwilling to accept the obligations of civility. A new version of this history is now being played out, in which the constraints of rule of law can be waived in order to confine risky individuals under a psychiatric mandate in the name of public defence—that is to say, not so much because of what they have done, but of what they are and what they might do.

Within these new configurations of control, what becomes of the classical question that psychiatry faced in the courtroom—the issue of criminal responsibility? The conception of 'the subject of law' that underpinned the insanity legislation of the mid-nineteenth century was one of a punctual, rational, choosing individual deemed responsible unless unable to appreciate the nature and quality of their acts or to know that they were wrong. This image never really captured the operative conceptions of female offenders, juvenile offenders or offenders after verdict being considered for sentence within the criminal justice complex. But contested murder trials in many jurisdictions are still played out in these terms. For reasons that are now familiar, psychiatric evidence of current mental disorder frequently fails to match the requirements and constraints of legal reasoning, which is concerned solely with whether an individual should be held responsible and thus culpable for the act committed. But one significant development is under way within psychiatry which may well have implications for the traditional dilemmas of the psychiatric expert when insanity is on trial.

After some decades of disrepute, biological explanations of the propensity for certain kinds of criminal behaviour have re-emerged (Wright and Miller 1998). As I have argued in more detail elsewhere (Rose 2000a), these new biological arguments do not concern themselves with crime in general or the biology of 'the criminal'. They accept, usually implicitly, sociological contentions concerning the heterogeneity and social relativity of those forms of conduct designated criminal and the fact that those convicted of crimes are by no means representative of those who have committed breaches of the law. Hence, rather than trying to account for some mythical 'criminal personality', the new criminological biology has come to focus on specific kinds of aggressive, impulsive, anti-social behaviour. Earlier arguments concerning the role of major genetic abnormalities such as XYY have been rejected. Defences based upon hormonal arguments, such as those mounted around pre-menstrual syndrome, have largely fallen into disuse. Contemporary biological criminologists draw on evidence from the new molecular genetics, neuroscience and brain imaging, to claim that there is a strong genetic component in such aggressive or impulsive behaviours, and that they are probably linked to abnormalities in the neurotransmitter system, perhaps related to serotonin. More significant for their role in the criminal justice system, they claim that such abnormalities are, in some circumstances, objectively detectable by the examination of family histories to show genetic linkages, by the analysis of samples of cerebro-spinal fluid to detect abnormal neurotransmitter levels and by the use of other investigative techniques—electro-encephalograms, computerised tomography, magnetic resonance imaging and so on—to show abnormal patterns of brain activity. The promise, therefore, is that the interpretative and 'subjective' difficulties of conventional psychiatric evidence of mental ill health will be soon overcome. Enthusiasts believe that it will soon be possible to demonstrate objectively and conclusively the biological correlates of offending behaviour in the abnormal brain of the offender.

Many question the validity of these hopes and beliefs. But my concern here is with their consequences. The courts in the USA, where such developments are most advanced, have proved remarkably resistant to genetic defences where a family history of disturbed conduct is claimed as contributing to the offending behaviour, or to accepting that abnormal brain scans should lead to the mitigation of responsibility. Defence lawyers have, of course, utilized such arguments as and when they suit their case. But neither the courts, not biological criminologists themselves, have regarded such evidence as undercutting the traditional ascription of free will. The move has been in precisely the reverse direction. Researchers in this area increasingly insist that while their research findings show a biological contribution to impulsivity and aggressiveness, the courts are concerned with a question at a different level. Courts, they suggest, must address a question of morality, and this must continue to be based on the moral premise that humans have free will. Such arguments fit well with current developments in judicial practice. Evidence that offending behaviour is a result of illness has traditionally been seen as mitigating culpability. Even if not sufficient to overturn the presumption of legal responsibility before conviction, such evidence has led to reduced sentences or diversion to treatment regimes. But, increasingly, courts are arguing that no appeal to 'causal factors'—sociological, psychological, biographical or biological—should be allowed mitigate the legal requirement to treat the offender as if he or she bore full *moral* responsibility for the actions in question. Indeed, in many American states, the insanity defence with its verdict of 'Not Guilty by Reason of Insanity' is being restricted or scrapped altogether. In the American courts, evidence that there are biological and psychiatric explanations of the offending behaviour of the accused do not mitigate culpability; quite the reverse. Such evidence convinces juries and judges that reform is unlikely, that anti-social conduct will persist and hence that harsh sanctions, up to and including the death penalty, are most appropriate. For evidence of biological propensities mandates almost any form of action that will meet the overriding 'need for public protection'.

Arguments from biological psychiatry are also being taken up within the other, preventive axes of risk thinking. This can be observed in strategies of risk reduction targeted upon the perceived problem of anti-social, amoral and aggressive conduct in inner city youth. If a proportion of the population can be seen as suffering from genetic or biological vulnerabilities that overwhelm most environments, then the appropriate crime control strategy appears to be preventive intervention, early identification, screening and presymptomatic treatment, possibly compulsorily. Once believed to have a predisposition to undesirable conduct on the basis of DNA testing or family history, the individual concerned may be treated as if they were certain to be affected in the severest fashion, even where they show no present signs of the problem in question, and even though the certainty, nature, timing or severity of any difficulty cannot be predicted (cf. Gostin, 1991). What we are seeing here is the emergence of a new problem and object for regulation: the person biologically 'at risk' of being the perpetrator of aggression or violence. As biological and genetic models of psychiatric disorder achieve intellectual hegemony, and as new diagnostic techniques are developed claiming to be able to make visible such biological abnormalities at the level of the DNA, the neurotransmitters or the brain, it seems likely that the predictive obligations associated with such biological and genetic risk thinking will penetrate, and perhaps even reshape, the work of many control professionals, not least the activities of psychiatrists.

Once more, developments in the USA are instructive. In the early 1990s, the United States National Institute of Mental Health launched a 'National Violence Initiative' in which psychiatrists would seek to identify children likely to develop criminal behaviour and to develop intervention strategies. The *Chicago Tribune* reported in 1993 that this programme raised the hope 'that violent behavior can eventually be curbed by manipulating the chemical and genetic keys to aggression … anti-violence medications conceivably could be given, perhaps forcibly, to people with abnormal levels' (cited in Citizen's Commission on Human Rights 1996). The report, issued in 1993 and 1994 in four volumes, called for more attention to biological and genetic factors in violent crime and for more research on new pharmaceuticals that reduce violent behaviour (Reiss and Roth 1994). At the same time the US Federal Government, in partnership with the private MacArthur Foundation, was sponsoring the 'Program on Human Development and Criminal Behavior', based on the view that 'advances in the fields of behavior genetics, neurobiology, and molecular biology are renewing the hope that the biological determinants of delinquent and criminal behavior may yet be discovered' (Earl 1991, quoted in Breggin 1995/6). Hence the project aimed at screening children for biological, psychological and social factors that may play a role in criminal behaviour and following subjects over an eight-year period with a view to ultimately identifying biological and biochemical markers for predicting criminality. There was much controversy over these developments. Opponents argued that they were racist, amounted to a new eugenics, and diverted attention from the urgent need for social reform in America's inner cities. Partly as a consequence, the violence initiatives were split up and scaled down. But research in this area continues apace. Diane Fishbein, of the US Department of Justice, is typical in arguing that 'Once prevalence rates are known for genetically influenced forms of psychopathology in relevant populations, we can better determine how substantially a prevention strategy that incorporates genetic findings may influence the problem of antisocial conduct' and considers that at a minimum, the evidence 'suggests the need for early identification and intervention' (Fishbein 1996). The hope is that neuro-genetic research might identify markers and genes associated with anti-social behaviour, allowing for programmes of screening to detect individuals carrying these markers and pre-emptive intervention. Biological information on criminal and violent propensities could thus be the basis of risk prevention strategies for a variety of agencies of social control. Full-scale screening of the inhabitants in the inner cities might be too controversial to contemplate in most jurisdictions. But one might expect to see the emergence of genetic screening of disruptive schoolchildren, with pre-emptive treatment made a condition of continuing schooling, Or one might imagine the development of postconviction screening of petty criminals, with genetic testing and compliance with treatment made a condition of probation or parole. Or one might imagine scenarios in which genetic therapy is offered to disruptive or delinquent employees as an alternative to termination. In the light of the fact that many psychiatric medications, for example antabuse for alcoholics and lithium for manic depression, were introduced in this way, one might expect some psychiatrists to see this as a central area for expansion. Such potential for the pre-emptive and compulsory use of psychiatric powers throws the conflict between the medical obligation of care and the political obligation of control into sharp focus.

Control and community

Contemporary demands upon psychiatry in the name of control clearly arise, in part, from psychiatry's rejection of the carceral strategies that dominated from the mid-nineteenth century in all western nations. It is not simply that much psychiatry is now practised outside the closed space of the hospital: even in the golden age of the asylum only a proportion of those receiving expert attention for afflictions of the mind were confined. More important, the asylum no longer acts as the integrating element in the complex map of psychiatric practices. In the postwar period, a new territory for psychiatry took shape: 'community'. As Castel has argued, the policies of 'sectorization' in France, of community mental health in the USA and of community care in the UK, irrespective of the specific political circumstances that produced them, shared a certain rationale—one of 'covering the maximum amount of ground, reaching the maximum number of people, through the deployment of a unified apparatus linked to the machinery of the state' (Castel 1991; cf. Castel 1981).

The notion of community had emerged within a variety of different attempts to reconfigure psychiatry. In the period immediately after the end of World War 2, community was proposed as the organizing theme for programmes for the reform of asylum psychiatry advocated by progressive psychiatrists. They argued that psychiatry should not be segregated from the places it serves, its institutions should be located in their communities, they should reach out into the community in terms of care for those who do not yet have to enter hospital, or those who are discharged from the hospital. At about the same time, the vocabulary of community became central to the critique of asylum psychiatry. Proponents argued that the asylum should not be a place of incarceration but a therapeutic community. This line was later developed by Franco Basaglia and others in Italy into a programme for the wholesale abolition of the asylum and its replacement by community mental health centres (cf. Lovell and Scheper-Hughes 1987). Over the course of the 1970s and 1980s, in the UK and the USA, community emerged as the key term in a set of national political policies and technologies. Community psychiatry was a way for psychiatry to modernize itself. Psychiatrists responded to critiques of their custodial and controlling role by seeking to divest their activities of their anti-liberal and 'carceral' features, sloughing these off to other forms of expertise so that psychiatry could become a liberal, open and curative medicine. But it was also an attempt to forge programmes that would 'simplify' and reintegrate the disparate elements of the psychiatric vocation that had taken shape for diverse forms of psychiatric expertise over the course of the twentieth century. In this new diagram, psychiatrists' role of curing illness would be supplemented, perhaps even supplanted, by the task of administering pathological individuals across a network of specialist institutions and locales. Simultaneously, psychiatrists would work with others in implementing prophylactic and preventive strategies to maximize public mental health.

The dream of community psychiatry in the UK—outlined in any number of policy documents, white papers and so forth across the 1970s and 1980s—was of a single organizational field that would mirror the complexity and diversity of the problems of mental ill health and the populations it was now seen as embracing:

> children and adolescents with psychological problems .... assessment and treatment of adults whose conditions require short term admission to hospital and for the longer term treatment, including asylum, of those for whom there is no realistic alternative ... places in hospitals and ... hostels, sheltered housing, supported lodgings ... for adults with a mental illness needing residential care outside hospital, together with an adequate range of day and respite services ... co-ordinated arrangements between health and social services, primary health care teams and voluntary agencies for the continuing health and social care of people with a mental illness living in their own homes or in residential facilities [including] domiciliary services, support to carers and the training and education of staff working in the community (Department of Health 1989).

Community psychiatry would bring together the diverse subjects of psychiatry—alcoholics, offenders, disturbed children, pathological parents as well as those suffering acute or chronic mental distress—the diverse sites in which it operated—hospitals, clinics, hostels, homes, schools, mental health centres, social workers' visits, general practitioners' surgeries—and the diverse professionals who staffed it—psychiatrists, primary care workers, nurses, occupational therapists, psychotherapists, clinical psychologists and so forth—into a coherent 'community care system'.

Of course there is nothing new in psychiatry assuming a predominantly administrative role. Indeed the growth of psychiatry as a profession in the mid-nineteenth century was linked to the administrative role that the asylums played in the containment of a motley assortment of socially undesirable or problematic individuals (Scull 1979; Rose 1996). Nonetheless, the diversity and range of the specialized institutions that made up community psychiatry shaped this administrative demand in a particular way. One of the central obligations of psychiatric professionals was to make diagnoses which would be performative, in the sense that they would determine where an individual would be directed within this archipelago of sites of professional–client interaction—half-way houses, concept houses, day-care centres, day hospitals etc. As this new diagram of psychiatry began to take shape, madness itself changed its significance. As mental ill health, madness became fully disenchanted. It was now seen as little more than the lack of the capacity to cope with the exigencies of a world outside the asylum. And where madness is seen as inability to cope, cure reciprocally becomes restoration of the capacity to cope. The role of therapeutic professionals undergoes a parallel transformation. Professionals now are required not so much to cure, as to teach the skills of coping, to inculcate the responsibility to cope, to identify failures of coping, to restore to the individual the capacity to cope and to return them to a coping life.

Once more, the idea of risk provides a useful perspective from which to examine these transformations of the relations between psychiatrists and the criminal justice system. In particular, we need to examine the significance of the shift from the problem of dangerousness to that of risk (in what follows I draw directly upon Rose 1999). The psychiatric debate about dangerousness recognized that, in practice, it was difficult if not impossible to draw a sharp dividing line between those mental patients who were or were not dangerous, and prediction was always uncertain. Nonetheless, up until around the mid-1960s, the issue of dangerousness arose only in relation to a small minority of actual or potential patients or prisoners. Dangerousness was understood as an internal quality of a few pathological individuals, even if it was a quality that was difficult to explain, diagnose or measure. Through the 1970s and 1980s, this understanding mutated. Dangerousness was increasingly understood not as a fixed internal quality, but as a matter of factors, of situations, of statistical probabilities. By the 1990s, risk had become naturalized as the organizing term of these debates (Potts 1995; Grounds 1995). As the *British Journal of Psychiatry* put it in 1997, in its special supplement on assessing risk in the mentally disordered: 'there has been a sea change ... away from assessing dangerousness to assessing (and managing) risk' (Duggan 1997). In the same publication, Snowden (1997) commenced his paper on practical aspects of clinical risk assessment and management in even clearer terms: 'It is debatable whether the notion of dangerousness now has any utilitarian value for psychiatry... dangerousness is [nothing] more than an adjective which has been elevated into a pseudoscientific construct whose definitions [here he refers to Scott 1977; Walker 1978; Home Office and Department of Health and Social Security 1975] amount to little more than "past harm predicts future behaviour" '. For Snowden, what does have such a value, however hard it is to assess, is risk. Risk, apparently 'does not contain pejorative connotations' and 'invites more objective and robust analysis'.

But when psychiatrists and other mental health professionals embraced risk thinking, they were not simply replacing an unscientific concept with a scientific one, or an ineffective strategy with an effective one. What was involved was a subtle but very significant mutation in our way of understanding and responding to almost all mental health problems. This shift in thinking owes something to the persistence, energy and persuasiveness of a small number of researchers and campaigners. In the USA, the key figures were John Monahan and Henry Steadman. Steadman's work in this area arose from concerns in the USA to protect people with mental health problems against excessive detention in the name of their civil rights. It was argued then that whilst detention and involuntary treatment was justified in terms of danger of harm to self or others, mental health professionals were very bad at making accurate and reliable predictions of future behaviour, and so were erring on the side of excessive caution leading to unwarranted detention. Steadman was amongst many who argued that assessments of dangerousness were inaccurate and unreliable, that psychiatrists tended to greatly overdiagnose offenders as dangerous, and that current psychiatric knowledge and procedures could provide no firm or legitimate basis for decisions about detention (Steadman and Cocozza 1974). Similarly, Monahan, at the start of the 1980s, drew attention to the inaccuracy of clinical predictions of violent behaviour, arguing that evidence from the best clinical research showed that psychiatrists and psychologists were accurate in no more than one out of three predictions of violent behaviour over a several year period, when their subjects were institutionalized populations with a history of violence and a mental illness diagnosis (Monahan 1981).

In subsequent years, in a number of very influential articles, Steadman, Monahan and their colleagues outlined an alternative approach: one whose object was defined not in terms of dangerousness but risk, and which argued that mental health professionals should frame predictions of future violence in probabilistic terms. In 1993, in a paper entitled 'from dangerousness to risk assessment', they set out what they considered to be the key characteristics of the shift in thinking, communicating and practising. Risk assessment, they argued, differs from previous assessments in three ways. First, it is not about legal categorization but administrative decision making. Second, it is not about binary distinctions but location on a continuum. Third, it does not identify something fixed, stable, inherent and hence predictable to all futures, but implies continuous day-to-day risk management of the potentially risky person (Steadman *et al.* 1993, cf. Crichton 1995). In practice, to put it crudely, all psychiatric patients can, and should, be allocated to a level of risk, risk assessed and risk re-assessed, risk classified, risk managed, risk monitored: high risk, medium risk, low risk —but rarely no risk. And risk management should not be confined to the question of whether or not a person should be detained in hospital or prison or to the mentally disordered offender: it should extend over the everyday life of all 'mental patients' and the everyday work of all psychiatric professionals.

It was through the notion of risk, and the techniques and practices to which it was linked, that care and control became inextricably linked in the community. In Britain in the 1990s, a whole series of official documents and guidelines stressed the centrality of risk management to all mental health practice, not just the activities of a few forensic specialists. Thus all patients referred to specialist psychiatric services were required to be risk assessed and allocated to one of three levels of care. Supervised discharge was introduced for some patients who had been detained in hospital for treatment, which meant that *all* patients for whom this was a possibility had to be assessed to see if they presented a substantial risk of serious harm to themselves or other people, or of being seriously exploited: the risk assessment was to be carried out before a patient was discharged from hospital. These risky persons were to be placed on supervision registers, along with all patients in the care of the psychiatric services who 'are, or are liable to be, at risk of committing serious violence or suicide, or of serious self neglect' whether they were existing patients or new patients to the psychiatric services (National Health Service (NHS) Executive 1994). As the Special Working Party on Clinical Assessment and Management of Risk, set up by The Royal College of Psychiatrists, made clear in its report entitled 'Assessment and clinical management of risk of harm to other people', risk assessment and risk management were to be 'of the highest priority for the allocation of resources' (Royal College of Psychiatrists 1996). Facilities, strategies, training and inter-agency collaboration were all to be rethought in terms of the management of risk. In thousands of offices, team meetings, ward rounds, case conferences and training programmes, techniques were devised and disseminated that aspired to be able to identify levels of risk, signs of risk, indicators of risk and the like, to measure risk levels, to document risk levels in case notes and care plans. All mental health professionals were now obliged to calculate risk and to manage individual patients or clients in the in the light of a calculation of their riskiness and in the name of risk reduction on the territory of the community.

What, then, are the implications of these mutations? First, risk thinking generates new dividing practices. In a political and cultural climate stressing the need for individuals to be prudent, to take responsibility for themselves, a new division appears between the prudent and the imprudent self, the self able to manage itself from the self who must be managed by others. The subjects of psychiatry are no longer unified by their institutional confinement, and the visibility which confinement conferred upon them, but by the fact that they are unable to manage themselves prudently in the matrix of encounters outside the asylum. Failures of management of the self, lack of skills of coping with family, with work, with money, with housing are now all, potentially, criteria for qualification as a psychiatric subject. Ideas of risk management also underpin new divisions within the subjects of psychiatry. Notably, they reshape the divide between those 'good subjects of psychiatry' who are 'medicine compliant', keep appointments, are able to assess their coping performance in a way that aligns with the assessment of professionals, and those who do not 'play the game' of community care. Professionals become tutors—sometimes gentle, sometimes harsh—in the arts of self-management: meet your appointments, take your medicine, do not get drunk or violent or you will be considered risky, and lose your place in this project or be returned to hospital or prison. The will to cure becomes little more that the inculcation of a particular type of relation to the self—prudent self-management, making contracts and abiding by them, setting reachable targets and achieving them, learning skills of management of everyday life.

Second, the logics of risk transform the act of diagnosis. Previously, one might say that there was a kind of division of labour in the management of the person who was mentally ill. Diagnosis and treatment was the responsibility of the doctor, care and control was the responsibility of the nurse, assistance was the responsibility of the social worker. The clinical diagnosis by the psychiatrist was the fulcrum of this division of labour, even if, on the territory of the community, the actual management of the patient was to be undertaken by other experts and in other sites. Diagnosis by a medically qualified expert was thus a condition of entry to the territory of psychiatry. Such diagnosis was performative: it mandated a certain regime of drugs, detention or referral to a particular specialist institution and so forth. However, new forms of diagnosis have emerged that challenge the pre-eminent role of the doctor. To quote Castel, 'The site of diagnostic synthesis is no longer that of the concrete relationship with a sick person, but a relationship constituted among the different expert assessments which make up the patient's dossier' (Castel 1991). The psychiatrist here loses his or her 'master status' as the locus of judgement. And judgement is, is in any event, carried out only partially in medical terms. Diagnosis comes to operate also in terms of a variety of other forms of expertise about such 'risk factors'—associated with undesirable outcomes either through probabilistic evidence or, more usually, through appeals to clinical experience—as employment history, family life, coping skills, capacity to cook, shop and manage money as well as information on past conduct and dangerous behaviour. Whilst the psychiatrist may formally remain in charge of the case—although even this is in doubt with the nomination of key workers from other disciplines—the terms of psychiatric judgement are no longer clinical (or even epidemiological, as Castel suggests) but what one might term 'quotidian'—to do with the management of the everyday.

The key question now asked of the psychiatrist is pragmatic: what should be done with this person? Should he or she be sent to this institution or to that, to this hostel or that sheltered housing scheme, back into the community or back into prison? The logic of prediction comes to replace the logic of diagnosis—but this is a logic at which the psychiatrist can claim no special competence. For the subjects of psychiatry must now be classified in terms of likely future conduct, their riskiness to the community and themselves and the identification of the steps necessary to manage that conduct. The psychiatric hospital is redefined. It is no longer a place of cure. It becomes little more than a container for the most risky until their riskiness can be fully assessed and controlled. The 'multi-disciplinary team', so beloved of the programmers as the solution to so many problems, does not actually emerge out of a recognition of the diagnostic and curative significance of different sorts of clinical and social expertise. It is the answer to a different problem, one of administration: what is to be done and how can we decide?

There is nothing particularly novel about the way in which psychiatry is applying the logic of risk to the problem of pathological conduct. The psychiatric risk registers under development in the UK reactivate a pattern that has been applied to child abuse since the 1970s without notable success. But new technologies of information recording and co-ordination embody the possibilities of new modes of surveillance. Unlike the forms of individualization which were born in the nineteenth century asylum— and the prison, school and hospital—they are not dependent upon the visibility conferred by the institution. Material gleaned from a whole variety of sources, designated by diverse experts as risk factors, may be brought together to individualize a subject in terms of the likelihood of future offending, mental breakdown, child abuse or whatever. Castel predicts the development of a general system for risk prediction which would record a whole array of factors shown to have a statistical, epidemiological connection with pathological conduct—age, nationality, previous history of illness and so forth—and where a certain combination of such factors will set off an automatic alert and result in the despatching of a professional to the individual concerned. Some foresee a kind of rationalized dystopia, where computers collate and interpret data from a whole variety of sources to identify risk levels and risk groups across a population, and engage in preventative targeting of particular sites and locales, and where unceasing administration assigns individuals to certain pathways on the basis of their risk categorization. But evidence from a string of enquiries into 'scandals' of risk management in child protection and psychiatry suggests that system failure is a more likely outcome than a 'Big Brother Society'. The real impact of risk thinking is a transformation of professional subjectivity. It is the individual professional who has to make the assessment and management of risk their central professional obligation. They have to assess the individual client in terms of the riskiness that they represent, to allocate each to a risk level, to put in place the appropriate administrative arrangements for the management of the individual in the light of the requirement to minimize risk, and to take responsibility —indeed blame—if an 'untoward incident' occurs. In a situation where the outcome of a mental health assessment may be an administrative decision to release a patient into the community, the risk assessment may be used, not so much in order to make accurate predictions, but to ensure that the decision made was defensible if something should go wrong. The psychiatrist is thus, as it were, to reflect upon the present decision making from the perspective of the need to defend it in some public tribunal in the future. Were all relevant factors taken into account? Were there sound reasons for the decision that can be adduced and justified? Would any other competent professional in the same position made a better decision? Would other colleagues consider the decision-making process as meeting standards of good practice? Despite the shift in current regulatory regimes towards market-based mechanisms, risk assessment is thus a powerful new way of regulating professional judgement. Professional practice is governed through enwrapping professionals in a bureaucratic nexus of reports, forms, monitoring, evaluation and audit, under the shadow of the law. Through such measures, psychiatric professionals are increasingly governed according to logics which are not their own, in the interests of community protection.

Conclusion

What general conclusions might one draw from this account of the role of psychiatry in contemporary regimes of control? It remains the case that the control functions of psychiatry focus disproportionately upon certain sectors of the population—those who are excluded from the wealth and opportunities of contemporary society, in particular upon ethnic minorities. However the criticisms made by an earlier generation of radicals about 'the medicalization of social control' do not help much in understanding the changing ways in which such control operates. I have argued that, in a variety of different ways, one of the principal tasks of psychiatry today relates to the problems of exercising and legitimating control over those individuals who appear to be unable or unwilling to control themselves appropriately according to the moral norms of our contemporary 'societies of freedom'. Psychiatry, that is to say, has a particular role within societies whose practices—employment and consumption, public order and private housing, health and education, sexuality and family life—are premised upon the capacities of individuals to conduct themselves according to the norms of regulated liberty.

On the one hand stand those individuals who appear to lack the capacities to manage themselves according to the norms of responsible autonomy required by these practices. Such individuals are the target of one face of risk thinking: the attempt to assess, quantify and record degrees of risk, to disseminate risk-related information across communication pathways with other professionals and the courts, to subject individuals to a regime of surveillance and continual judgement. Perhaps psychiatrists here would be wise to question the dynamics that generate such risk management programmes, not merely because of the difficulties of defining and assessing risk, nor simply because such dreams of complete and continuous surveillance are always likely to fail in practice for a multitude of reasons, or even because of the net widening consequences that are the consequence of such endeavours. More fundamentally, such programmes of risk management reinforce a highly skewed perception of risk and a prejudicial belief that individuals with mental health problems are distinct from, and a threat to the 'the general public'. On the other hand, the other face of risk thinking separates out a set of individuals who appear to violate the very bases of self-control upon which such societies depend—the impulsive, the amoral, the intractably different. Perhaps psychiatrists here would be wise to question the symbolic processes that try to distinguish and demonize certain individuals, to render them monstrous and thus to remove from them the rights and powers of 'normal citizens'—to proportionality in treatment, to the safeguards of legal rights and the rule of law.

These problems that face contemporary psychiatry arise from the problems of order thrown up by our contemporary notions of freedom, by the celebration of the rights of the majority to enjoy all the benefits of consumption and wealth and to be protected from their downsides by the symbolic and real process of exclusion. They expose all the dilemmas, contradictions and limits that characterize prevailing, and highly moralistic, notions of freedom and citizenship. One may be cynical about the eagerness with which some psychiatric practitioners have welcomed their new role, given that their strong powers are grounded upon such a weak knowledge base. But what one sees here is not simply a consequence of moral entrepreneurship or professional imperialism—it is made possible by recent shifts in rationalities and strategies of control. And many psychiatrists have themselves highlighted these difficulties: they have refused to overrate their own capacities to undertake the tasks thrust upon them by the risk-control agenda; they have pointed to the lack of evidence for the fears of violent madmen and the moral panics that have led to demands for preventive detention and a return to a more carceral psychiatric system; in the USA they have publicly aired their doubts about being involved in the assessment of individuals facing capital punishment; and in many jurisdictions they have sought to switch the focus of concern to the damaging effect of contemporary penal institutions on the mental health of all inmates. And it thus becomes clear that contemporary psychiatric dilemmas about control are not so much medical and scientific as ethical and political.

References

Beck, U. (1992) Risk society: towards a new modernity. London: Sage.

Bluglass, R. (1990) The scope of forensic psychiatry. *Journal of Forensic Psychiatry*, **1**, 5–9.

Bock, G.R. and Goode, J. A. (1996) *Genetics of criminal and anti-social behaviour: Ciba Foundation Symposium 194*. Chichester: John Wiley.

Breggin, P. (1995/6) Campaigns against racist federal programs by the Center for the Study of Psychiatry and Psychology. *Journal of African American Men*, **1**(3), 3–22.

Brown, M. and Pratt, J. (ed.) (2000) Dangerous offenders: punishment and social order. London: Routledge.

Castel, R. (1981) La Gestion des risques: de l'anti-psychiatrie a l'apres-psychanalyse. Paris: Edition de Minuit.

Castel, R. (1991) From dangerousness to risk. In *The Foucault Effect: studies in governmentality* (ed. G. Burchell, C. Gordon and P. Miller). Hemel Hempstead: Harvester Wheatsheaf.

Citizen's Commission on Human Rights (1996) The violence initiative— http://www.cchr.org/racism/pooaa3.htm.

Cocozza, J. and Steadman, H. J. (1976) The failure of psychiatric predictions of dangerousness: Clear and convincing evidence. *Rutgers Law Review*, **29**, 1084–101.

Cohen, S. (1985) *Visions of social control*. Cambridge: Polity.

Crichton, J. ed. (1995) *Psychiatric Patient Violence: Risk and Response*, London: Duckworth.

Department of Health (1989) Caring for people: community care in the next decade and beyond, Cm 849. London: HMSO.

Duggan, C. (1997) Introduction. In: *Assessing risk in the mentally disordered* (ed. C. Duggan) (Suppl. 32 to the *British Journal of Psychiatry*), pp. 1–3. London: Royal College of Psychiatrists.

Earl, F. (1991) A developmental approach to understanding and controlling violence. *Pediatrics*, **5**, 61–88.

Ericson, R. and Haggerty, K. (1997) *Policing the risk society*. Toronto: University of Toronto Press.

Feely, M. and Simon, J. (1992) The new penology: notes on the emerging strategy of corrections and its implications. *Criminology*, **30**(4), 449–74.

Feeley, M. and Simon, J. (1994) Actuarial justice: power/knowledge in contemporary criminal justice. In *The futures of criminology* (ed. D. Nelken). London: Sage.

Fishbein, D. (1996) Prospects for the application of genetic findings to crime and violence prevention. *Politics and the Life Sciences (Symposium on Genetics and Crime)*, **15**(1), 91–4.

Foucault, M. (1978) About the concept of the "dangerous individual" in 19th-century legal psychiatry (trans. A. Baudot and J. Couchman). *International Journal of Law and Psychiatry*, **1**, 1–18; reprinted 1988 in *Michel Foucault: Politics, Philosophy, Culture* (ed. L. D. Kritzman). London: Routledge.

Garland, D. (1994) Of crime and criminals: the development of criminology in Britain. In *The Oxford handbook of criminology* (ed. M. Maguire, R. Morgan and R. Reiner), pp. 17–69. Oxford: Oxford University Press.

Garland, D. (1996) The limits of the sovereign state: strategies of crime control in contemporary society. *British Journal of Criminology*, **36**(4), 445–71.

Garland, D. (2001) *The culture of control.* Oxford: Oxford University Press.

Garland, D. (ed.) (in press) *Mass imprisonment in the USA: social causes and consequences.* London: Sage.

Gostin, L. (1991) 'Genetic discrimination: the use of genetically based diagnostic tests by employers and insurers'. *American journal of law and medicine* **17**(1–2): 109–144

Grounds, A. (1995) Risk assessment and management in a clinical context. In *Psychiatric patient violence: risk and response* (ed. J. Crichton). London: Duckworth.

Hacking, I. (1991) *The taming of chance.* Cambridge: Cambridge University Press.

Home Office and Department of Health and Social Security (1975) Report of the Committee on mentally abnormal offenders, Cmnd. 6244. London: HMSO.

Johnstone, G. (1996) *Medical concepts and penal policy.* London: Cavendish.

Lovell, A. and Scheper-Hughes, N. (1987) *Psychiatry inside out: selected writings of Franco Basaglia.* New York: Columbia University Press.

MacArthur (1998) The MacArthur research network on mental health and the law web site— http://ness.sys.virginia.edu/macarthur/violence.html.

Monahan, J. (1981) *The clinical prediction of violent behavior.* Washington, DC: Government Printing Office.

NHS Executive (1994) *Guidance on the discharge of mentally disordered people and their continuing care in the community*, HSG(94)27. London: Department of Health.

Owen, D. (1991) Foucault, psychiatry and the spectre of dangerousness. *Journal of Forensic Psychiatry*, **2** (3), 238–41.

Pasquino, P. (1991) Criminology: the birth of a special knowledge. In *The Foucault effect: studies in governmentality* (ed. G. Burchell, C. Gordon and P. Miller). Hemel Hempstead: Harvester Wheatsheaf.

Peay, J. (1994) Mentally disordered offenders. In *The Oxford handbook of criminology* (ed. M. Maguire, R. Morgan and R. Reiner), pp. 1119–60. Oxford: Oxford University Press.

Potts, J. (1995) Risk assessment and management: A Home Office perspective. In *Psychiatric patient violence: risk and response* (ed. J. Crichton). London: Duckworth.

Pratt, J. (1995) Dangerousness, risk and technologies of power. *Australian and New Zealand Journal of Criminology*, **28**(1), 3–31.

Pratt, J. (2000) Sex crime and the new punitiveness. *Behavioural Sciences and Law*, **18,** 135–57.

Reiss, A. J. and Roth, J. A. (1994) *Understanding and preventing violence* (4 volumes). Washington, DC: National Academy Press.

Rose, N. (1989) *Governing the soul: the shaping of the private self.* London: Routledge (2nd edn, 1999, London: Free Associations).

Rose, N. (1996) Psychiatry as a political science: advanced liberalism and the administration of risk. *History of the Human Sciences*, **2,** 1–23.

Rose, N. (1998) Governing risky individuals: the role of psychiatry in new regimes of control. *Psychiatry, Psychology and Law*, **5**(2), 177–95.

Rose, N. (1999) *Powers of freedom: reframing political thought*. Cambridge: Cambridge University Press.

Rose, N. (2000*a*) The biology of culpability: pathological identities in a biological culture. *Theoretical Criminology*, **4**(1), 5–34.

Rose, N. (2000*b*) Government and control. *British Journal of Criminology*, special issue on criminology and social theory (ed. D. Garland and C. Sparks), **40**, 321–39.

Royal College of Psychiatrists (1996) *Assessment and clinical management of risk of harm to other people*. London: Royal College of Psychiatrists.

Scott, P. (1977) Assessing dangerousness in criminals. *British Journal of Psychiatry*, **131**, 127–42.

Scull, A. (1979) *Museums of madness*. London: Allen Lane.

Scull, A. (1984) *Decarceration: community treatment and the deviant* (2nd edn). Cambridge: Polity Press.

Simon, J. (1998) Managing the monstrous: sex offenders and the new penology. *Psychology, Public Policy and Law*, **4**, 1–16.

Smith, R. (1981) *Trial by medicine: insanity and responsibility in Victiorian trials*. Edinburgh: Edinburgh University Press.

Snowden, P. (1997) Practical aspects of clinical risk assessment and management. In *Assessing risk in the mentally disordered* (ed. Duggan, C.), Suppl. 32 to the *British Journal of Psychiatry*, pp. 32–4). London: Royal College of Psychiatrists.

Steadman, H. J. (1973) Some evidence on the inadequacy of the concept and determination of dangerousness in psychiatry and law. *Journal of Psychiatry and Law*, **1**, 409–26.

Steadman, H. J. and C., John (1974) *Careers of the criminally insane: excessive social control of deviance*. Lexington, DC: Heath.

Steadman, H. J., Monahan, J., Clark Robbins, P., et al (1993) From dangerousness to risk assessment: implications for appropriate research strategies. In *Mental disorder and crime* (ed. S. Hodgins). Newbury Park, CA: Sage.

Walker, N. (1978) Dangerous people. *International Journal of Law and Psychiatry*, **11**, 37–50.

Wasserman, D. (1996) Research into genetics and crime: consensus and controversy. *Politics and the Life Sciences (Symposium on Genetics and Crime)*, **15**(1), 107–9.

Wright, R. A. and Miller, J. M. (1998) Taboo until today? The coverage of biological arguments in criminology textbooks, 1961 to 1970 and 1987 to 1996. *Journal of Criminal Justice*, **26**(1), 1–19.

Chapter 2

The level of risk posed

David Tidmarsh

Citizens of the western world who are coming to maturity at the beginning of the third millennium expect to be protected from risk from any source other than their own deliberate choice and behave on the assumption that the biblical three score years and ten are theirs by right. It is hard for them to imagine how society faced the hazards of life in former times or even one century ago. Mining disasters and shipwrecks were accepted with equanimity, at least by those not directly involved, while factories and civil engineering took a steady toll. In the medical arena, childbirth was anticipated with as much fear as joy while death in childhood and a host of lethal infections were commonplace and surgery a dreaded last resort. Fatalism, however, is not a defining characteristic of western society: the moral climate changes and even *laissez-faire* has its limits, so that one by one hazards were seen as unacceptable and reduced by the actions of crusading politicians or the impact of scientific discovery. In addition there comes a time when life is no longer cheap and financial pressures dictate that safety has to be a priority. It becomes cheaper to redesign a product or alter procedures than it is to pay compensation if deaths can be attributed to faulty design or practice. Traditional and familiar practices are re-evaluated while nothing new can be introduced to an increasingly sceptical and sophisticated public unless it is safe and believed to be safe. Even wars must be fought with no casualties.

The overall result of a myriad of technological, organizational and political improvements is that we now live in a society safer than the world has ever known. If an accident occurs, and the very word is nowadays suspect, we are no longer prepared to attribute it to divine displeasure, call it an Act of God or blame uncontrollable social forces. We instead try to lay the responsibility on organizations or individuals and seek compensation or punishment, goals far more attainable now than they were even a few decades ago. Whether the organization is a supermarket, a car manufacturer or a hospital, the public now assumes that it will operate with a proper standard of care and expertise. *E. coli* in meat, potentially lethal mechanical defects in cars and surgical incompetence are no longer acceptable.

The path from courageous pioneering to an acceptable level of safety may be a tortuous one of trial and error and bitter experience but with growing knowledge it will normally lead to increasing degrees of proceduralization, the setting of standards, mechanisms to ensure compliance with policies and guidelines, inspectorates, disciplin-ary procedures and inquiries when things go badly wrong. Training and education become inevitable, individuality restricted and freedom for practitioners to do as they would like curtailed. Nowadays one is taught to drive a car, one's competence is tested, there is a highway code it is foolish to ignore, seat belts are compulsory, at least in the UK, there are regular rigorous tests of the functioning of one's vehicle and the threat of breath testing reduces one variety of driving impairment. All this is reinforced by severe penalties for breaking the law. Much of this would have been unacceptable, if not unthinkable, in the 1930s but it is accepted now and it has led to a dramatic decrease in fatal road accidents.

These accidents are, by and large, accidents to other people—drivers are less at risk than pedestrians. This is of course not the usual situation in medicine where inter-ventions, however risky in themselves, are intended only to reduce the greater risk to the patient himself posed by the condition from which he is suffering. It is, however, the situation in two branches of medicine—infectious diseases and psychiatry, particu-larly forensic psychiatry where doctors carry the main responsibility and in other areas, for instance child protection, where the opinions of doctors may lead to a con-siderable interference with civil liberties. In the case of infectious disease the current concern is drug-resistant tuberculosis and for this Section 37 of the Public Health (Control of Disease) Act allows a patient to be detained for treatment, though this happens only rarely (Coker 1999). Psychiatrists likewise have a responsibility to ensure that their patients' illnesses do not lead them to harm anyone. The possibility that the mentally ill might do so is encapsulated in legislation stretching back from the 1983 Mental Health Act at least to the 1744 Vagrancy Act. Part II of the 1983 Act, which deals with civil procedures, states quite clearly that admission to hospital and detention there is possible for a patient suffering from mental disorder for assessment or treat-ment either 'in the interests of his own health or safety or with a view to the protection of other persons'. Nothing more is said in this part of the act about the protection of other persons and one can only assume the legislators believed that patients would be treated and kept in hospital until they were safe. Under Part III of the act, which deals with patients concerned in criminal proceedings or under sentence, the criterion for admission is whether the offence committed is punishable with imprisonment and then if 'it appears to the court, having regard to the nature of the offence, the ante-cedents of the offender and the risk of his committing further offences if set at large, that it is necessary for the protection of the public from serious harm' the court may impose a restriction order which means that a patient may only be discharged from hospital by the Secretary of State or by a Mental Health Review Tribunal chaired by a judge. Again nothing is said about the criteria for discharge but the possibility that risk may remain is covered by the power of the Secretary of State to set conditions for a conditional discharge and to recall a patient to hospital. The possibility that patients might need maximum security is recognized by the existence of the Special Hospitals, so designated by Section 97 of the 1959 Mental Health Act for patients 'who, in the opinion of the Minister, require treatment under conditions of special security on account of their dangerous, violent or criminal propensities'.

Fears about the dangerousness of psychiatric patients were more justified before the advent of sedatives and tranquillizers but even in 1922 Ashley could report an annual arrest rate of only 2.4 per thousand and no serious violence amongst patients paroled from the Middletown State Homeopathic Hospital (Ashley 1922). Sporadic follow-up studies of patients discharged from hospitals in the USA showed arrest rates that gradually increased to reach that for the normal population only in the 1970s. Then in 1974 Steadman and Cocozza published their follow-up study of the 967 patients transferred from maximum security to conventional hospitals in the wake of the Baxstrom decision. Of a sub-sample of 121 who reached the community only 16 were convicted in the next four years, demonstrating the safety even of patients who had been identified as dangerous. However, the authors themselves pointed out that these patients had been in prison or hospital for an average of 18 years and were 46 years old when released. One could add that the offences they had originally committed were not comparable with those of Special Hospital patients in the UK and during the follow-up period three patients out of the whole cohort of 967 did commit a homicide. Nevertheless, even when patients make threats to kill the outcome is surprisingly benign. Macdonald (1968) found that only 1% went on to do so. These and similar findings undoubtedly added force to the view that psychiatrists overpredicted dangerousness and, when this was perceived as leading to the unnecessary locking up of large numbers of people in sordid surroundings with inadequate treatment at great cost to society, politicians supported policies of deinstitutionalization and decarceration though not necessarily the provision of good care in the community (Tidmarsh 1982).

For many years even psychiatric text books were virtually silent on the subject of the risks posed by psychiatric patients. Then came the case of Graham Young, who in 1971 poisoned two of his workmates only months after being conditionally discharged from Broadmoor (Holden 1974). This discharge took place at a time when the gross overcrowding there was being rapidly reduced and owed more to humanity and therapeutic optimism than diagnostic and prognostic accuracy. Concern about risk was rekindled but only in the context of the Special Hospitals. The Aarvold Committee recommended additional procedures to make discharge safer but the Butler Committee's recommendation in 1974 that medium secure units should be set up in every regional health authority had as much to do with overcrowding in the Special Hospitals as with the risks posed by their patients (Home Office and Department of Health and Social Security (DHSS) 1974). This renewed interest certainly surprised Professor Bottoms to the point that he found it appropriate to entitle his inaugural lecture in 1977, 'Reflections on the renaissance of dangerousness'. However the Special Hospitals and the Regional Secure Units form only a small part of the psychiatric services and even in 1997 Grounds could still write in the context of homicide inquiries, 'The truth is that contemporary psychiatric services are not primarily designed to protect the public'.

Before considering what the level of risk to the public might be, it is worth digressing into what Sir Kenneth Calman, then the Chief Medical Officer at the Department of Health, called the language of risk (Department of Health 1996). He talked of the value-laden dichotomies, justifiable–unjustifiable and acceptable–unacceptable and the more mundane, avoidable–unavoidable. He then suggested labels for various levels of risk of an adverse event:

Frequency below one per million	Negligible
Between one in a million and one in 100 000	Minimal
Between one in 100 000 and one in 10 000	Very low
Between one in 10 000 and one in 1000	Low
Between one in 1000 and one in 100	Moderate
Frequency more than one in 100	High

As an example of a negligible risk he gave being killed by lightning, but one must remember that this low figure has a lot to do with the invention of lightning conductors. There are therefore risks that would be high in a state of nature but for which society has found defences that come to be taken for granted. Again, a negligible single risk to one individual can be translated into a significant risk if enough individual risks are summated. Thus the risk of an individual lorry bursting into flames must be very low indeed but multiply this by the millions of lorries using the Mont Blanc tunnel and the stage was set for disaster. The problem is how to relate the actual risk to subjective views about it.

What is an acceptable risk in psychiatry? Lewis, in 1982, commenting on a survey of mortality associated with anaesthesia which had shown one death in 10 000 applications or perhaps 280 deaths a year in England and Wales (Lunn and Mushin 1982), wrote 'To all other disciplines, in fact to all who make decisions, it presents the challenge: can you demonstrate that your disaster rate is as low as 1 in 10 000?'. This corresponds to the 'Very low' level of risk in Calman's classification. Since then, despite the ever-increasing problems which anaesthetists face, the mortality associated with anaesthesia has fallen. Even by 1986 it had fallen to 0.5 per 100 000 applications, that is to Calman's 'Minimal' level (Lunn and Devlin 1987).

What counts as a disaster in psychiatry? I suggest that the most obvious is a homicide by a psychiatric patient. How does psychiatry measure up to Lewis's challenge? Information about deaths caused by discharged psychiatric patients are hard to come by because of their rarity and for understandable political reasons. Thus comprehensive statistics of homicides committed by patients discharged from the Special Hospitals are not available, despite the existence of a case register started in 1972. McGrath (1968) was able to report that of 293 murderers released from Broadmoor none had killed again and only 4% had had to be recalled. His concern was that Broadmoor had been over cautious. As patients with the legal classification of Psychopathic Disorder were only admitted in 1960 when the 1959 Mental Health Act was implemented, the overwhelming majority of these patients would have been schizophrenic or depressed. Perhaps as a result of his findings, depressed patients who have committed homicide, usually as part of an extended suicide, are no longer considered dangerous and, being easily treated elsewhere, are now seldom admitted to Special Hospitals. However, 10 years after this report the author found that the situation had changed. Between 1960 and the end of 1978, 1946 patients had left Broadmoor, either as transfers to conventional National Health Service (NHS) hospitals, discharged to the community or returned to prison. Of these, 20, of whom 12 were classified as Psychopathic Disorder, had committed homicide by the end of 1978 (Tidmarsh 1982). By Calman's criteria this rate was moderate or high. I suggest it was acceptable only because the media and the general public knew nothing about it. Tennent and Way (1984) followed up a cohort of 1001 patients admitted to Special Hospitals between 1961 and 1965. Of these, 617 had been discharged by the end of 1977 and were responsible for six murders and two cases of manslaughter. Bailey and MacCulloch (1992) found one homicide in a sample of 106 patients discharged directly to the community from the new Park Lane Hospital between 1974 and 1989. The most recent follow-up study of Special Hospital patients was of 425 patients discharged in 1982 and 1983 (Buchanan 1998). By the end of 10 years 14% had been convicted of a violent offence and 7% of a sexual offence. Again, it was those classified as Psychopathic Disorder who were more likely to be convicted. These figures are lower than those found in 1984 by Tennent and Way. However homicide is not mentioned and whether the 1% rate for the 1960s and 1970s still applies to Special Hospital discharges is unknown. Unfortunately the Home Office statistics on discharged restricted patients are silent on this point but 5.3% of those released between 1972 and 1990 were reconvicted within five years of a grave offence, that is one that carries a maximum sentence of life imprisonment, a figure higher than the 3% for life sentenced prisoners (Kershaw et al. 1997a; Kershaw 1999)[1].

Even more obscure are the statistics for Medium Secure Units. Because they are small they need to be considered together for statistical purposes but there is no mechanism in place to do this. It appears that there have been only two long-term follow-up studies of patients from such a unit, by Baxter et al. (1999) and Maden et al. (1999). In the first, of a cohort of 63 schizophrenic patients followed up for 10 years 30% were reconvicted of at least one violent offence and, significantly, episodes of violent reoffending, which did not result in reconviction, were four times as frequent. No homicides were reported. In the second, 20% were convicted of a violent, sexual or

[1] The presentation of statistics by the Home Office team is a model of clarity. It is a great pity that there is no agreement about how further offences should be classified and that other studies of this population have not been presented in the same way. Comparisons between studies remain impossible.

arson offence over a 6.6 year follow- up. These failure rates are high by any standards and, even if the rate of violent offending was lower than before treatment, is it acceptable or, as with the Special Hospitals, is it accepted only because the public is unaware of the statistics?

What about non-secure hospitals and the psychiatric services more generally? In 1996 Bennett published the number of patients admitted to Special Hospitals between 1972 and 1992 convicted of murder or manslaughter. Probably two-thirds of these would have had previous admissions to ordinary NHS hospitals. The average was 33 a year with no sign of any trend. Patients who were not considered a continuing danger, for instance those who were depressed when they committed homicide, would have been admitted elsewhere so that these figures are not complete. Taylor and Gunn (1999), basing their calculations on nearly 40 years of Home Office statistics, concluded that people with schizophrenia were responsible for 40–50 homicides each year. They also concluded that the number had been falling but their assumption that the proportion of mentally ill amongst the falling number of diminished responsibility cases has not changed may not be justified. A more detailed analysis of 718 cases of homicide in the 18 months between April 1996 and November 1997 by the National Confidential Inquiry into Suicide and Homicide by People with Mental Illness in England and Wales found that 220 of the perpetrators had a lifetime history of mental disorder. The commonest diagnosis was personality disorder and substance abuse was frequent but schizophrenia was the diagnosis in 30 cases. One-hundred-and-two had been in contact with the psychiatric services at some time and 58 in the year before the homicide. Seventy-one were said to have had symptoms of mental illness at the time of the offence, 27 with delusions or hallucinations. The authors concluded that 40 homicides a year are committed by people who have been in contact with the psychiatric services in the year before the offence and that of these 12 are schizophrenic and four have affective disorders (Shaw *et al.* 1999a,b). In 1995/96 there were 45 780 'finished consultant episodes' for patients suffering from schizophrenia and related conditions (personal communication from DHSS Hospital Episode Statistics) so that these 12 represent one in about 4000 admissions and discharges. It is, according to Dr Calman, a low risk, and one which has not risen as the number of psychiatric hospital beds has declined, but higher than Lewis's challenge.

There are those who, by comparing the very few homicides by the mentally disordered with the much larger number of homicides by more normal people or with the number of people dying in other circumstances, for instance on the roads or by suicide, come close to saying that public and political concern is misplaced (Taylor and Gunn 1999). However, to take a view from outside psychiatry, the working rule of the Health and Safety Executive is that a risk of death to a member of the public above 1 in 10 000 is intolerable and calls for immediate action to reduce it regardless of cost (Royal Society Study Group 1992). This study group quoted a list of 11 negative attributes of hazards that influence the perception and therefore the acceptance of risk. No fewer than 8 of these are relevant to psychotic homicide and explain why the general public is disinclined to ignore this small risk. The perception of this small risk is no doubt reinforced by the violence that schizophrenics may display before admission. Humphreys *et al.* (1992) found that a fifth behaved in a potentially life-threatening way immediately before their first admission to hospital. That the managers of the psychiatric services have been slow to accept the need for clinical guidelines or to examine the processes by which treatment is given has been shown by recent surveys of what goes on, or perhaps more accurately, what does not go on, in psychiatric hospitals (Beardsmoore *et al.* 1998). Risk assessment and the concept of maintaining a culture of safety are still unusual and conflicts with civil liberties are unresolved. They have also, perhaps, taken little note of what others have been doing. It might be useful, therefore, to give some examples of how rare, but potentially avoidable, hazards are being recognized and managed in other medical or related areas.

My first example is maternal mortality and the part played by the Confidential Enquiry into Maternal Deaths in its reduction. In 1951 there were 686 maternal deaths, a mortality rate of 98.9 per 100000 births or 1 in 1011 (Cloake 1986). From 1994 to 1996 there were 134 deaths directly due to pregnancy (including abortion), about 45 a year, a rate of 6.1 per 100 000 or 1 per 16 393 births (Tomkinson 1979; Department of Health 1998). In Calman's terms the risk has fallen from low to very low and this reduction has obviously been associated with a host of clinical advances. In 1952 this 'low' risk was not acceptable and one of the strategies intended to reduce it was the setting up of the Confidential Enquiry into Maternal Deaths in England and Wales. Its remit was to identify avoidable factors in the sequence of events associated with a maternal death, an avoidable factor being defined as a departure from the accepted standard of satisfactory clinical and administrative care which may have played a part in the ensuing death. These avoidable factors may not have caused the death but may have increased its probability. The success of this enquiry has been due to its methodology and very largely to the trust fostered by the strict anonymity given to its informants which soon ensured honest and almost complete reporting. By the 1976–8 triennium only 1% of cases were missing. The information provided is assessed by three obstetricians working independently assisted where appropriate by an anaesthetist and a pathologist. Avoidable factors are classified as administrative, clinical and failures of co-operation on the part of the patient and have been found in rather over half the cases. They range from individual clinical failures at one extreme to administrative decisions at the other. The triennial reports have highlighted the uneven geographical distribution of mortality and resources, identified failures to introduce clinical advances, reinforced good practice, investigated and publicized rare problems, set standards and educated all concerned. More specifically, the 1967–9 report attributed 32 caesarean section deaths to anaesthesia: there was only one death in 1994–6. The enquiry has credibility and authority so that its recommendations are likely to be implemented and, though it can never be proved, it seems likely that without it mortality would have fallen more slowly and more unevenly than it has.

The inquiry has had its critics, for instance Beavis *et al.* (1993), but is set to continue and one notes that the number of deaths with which it is now concerned, 40–50 a year, is very similar to that for homicides by the mentally ill. Some findings have a relevance outside the specialty and will ring bells for psychiatrists, for instance, shortage of resources, non-availability of consultant staff, junior staff dealing with cases beyond their capabilities, lack of protocols, lack of team work and lack of co-operation on the part of the patient but it is its philosophy and methodology, now much copied by other specialties and by the National Confidential Inquiry into Suicide and Homicide by People with Mental Illness, that are of most relevance to psychiatrists. Where there have been avoidable factors or sub-standard care there has often been a failure to recognize a hazard, to assess risk and to manage that risk appropriately.

Recent developments in psychiatry have a lot in common with developments in the services for child protection that occurred a few years earlier and are now described in detail by Reder and Duncan (1999). Social workers and the National Society for the Prevention of Cruelty to Children (NSPCC) have long had the thankless task and the statutory duty to protect children. Their failure to do so adequately was highlighted in the reports of cases such as that of Maria Colwell (DHSS 1974). One response to these cases was that social work departments, following the example of the NSPCC, began setting up Child Abuse (now Child Protection) Registers as part of their multi-disciplinary management of cases of non-accidental injury. In the late 1970s there were reports of children dying of neglect which led to the recommendation that children who had been physically neglected, were failing to thrive or had been emotionally abused should be added to the register. In the 1980s there were reports of the deaths of children already statutorily in the care of local authorities. Then in 1987 came the juxtaposition of the Cleveland child sexual abuse scandal, where children had been taken from their parents without good reason (Butler-Sloss 1988), and the death of Kimberley Carlile, who had not been removed (Blom-Cooper *et al.* 1987). The dilemma was similar to that facing psychiatrists making decisions about patients at risk of violence, but with even more public obloquy. The subsequent 1989 Children Act was accompanied by guidance—'Working together under the Children Act 1989' (Home Office *et al.* 1991). This formalized the setting up of a case conference whenever abuse is reported, a decision whether or not to place the child on the register, the formulation of a care plan and the allocation of a key worker. Part 8 of this set out the procedures for conducting multi-agency reviews of child deaths by Area Child Protection Committees. These reviews, now known as Part 8 reviews, were therefore in place five years before the equivalent procedures for psychiatric homicides.

What then are the risks that social workers have to manage? Creighton (1992) estimated that 1–2 children in Britain died at the hands of their parents or relatives each week or 50–100 each year, a figure not entirely dissimilar from that of homicides by the mentally ill. Wilczynski (1997), quoting Home Office figures of 87 homicides of children under 16 annually, estimated that 58 would be filicides. These figures were for cases proved beyond reasonable doubt but after an examination of files from the Director of Public Prosecutions she estimated that the true figure could be 308 child deaths caused by abuse or neglect annually of which 275 would be filicides, almost five times higher than the official figure. If one accepts a figure of 300 deaths and the number of children at risk as 11 million this comes to a rate of 2–3 per 100 000 per year. Similar doubts about unidentified cases were expressed by Hobbs *et al.* (1995) following a confidential inquiry in Hull of 37 unexpected deaths in infancy. The social services had been involved in 11 cases but in only three had child protection case conferences been held. Though this study was modelled on the Confidential Enquiry into Maternal Deaths the report does not mention avoidable factors.

Both the earlier and the more recent Part 8 reports have been reviewed (DHSS 1982; Department of Health 1991; Reder *et al.* 1993; Falkov 1996; Reder and Duncan 1997). Their methodology, and in particular the haste in which they have to be produced, have been criticized by Wilczynski (1997) and by Reder and Duncan (1996*a*) who later made suggestions for their improvement (Reder and Duncan 1996*b*). General problems that cannot be deduced from single cases have emerged from these reviews. Thus Falkov found that in 32 of 100 cases there was clear evidence of parental psychiatric morbidity and in 10 cases psychosis, suggesting an overlap with patients involved in psychiatric homicide inquiries. Surprisingly, there were more psychotic parents than personality disordered or addicted ones. He recommended much greater co-operation between the child protection and the adult psychiatric services, a theme now all too familiar from psychiatric homicide inquiries. James (1994) too found that of 30 children, eight had been killed as a result of mental illness in a parent. He also found 11 cases in which men with known records of violence had joined the family. Twenty-six of these families were known to the social services, 12 had been subject to a case conference and 10 were on a register, but there is no way of knowing whether his sample is representative. Thus despite the fact that the Department of Health is notified of 120 cases a year and receives one case review each week, it is not possible to discover how many of the children killed were known to the social services before their deaths or in how many cases there were known risk factors.

There are doubts as to whether fatal child abuse is preventable by existing procedures. Despite the policies introduced by the 1989 Act, the child homicide rate has not fallen in the last 20 years, at least according to the official figures, despite, or perhaps because of, the large number of children on the registers (Creighton 1995). Thus statistics for the year ending 31 March 1993 show that 42 600 children were subject to case conferences of whom 24 700 were placed on the register. On that date there were 32 500 children on the register, which by then included sexual abuse cases, or 29.6 children per 10 000 of the population under 18 years of age (Department of Health 1994). If one uses Wilczynski's estimate, this means that about 1% of the number registered each year would be killed, a figure also suggested by Reder and Duncan (1999) and similar to that for Georgia where Jason and Andereck (1983) claimed that the fatality rate was 12 in every 1000 cases of physical abuse. This rate of 1% of cases would be called moderate to high by Calman but would not be acceptable in most circumstances. It is also a rate surprisingly similar to that for homicide among discharged Special Hospital patients. However, many of the children killed are not on the register, particularly infants, and older children are more often killed by friends, relatives or strangers. There are thus those at risk who are identified and protected, those who are identified but not protected, others who are not identified and some who could neither be identified nor protected. It would be interesting to see what the risks are for those who have case conferences but are not registered. One may conclude that though the system has many benefits, it is by no means certain that protection of children from homicide is one of them. The situation in psychiatry with respect to risk registers is, of course, similar.

My next example is the Parole Board and in particular its responsibilities for life sentence prisoners, responsibilities shared by forensic psychiatrists who are involved with a substantial minority of these cases. Since the implementation of the 1991 Criminal Justice Act, the numerically greater part of the Board's work has concerned prisoners serving determinate sentences of four years or longer. Those serving shorter sentences are released automatically with compulsory supervision for those serving one to four years. Those serving four years and over are also now subject to compulsory supervision and the rules are such that for many the granting of parole does not increase their time at risk in the community by very much. The Parole Board was set up following the 1967 Criminal Justice Act and has therefore had time to develop its procedures and monitor its results. It is of course only part of a process that starts with sentencing. The risk that concerns Parole Board panels is the risk of reoffending during the period of parole licence and here the maxim 'a small risk of violent offending is to be treated as more serious than a larger risk of non-violent offending' applies. The dossiers considered by panels come complete with predictions of reoffending generated using models described by Nuttall *et al.* (1977) and, more recently, Copas *et al.* (1996). The calculated risks of reoffending are based almost entirely on criminological data and not at all on behaviour or response to treatment packages in prison and may range from almost zero to over 80% in the two years after release. It has been found that they are bad predictors of reoffending by sex offenders and for them another instrument is available (Thornton 1995). Here again the predicted risk ranges widely from 2% to at least 36% in two years. The problem with these predictors is how to respond to them. Keeping a high-risk prisoner in prison will certainly prevent him offending during the possible parole period but it may only postpone his offending. However, knowing that a prisoner is a high risk on criminological grounds will certainly lead to a close scrutiny of his record in prison and his release plan. It is perhaps selecting those with a good response to treatment programmes and realistic after-care plans that has enabled the parole board to do rather better than these predictions would lead one to expect.

Less important numerically but more so politically are the life sentence prisoners. For mandatory lifers, that is, those convicted of murder, the Parole Board advises the Secretary of State who remains responsible for the decision to release on life licence. For discretionary lifers, that is, those convicted of other very serious offences, it has since the 1991 Criminal Justice Act been the Parole Board which takes the decision. There are three criteria for these discretionary life sentences: (1) the offence is a grave one and requires a long sentence; (2) the defendant is a person of unstable character and likely to commit such offences in the future; and (3) the consequences of such offences may be specially injurious. The Home Office collects statistics of reoffending for both kinds of lifers (Kershaw et al. 1997b). Between 1972 and 1994 there were 1687 people released on licence averaging about 73 a year. Of these, 362 (21%) have since been convicted of a standard list offence and 66 (3.9%) of a grave offence, though in only 28 of these was another life sentence given, the rates for the first five years at liberty being 19% for conviction for a standard list offence and 3% for a grave offence, a high risk in Calman's terms. In these first five years, 17% were recalled, only some of whom had committed offences. Recall is a failure for the individual but a success for the system as it means that the supervising probation officer has become aware of signs of relapse or decompensation and acted upon them. Indeed it may be the case that a high ratio of recalls to serious reoffending is a mark of a safe system and even perhaps that a system that allows rapid recall is one that can allow those at higher risk to be released. It will therefore depend in practice on the vigilance and professionalism of the Probation Service.

As one would expect from the reasons for their sentences, the reconviction rates for discretionary lifers are somewhat higher than for mandatory. After the Parole Board became responsible for these cases in 1992 the high rate of recall gave rise to some concern though there is no evidence of any increase above the 3% rate for grave offending. The systems for predicting the reoffending of determinate prisoners were not designed to predict violent or grave offences and no prediction scales for lifers have been worked out so that decisions have to be made on an individual basis for which the system in operation does at least provide plenty of information.

My fourth example concerns blood transfusion. In the U.K. the risks of transfusion are now very low indeed. Nevertheless even these very low rates were considered worrying and, following the lead of the Confidential Inquiry into Maternal Deaths, the Serious Hazards of Transfusion Committee was set up in 1996 to manage an anonymous system for reporting transfusion incidents aimed at improving safety still further. The findings of its very first report stimulated the Department of Health to issue a circular detailing appropriate action (Provan 1999; NHS Executive 1998). The most recent figures show that in the UK in 1997/8 major morbidity occurred 42 times and there were nine deaths—a rate of one in over 200 000 transfusions (SHOT Steering

Group 1999; personal communication from SHOT). In addition to these quantifiable risks, anxieties about the unknown risk of the transmission of new variant Creutzfeldt–Jacob disease are driving technical changes which will more than double the cost of transfusion.

Dental anaesthesia is my fifth example. For various reasons this country had an unusually and unnecessarily high rate of general anaesthesia given for dental procedures, there being two million general anaesthetics administered in 1967. Forty-four people died between 1979 and 1987, an average of 5.5 a year, giving a rate of perhaps 1.5 per 100 000 anaesthetics (Woodman 1998; British Dental Association 1998). In 1991 the report of the Poswillo Committee was published. Its recommendations accelerated the fall in these anaesthetics to 350 000 in 1997 and even fewer since then and deaths have fallen to two a year. In the present context it is interesting that this committee recommended the setting up of an ongoing inquiry into morbidity in relation to general anaesthesia and sedation. This, however, was not accepted. Concern remained and in November 1998 the General Dental Council, acting on the philosophy that 'any death is one too many', issued stringent new guidance to ensure that only properly trained and supervised anaesthetists should give general anaesthesia to dental patients, and that this should only take place in properly equipped premises supported by trained staff (General Dental Council 1998). The Department of Health has now gone further, recommending that by 31 December 2001 all general anaesthesia for dental treatment be provided in hospital (Department of Health 2000). One has to remember, however, that even in hospital dental anaesthesia has had its tragedies.

My final example is epilepsy and driving. Epilepsy shares with mental illness the fact that the illness frightens the general public, is stigmatized and may lead to restrictions. It appears obvious that a seizure while at the wheel of a vehicle is likely to lead to an accident and in the early part of the century many countries banned any person with a history of epilepsy from driving. Since then research has shown that the risks are not particularly high. Thus it was estimated in 1966 that 0.3–1 per thousand traffic accidents were attributable to epilepsy, causing perhaps between 2 and 8 deaths each year (Maxwell and Leyshon 1971). Taylor (1983) reported on 1605 accidents where the driver had collapsed at the wheel but had survived. Of these no less than 38% were due to a witnessed general seizure. In 12% of these it was a first seizure but 70% of the others had not declared their condition to the Licensing Authority. It was suggested that accidents caused by people who collapse at the wheel do not usually involve others but when they do and the driver is killed the cause of any collapse is hard to determine and these figures are therefore taken seriously. It is believed that the accident rate amongst licensed drivers with epilepsy is 1.3–2 times that of age-matched controls but perhaps three times as high when their epilepsy is undisclosed (Harvey and Hopkins 1983) but Taylor *et al.* (1996) found no difference in accident rates between patients with active epilepsy and estimates provided by the Transport and Road Research Laboratory for people without epilepsy. However a further large survey of drivers who had had a single seizure and had then had their licence restored after a seizure-free period of two years found that they had no more accidents than a population sample. They did appear to cause more non-driver fatalities, an increase of the order of 40–100%. There were in fact 12 deaths in three years caused by 16 958 drivers with epilepsy, an annual risk of about one in 4000. This risk is presumably considered acceptable if only because driving licences may now be restored after a seizure-free period of one year.

Because the potential damage is so much greater, the law debarred people who had had even one epileptic attack since the age of three from driving a Heavy Goods Vehicle or a Public Service Vehicle. As a result, probable epilepsy was responsible for only 17 accidents by London Transport drivers between 1953 and 1977, that is about one a year, but even so there were two fatalities (Raffle 1983). Medical supervision of these drivers is strict and the author ends his contribution: 'One can only speculate what might happen without this surveillance'.

Improvements in the treatment of epilepsy, a greater understanding of the prognosis and more information about the risks have led from a total prohibition to a gradual relaxation of the regulations for private motorists so that since 1994 one may start driving again after a seizure-free period of one year. The rules for heavy goods and public service vehicles have also been relaxed so that it is possible to drive these vehicles after a seizure-free period of 10 years. No recent estimates of the total number of fatal accidents caused by drivers who have seizures at the wheel are available.

Through these examples of responses to low risks runs a theme, though one not always played in the same sequence or with the same emphasis on its components. First there is a high-profile case spotlighted by the media and taken up by politicians, then a reluctant realization by the professions that such cases are no longer acceptable to the general public, the recognition and definition of a hazard, an examination of existing practices which are found wanting, a flurry of guidelines and perhaps legislation, changes in procedures at times actively opposed by practitioners, the enforcement (and perhaps even ritualization) of these procedures, the introduction of a system to inquire into further tragedies, the collation of these reports and identification of avoidable factors, and finally the implementation of improvements to the service so that it operates at a safer level. In short, the elements of audit but on a large scale. Over the last 15 years psychiatry in the U.K. has followed the same pattern.

In 1984 Sharon Campbell, a schizophrenic, killed Isabel Schwarz, her social worker. At a stroke this tragedy destroyed the myth of the invulnerability of those working with the mentally ill and demonstrated that it was not only Special Hospital or 'forensic' patients who could be dangerous. Until then, when the subject was not taboo, it was the prevailing belief amongst social workers that violence against them was due to their own failings. I believe that it was this case that initiated the changes that have led to our current policies and concern about risk and its management. The inquiry into the case (DHSS 1988) was only set up after prolonged pressure from the victim's father who continued to press for action after its publication[2]. In October 1991, after discussions with the Royal College of Psychiatrists and the National Schizophrenia Fellowship (which had proposed that there should be an inquiry covering all cases where serious harm had occurred), Mr Stephen Dorrell, then Parliamentary Under Secretary of State for Health, announced the setting up of a confidential inquiry covering homicides committed by discharged patients. Only later were suicides added but cases of serious harm, and other 'near misses', were never included. The inquiry was modelled closely on the Confidential Enquiry into Maternal Deaths. The first report appeared in 1994 and the most recent in 1999 (Steering Committee of the Confidential Inquiry into Homicides and Suicides by Mentally Abnormal People 1994; Shaw *et al.* 1999).

This measure was not enough to allay public anxieties about psychiatric homicides, partly no doubt because of a lack of openness over certain cases. Thus the report of the inquiry into the case of Larkland Francis, who in 1988 killed a neighbour's baby while he was part of a trial of community care, was never published (Connolly *et al.* 1996; Cowdry 1989), nor was the report of an inquiry into the case of Catherine Sullivan, who in 1992 killed a care worker while a patient in a MIND hostel in Kingston. It was, however, the reports that were published of the high-profile cases of Christopher Clunis, who killed Jonathan Zito at an underground station, and of Michael Buchanan that demonstrated just how meaningless the concept of community care could be for unstable patients, despite the Department's attempt to introduce the Care Programme Approach in 1990 (Ritchie *et al.* 1994; Heginbotham *et al.* 1994; Department of Health 1990). It was these cases that prompted the Department of Health to reinforce its commitment to the Care Programme Approach, issue its first tentative guidelines on risk assessment, introduce supervision registers and insist on the setting up of independent inquiries in cases of homicide (NHS Management Executive 1994; NHS Executive 1994). The hope is that risk assessment will identify the patients at risk of harming themselves and others and that the risks identified can be managed outside hospital. If not, these patients will not be discharged. Unfortunately nobody has suggested what level of risk is acceptable, and in any case assessment is an uncertain process. Furthermore, the pressure on psychiatric beds has already reached crisis point and it is difficult to see how these patients will be accommodated.

It is too early for official statistics to show whether the introduction of the practice guidelines has reduced risk. Neither the Confidential Inquiry nor the accumulating individual homicide inquiries have been in existence long enough to identify relevant avoidable factors in these deaths, still less whether they are diminishing. It is of course only too easy to equate an error in procedure to the cause of a homicide and to over-

---

[2] Interestingly, in the light of recent Department of Health circulars, one of the key objectives in her job description was to prevent admission of patients/clients from the community. One of her father's proposals was that psychiatric patients should be given a dangerousness rating, an idea which foreshadowed the Department's circular HSG(94)5 on risk assessment and supervision registers for patients.

look the importance of softer clinical data. Individual homicide inquiries are good at identifying local problems and individual failings but they are not good at looking at resource and organizational factors or assessing whether the problems they uncover have a more general significance. For this a series needs to be analysed and as yet there is no official procedure for doing this. Unofficial analyses have however suggested the importance of two clinical risk factors, substance abuse in combination with psychosis (Ward and Applin 1998) and non-compliance with medication (Howlett 1998). No doubt others will emerge.

Conclusion

The social and political climate is now such that avoidable risks to life have to be reduced to what historically is a very low level indeed. The risks that have prompted responses from the various organizations and professions described above have varied widely, from fewer than five deaths a year for dental anaesthesia and nine for blood transfusion to as many as 2–300 for child protection. The responses to these low risks have also varied, ranging from a total change in practice in the case of dental anaesthesia to the incremental changes in procedure that have characterized the management of life sentence prisoners.

There are many reasons why mortality is not reduced, lack of awareness of a risk being the first. Then there is the ascertainment of the outcome one is wanting to avoid. This may be easy, as for instance a death from dental anaesthesia, or uncertain, as, for instance, where a fatal accident has been caused by an epileptic fit or where a child has died in suspicious circumstances. A homicide by a psychotic patient is not difficult to identify but until recently there was no system to collect national statistics. Then there is the elucidation of the links in the causal chain which have led to the outcome. It may be impossible to prove their relevance, however, and perhaps the best one can hope for is the identification of avoidable factors which may have increased the probability of the fatal outcome. The exact weight one puts on these factors is unimportant: what is important is to discover their existence and thus provide the basis for remedial action, this being the philosophy which has always guided the Inquiry into Maternal Deaths. Once identified, there is no escaping the pressure to reduce a risk. The remedy may take many forms, for instance changing the organization as with dental anaesthesia or changing technical procedures as with blood transfusion. Inevitably, however, there is the hard fact, spelled out in the reports of the Enquiry into Maternal Deaths, that there are some hazards for which there are still no answers. One of these, which is of particular relevance to psychiatrists, but also to those involved with child protection and even obstetricians, is neither technological nor a matter of organization. It is the unco-operative patient who may have every right not to co-operate and whose altruism does not extend to taking every precaution necessary to insure himself against doing harm. The current debate about community treatment orders suggests that where the limits to the responsibilities of the psychiatric profession are to be drawn in these cases is debatable, but they may in time go beyond the mentally ill as indeed they already have for the probation service in their dealings with the many personality disordered people on life licence.

It is inevitable that psychiatry will follow the pattern set by other disciplines. Bennett (1996), on the grounds that policy changes in the last 30 years have not led to an increase of homicide patients admitted to Special Hospitals, was concerned about the scapegoating of psychiatric patients and, by implication, psychiatrists while others have compared the small number of psychiatric homicides with the much larger numbers of those succumbing for other reasons such as road accidents. It is, however, the case that other professions are concerned about risks that are much lower than those that have until now been accepted by psychiatrists. It is the author's belief that the current static level of risk of homicide is unacceptable, as was the static risk of death in childbirth between the wars, and that to compare it with greater risks in other fields is a poor excuse for maintaining the status quo; in any case, the changes that that are designed to reduce the risk of homicide will also reduce the risk of other kinds of harm. The political climate in which psychiatrists work has changed. In the 1970s, when this author started his career in forensic psychiatry, there were no more than 20 forensic psychiatrists in the UK. To psychiatrists in general, forensic psychiatry was another country. There were no textbooks, no training schemes, no diplomas, very little research and no information about risk. There is now an establishment for 158 consultant forensic psychiatrists in England and Wales and 22 in Scotland and this branch of the profession is identified as a sub-specialty or discipline. As with other disciplines, it cannot now escape a close and public inspection of its results and procedures. I believe that psychiatrists in general and forensic psychiatrists in particular will have to accept the kind of scrutiny that has been accepted by other professions and medical specialties and will have to be seen to be doing all that is possible to reduce the risks associated with their patients.

References

Aarvold Committee (1973) Report of the review of the procedures for the discharge and supervision of psychiatric patients subject to special restrictions, Cmnd. 5191. London: HMSO.

Ashley, M. C. (1922) Outcome of 1,000 cases paroled from Middletown State Homeopathic Hospital. *New York State Hospital Quarterly*, **8**, 64–70.

Bailey, J. and MacCulloch, M. (1992) Characteristics of 112 cases discharged directly to the community from a new Special Hospital and some comparison of performance. *Journal of Forensic Psychiatry*, **3**, 91–112.

Baxter, R., Rabe-Hesketh, S. and Parrott, J. (1999) Characteristics, needs and reoffending in a group of patients with schizophrenia formerly treated in medium security. *Journal of Forensic Psychiatry*, **10**, 69–83.

Beardsmoore, A., Moore, C., Muijen, M. *et al.* (1998) *Acute problems. A survey of the quality of care in acute psychiatric wards.* London: Sainsbury Centre for Mental Health.

Beavis, J., Keene, G. and Dunling, C. (1993) Value of confidential inquiries. *British Medical Journal,* **307,** 1426–7.

Bennett, D. (1996) Homicide, inquiries and scapegoating. *Psychiatric Bulletin,* **20,** 298–300.

Blom-Cooper, L., Harding, J. and Milton, E. (1987) A child in mind: protection of children in a responsible society. The report of the commission of inquiry into the circumstances surrounding the death of Kimberley Carlile. London Borough of Greenwich.

Bottoms, A. E. (1977) Reflection on the renaissance of dangerousness. *Howard Journal of Penology and Crime Prevention,* **16,** 70–96.

British Dental Association (1998) *General anaesthesia in the GDS.* London: British Dental Association.

Buchanan, A. (1998) Criminal conviction after discharge from special (high security) hospital. *British Journal of Psychiatry,* **172,** 472–6.

Butler-Sloss, E. (1988) Report of the inquiry into child abuse in Cleveland, Cm 412. London: HMSO.

Cloake E. (1986) Report on confidential enquiries into maternal deaths in England and Wales 1979–81. *Health Trends,* **18,** 40–3.

Coker, R. (1999) Public health, civil liberties, and tuberculosis. *British Medical Journal,* **318,** 1434–5.

Connolly, J., Marks, I., Lawrence, R. *et al.* (1996) Observations from community care for serious mental illness during a controlled study. *Psychiatric Bulletin,* **20,** 3–7.

Copas, J.B., Marshall, P. and Tarling, R. (1996) Predicting reoffending for discretionary conditional release (Home Office Research Study 150). London: HMSO.

Cowdry, Q. (1989) Killing triggers call to block release of mentally ill patients. *The Times,* November 2 1989.

Creighton, S. J. (1992) Child abuse trends in England and Wales 1988–1990. London: NSPCC.

Creighton, S. J. (1995) Fatal child abuse—how preventable is it? *Child Abuse Review,* **4,** 318–28.

Department of Health (1990) The Care Programme Approach for people with mental illness referred to the specialist psychiatric services, HC (90)23/LASSL(90)11. London: Department of Health.

Department of Health (1991) Child abuse: a study of inquiry reports 1980–1989. London: HMSO.

Department of Health (1994) Children and young people on child protection registers. Year ending 31 March 1993. London: Government Statistical Service.

Department of Health (1996) On the state of the public health: the annual report of the Chief Medical officer of the Department of Health for the year 1995. London: HMSO.

Department of Health (1998) Confidential enquiries into maternal deaths. 1994–6, HSC 1998/211. London: Department of Health.

Department of Health (2000) A conscious decision. A review of the use of general anaesthesia and conscious sedation in primary dental care. London: Department of Health.

DHSS (1974) Report of the committee of inquiry into the care and supervision provided in relation to Maria Colwell. London: HMSO.

DHSS (1982) Child abuse: a study of inquiry reports 1973–1981. London: HMSO.

DHSS (1988) Report of the committee of inquiry into the care and after-care of Miss Sharon Campbell, Cm 440. London: HMSO.

Falkov, A. (1996) Study of Working Together "Part 8" reports. Fatal child abuse and parental psychiatric disorder: an analysis of 100 area child protection committee case reviews conducted under the terms of Part 8 of Working Together Under the Children Act 1989. London: Department of Health.

General Dental Council (1998) *Maintaining standards. Guidance to dentists on professional and personal conduct.* London: General Dental Council.

Harvey, P. and Hopkins, A. (1983) Neurologists, epilepsy and driving. In *Driving and epilepsy—and other causes of impaired consciousness* (ed. R.B. Godmin-Austen and M.L.E. Espir), International Congress and Symposium Series, No. 60. London: Royal Society of Medicine.

Heginbotham, C. J., Carr, J., Hale, R. *et al.* (1994) The report of the independent panel of inquiry examining the case of Michael Buchanan. London: North West London Mental Health NHS Trust.

Hobbs, C. J., Wynne, J. M. and Gelletlie, R. (1995) Leeds inquiry into infant deaths. The importance of abuse and neglect in sudden infant death. *Child Abuse Review,* **4,** 329–39.

Holden, A. (1974) *The St Albans poisoner.* London: Hodder and Stoughton.

Home Office and DHSS (1974) Interim report of the committee on mentally abnormal offenders, Cmnd 5698. London: HMSO.

Home Office, Department of Health, Department of Education and Science and Welsh Office (1991) Working together under the Children Act 1989. London: HMSO.

Howlett, M. (1998). Medication, non-compliance and mentally disordered offenders. A study of independent inquiry reports. London: Zito Trust.

Humphreys, M. S., Johnstone, E. C., MacMillan, J. F. *et al.* (1992) Dangerous behaviour preceding first admissions for schizophrenia. *British Journal of Psychiatry,* **161,** 501–5.

James, G. (1994) Study of Working Together "Part 8" reports. Discussion report for ACPC national conference. London: Department of Health.

Jason, J. and Andereck, N. (1983).Fatal child abuse in Georgia: the epidemiology of severe physical child abuse. *Child Abuse and Neglect,* **7,** 1–9.

Kershaw, C. (1999) Reconvictions of offenders sentenced or discharged from prison in 1994, England and Wales, Home Office Statistical Bulletin. London: Government Statistical Service.

Kershaw, C., Dowdeswell, P. and Goodman, J. (1997*a*) Restricted patients—reconvictions and recalls by the end of 1995: England and Wales, Home Office Statistical Bulletin. London: Government Statistical Service.

Kershaw, C., Dowdeswell, P. and Goodman, J. (1997*b*) Life Licensees—reconvictions and recalls by the end of 1995: England and Wales, Home Office Statistical Bulletin. London: Government Statistical Service.

Lewis, A. F. (1982) Mortality associated with anaesthesia. *Health Trends,* **14,** 110.

Lunn, J. N. and Devlin, H. B. (1987) Lessons from the confidential inquiry into perioperative deaths in three NHS regions. *Lancet,* 12 December, 1384–6.

Lunn, J. N. and Mushin, W. W. (1982) Mortality associated with anaesthesia. London: Nuffield Provincial Hospitals Trust.

Macdonald, J. M. (1968) *Homicidal threats.* Springfield, IL: Charles Thomas.

Maden, A., Rutter, S., McClintock, T. *et al.* (1999) Outcome of admission to a medium secure psychiatric unit. 1. Short- and long-term outcome. *British Journal of Psychiatry,* **175,** 313–16.

McGrath, P.G. (1968) Custody and release of dangerous offenders. In *The mentally abnormal offender* (ed. A.V.S. de Reuck and R. Porter). London: Churchill.

Maxwell, R.D.H. and Leyshon, G.E. (1971) Epilepsy and driving. *British Medical Journal,* **3,** 12–15.

NHS Executive (1994) Guidance on the discharge of mentally disordered people and their continuing care in the community, HSG(94)27.

NHS Executive (1998) Better blood transfusion, HSC 1998/224.

NHS Management Executive (1994) Introduction of supervision registers for mentally ill people from 1 April 1994, HSG(94)5.

Nuttall, C. P., Barnard, E. E., Fowles, A. J. *et al.* (1977) Parole in England and Wales, Home Office Research Study No. 38. London: HMSO.

Provan, D. (1999) Better blood transfusion. *British Medical Journal*, **318,** 1435–6.

Raffle, P. A. B. (1983) The HGV/PSV driver and loss or impairment of consciousness. In *Driving and epilepsy—and other causes of impaired consciousness* (ed. R.B. Godmin-Austen and M. L. E. Espir), International Congress and Symposium Series. No. 60, London: Royal Society of Medicine.

Reder, P. and Duncan, S. (1996*a*).Reflections on child abuse inquiries. In *Inquiries after homicide.* London: Duckworth.

Reder, P. and Duncan, S. (1996*b*) A proposed system for reviewing child abuse deaths. *Child abuse and neglect,* **7,** 280–6.

Reder, P. and Duncan, S. (1997) Study of working together "Part 8" reports. Practice implications from a review of cases, report to the Department of Health.

Reder, P. and Duncan, S. (1999) *Lost innocents.* London: Routledge.

Reder, P., Duncan, S. and Gray, M. (1993) *Beyond blame: child abuse tragedies revisited.* London: Routledge.

Ritchie, J. H., Dick, D. and Lingham, R. (1994) The report of the inquiry into the care and treatment of Christopher Clunis. London: HMSO.

Royal Society Study Group (1992) Risk: analysis, perception and management. London: Royal Society.

Shaw, J., Appleby, L., Amos, T. *et al.* (1999*a*) Mental disorder and clinical care in people convicted of homicide: national clinical survey. *British Medical Journal*, **318,** 1240–4.

Shaw, J., Appleby, L., Amos, T. *et al.* (1999*b*) Report of the National Confidential Inquiry into suicide and homicide by people with mental illness. London: Stationery Office.

SHOT Steering Group (1999) Summary of Annual Report 1997–98. Manchester: SHOT Office, Manchester Blood Centre.

Steadman, H. J. and Cocozza, J.J. (1974) *Careers of the criminally insane.* Lexington: Lexington Books.

Steering Committee of the Confidential Inquiry into Homicides and Suicides by Mentally Abnormal People (1994) A preliminary report on homicide. Steering Committee of the Confidential Inquiry into Homicides and Suicides by Mentally Ill People.

Taylor, J. F. (1983) Epilepsy and other causes of collapse at the wheel. In *Driving and Epilepsy – and other causes of impaired consciousness* (ed. R. B. Godmin-Austen and M. L. E. Espir), International Congress and Symposium Series, No. 60. London: Royal Society of Medicine.

Taylor, J., Chadwick, D. and Johnson T. (1996) Risk of accidents in drivers with epilepsy. *Journal of Neurology, Neurosurgery and Psychiatry,* **60,** 621–7.

Taylor, P. J. and Gunn, J. (1999) Homicides by people with mental illness: myth and reality. *British Journal of Psychiatry,* **174,** 9–14.

Tennent, G. and Way, C. (1984) The English Special Hospital— a 12–17 year follow-up study: a comparison of violent and non-violent re-offenders and non-offenders. *Medicine, Science and the Law,* **24,** 81–91.

Thornton, D. (1995) Guidance on assessing the risk presented by sex offenders. Unpublished internal Prison Service document.

Tidmarsh, D. (1982) Implications from research studies. In *Dangerousness: psychiatric assessment and management* (ed. J.R. Hamilton and H. Freeman), pp. 12–20. London: Gaskell.

Tomkinson, J.S. (1979) An assessment of the enquiries into maternal mortality in England and Wales from 1952 to 1975. *Health Trends,* **11,** 77–80.

Ward, M. and Applin, C. (1998) *The unlearned lesson. The role of alcohol and drug misuse in homicides perpetrated by people with mental health problems.* London: Wynne Howard.

Wilczynski, A. (1997) *Child homicide.* London: Greenwich Medical Media.

Woodman, R. (1998) Dental Council aims to cut anaesthetic rate. *British Medical Journal,* **317,** 1407.

Chapter 3

Public policy and mentally disordered offenders in the UK

Ian Jewesbury and Andrew McCulloch

Introduction

In the second half of the twentieth century the main focus of general mental health policy has been on looking after mentally ill people within the communities where the rest of the population lives. In later years the idea of 'community care' has itself come under attack. The phrase has often been used ironically as a synonym for 'no care at all'. The foreword to the Labour Government's policy document 'Modernising mental health services' (see below) states that 'Care in the community has failed because, while it improved the treatment of many people who were mentally ill, it left far too many walking the streets, often at risk to themselves and a nuisance to others. A small but significant minority have been a threat to others or themselves'. However the reference to the 'many people' whose treatment has improved indicates that the approach is not, after all, being rejected out of hand. As will be seen in this chapter, there are separate questions about the definition of the 'community care' policy, about its validity, and about the adequacy of the resources devoted to it.

Legal framework

At the time of writing the main legislation governing the care and treatment of people suffering from mental disorder in England and Wales, including those who have committed offences, is the 1983 Mental Health Act. Its main focus is on the arrangements for compulsory admission to hospital of those suffering from serious mental disorders. An important point is that the power to treat patients against their will is limited to those who are detained in hospital. Although the act does provide for patients to be subject to a form of community supervision known as 'guardianship'——and, since 1996, to 'supervised discharge' or 'after-care under supervision'—there is then no power to compel them to undergo treatment.

The main provisions dealing with the compulsory admission and detention of non-offender patients are in Part II of the 1983 act—sometimes known as the 'civil sections' to differentiate them from those dealing with offenders. Generally speaking patients may be admitted to hospital on an application by their nearest relative or (more usually) a social worker approved under the act. The application must be supported by two medical recommendations.

Part III of the 1983 act contains the equivalent provisions for mentally disordered offenders, described as 'patients concerned in criminal proceedings or under sentence'. These sections deal with admission to hospital under a court order or (for those already in prison) a direction made by the Home Secretary. Like an admission under the civil powers, a court order or direction must be supported by two medical recommendations.

Once they have been admitted to hospital, mentally disordered offenders are subject largely to the same powers as those admitted under Part II—though they may be subject to a restriction order or direction giving the Home Secretary powers over their discharge, leave of absence or transfer to other hospitals. A restriction order may be made by a court at the same time as a hospital order on the grounds that it is 'necessary for the protection of the public from serious harm'. A restriction direction is made by the Home Secretary when a sentenced prisoner is transferred to hospital (whether or not that person is thought to present a serious risk).

The 1983 act also contains a number of provisions designed to protect the rights of patients, including the system of tribunals to consider appeals against detention and the definition of forms of treatment for which the patient's consent or a second opinion (or in some instances both) is required. The criteria for compulsory admission under the 'civil' powers reflect a general preference for non-compulsory approaches: a patient may only be detained for treatment if that treatment 'cannot be provided unless he is detained under this section'. This particular limitation does not apply to mentally disordered offenders, for whom the alternative to enforced hospital admission may be a prison sentence.

The Labour Government's proposals, published in 1999, for replacing the 1983 act are described later in this chapter.

Care in the community

At the start of the twentieth century it was usual for seriously mentally ill or disturbed people to be detained for care and treatment in large hospitals or asylums. From the 1950s onwards the movement away from this approach—initially driven by advances in medical treatment—became the dominant force in mental health policy and legislation. The 1959 Mental Health Act, which gave effect to the proposals of the Royal Commission on the Law Relating to Mental Illness and Mental Deficiency (the Percy Commission) (Royal Commission on the Law Relating to Mental Illness and Mental Deficiency 1954–57) had removed statutory controls from the great majority of mental patients, and provided a clearer statutory framework, including new safeguards for those patients who would still be subject to legal restrictions. These procedures were largely retained when a new Mental Health Act was introduced in 1983. The 1959 act also provided for the 1946 National Health Service Act and the 1948 National Assistance Act to apply to people with a mental disorder, so establishing the principle that general health and social services should be available to them as they were to those with a physical illness. In 1961 the then Minister of Health, Enoch Powell, declared the Government's commitment to the eventual closure of the old mental hospitals (Powell 1961).

Part of the dynamic which drove the move away from institutional care was the conviction that mentally ill people as a group were not especially dangerous. As Taylor and others have recorded (Taylor *et al.* 1993): 'Virtually all the work from the first half of this century showed that mental hospital patients were less likely to commit violent acts than the general population'. The influence of this belief is clearly apparent in the 1975 White Paper 'Better services for the mentally ill' (Department of Health and Social Security (DHSS) 1975). While this recognized violent or disruptive behaviour as a serious issue for mental health services, it was seen essentially as a problem at the margin of mental health care: 'adequate supervision *of the relatively few patients who require it* is important for public trust and confidence in the overall pattern of care' (italics added).

The Butler and Glancy reports

The belief in a community-based model of care as it developed in the 1960s and 1970s stopped short of including those patients who fell within the remit of the three special (high security) hospitals. But if providing physical security was no longer to be a function of the local mental health services the question was left of what to do about those patients who really did need it. This was considered in the reports of two separate Government committees.

The first was the Butler Committee on Mentally Abnormal Offenders. The Committee was appointed in September 1972 with a wide-ranging remit:

(1) To consider to what extent and on what criteria the law should recognize mental disorder or abnormality in a person accused of a criminal offence as a factor affecting his liability to be tried and convicted, and his disposal.

(2) To consider what, if any, changes are necessary in the powers, procedure and facilities relating to appropriate treatment, in prison, hospital or the community, for offenders suffering from mental disorder or abnormality, and to their discharge and aftercare; and to make recommendations.

The committee's appointment was prompted by the case of a notorious poisoner, Graham Young, who had been released with little or no supervision after eight years in Broadmoor special hospital and had gone on to commit two murders and another attempted murder. While the committee was not directly concerned with changes in the broader shape of mental health services, it identified an urgent need for secure hospital units to be established in each National Health Service (NHS) region. Indeed, the perceived urgency was such that the committee made this the subject of an interim report published in advance of its main report in 1974. This recommended a level of 40 beds per million total population, or a total of 2000 for England and Wales, to cater for those mentally disordered people (both offenders and non-offenders) who needed to be looked after in conditions of security but not at the level provided by the special hospitals.

The Butler Committee's main report, published in 1975 (Home Office/DHSS 1975), also included important recommendations on the law relating to psychopathic disorder and the management of those suffering from it. This is considered later in this chapter.

The second report to consider the subject of secure hospital provision, also published in 1974, was that of a working party chaired by Dr James Glancy of the DHSS (DHSS 1974). The Glancy report estimated the need at 20 places per million total population or 1000 nationally—only half the level proposed by Butler. However, this took account only of patients already in NHS hospitals, while the Butler Committee's estimate also included those unsuitably placed in prison. Moreover, the Glancy working party emphasized that theirs was a provisional figure which would need to be reappraised in the light of experience. The Government of the day adopted the Glancy figure as an interim target, to be reviewed when the first 1000 beds were in place.

The units which were to provide the new secure places were termed 'regional secure units'. In later years the terms 'medium secure units' and 'medium security' became more usual. These imply a level between the 'special' high security hospitals and more local, lower, security provision. But this is not how it was seen in the mid 1970s. Neither the Glancy report nor 'Better services for the mentally ill' saw physical security as having any real place in a local psychiatric service. The Glancy report made it clear that locked wards were seen as a negative performance measure. The report records that in 1971 'some 13 000 (7.6%) of the total [patients] in psychiatric hospitals were in wards that were regularly locked by day'. It goes on to say that this was largely accounted for by 'practices which in varying degrees constitute a mistaken and negative use of security—the application of the principles laid down in the later part of this report would have resulted in the great majority of the 13 000 being treated without secure accommodation'. The aim in recommending the 1000 regional secure beds was to obviate entirely the need for physical security in local psychiatric services. By contrast, in 1992 the final report of the Reed review of services for mentally disordered offenders (see below) was to record that the number of beds in locked or lockable mental illness wards at local level had fallen by 45% between 1986 and 1991 (the fall for learning disabilities had been even sharper) and that this needed to be restored to somewhere near the 1986 total.

The general messages of the Glancy report and 'Better services for the mentally ill' can be summed up as:

(1) Violence by psychiatric patients, though an important issue in its own right, did not rank among the major problems confronting psychiatric services; possibly more of a challenge for the services was to dispel popular stereotypes about mentally ill people being violent.

(2) The small minority of mentally ill people who were found to be 'continuously difficult or unpredictably violent' were not the responsibility of local district services but should be looked after by a separate service (regional secure unit or special hospital, according to the level of violence and dangerousness) which had the special expertise necessary to deal with the problems they presented. However, the importance of co-operation between the different services was emphasized.

In the event the 'interim target ' of 1000 medium secure places adopted in 1974 took more than 20 years to achieve. This failure was central to the problems identified in the 1990s by the Reed review.

The Reed review

At the end of 1990 the Department of Health and Home Office embarked on a joint review of health and social services for mentally disordered offenders (Department of Health and Home Office 1992). The review was chaired by Dr John Reed of the Department of Health by whose name it became known. It was to be a watershed in the development of Government policy for forensic services. Its remit was:

> To plan, co-ordinate and direct a review of the health and social services provided in England by the NHS, Special Hospitals Service Authority and local authorities for mentally disordered offenders (and others requiring similar services without having come before the courts), with a view to determining whether changes are needed in the current level, pattern, or operation of services and identifying ways of promoting such changes …

Among other things the review was to take account of the new management arrangements being introduced for the NHS, the way different services were funded and how this might be improved, and relevant research and studies.

The establishment of the review reflected a climate of growing concern about the problems of dealing with mentally disordered offenders and the difficulty of securing co-operation between the agencies concerned in the health and social services and the criminal justice system. A Home Office circular issued in 1990 (with the Department of Health's co-operation) had encouraged diversion of mentally disordered offenders from criminal proceedings at the earliest possible stage (Home Office 1990). An element of this was the high proportion of prisoners suffering from serious mental disorder. Contemporary research by Gunn and others had shown that between 750 and 1400 sentenced prisoners might require transfer to hospital for psychiatric treatment (Gunn *et al.* 1991). The review's terms of reference referred specifically to the reports of the Woolf inquiry into disturbances in 1990 at Strangeways prison and of a recent efficiency scrutiny of the Prison Medical Service.

On the health service side of this equation the number of places in regional secure units had only reached 600 against the 'interim' Glancy target of 1000 adopted in 1974. Concern about this was sharpened by the separation of NHS purchaser and provider functions from 1991, which it was feared would put services for mentally disordered offenders in direct competition with other local services.

The Reed review was mainly conducted over the period 1990–92 but provided the starting point for work on a number of specific issues which continued in the following years. As the foundation for their work the review team formulated a set of 'guiding principles' which should govern the way mentally disordered offenders are cared for. To some extent these can be seen as a reaffirmation of the philosophy of community-based care: patients should be cared for 'as far as possible, in the community, rather than in institutional settings', 'under conditions of no greater security than is justified by the danger they present to themselves or others', and 'as near as possible to their own homes or families, if they have them'.

These principles could have been applied almost equally to general mental health services and their adoption by the review reflects the fact that the term 'mentally disordered offenders' covers a very broad range of individuals, not all of whom represent a physical danger to other people. The same thinking is reflected in the Reed review's detailed recommendations—of which there were nearly 300 in total. The key elements included the following.

(1) There should be formal arrangements for co-operation between agencies concerned with mentally disordered offenders, including those in the criminal justice system as well as the health and social services. These arrangements should include regular assessments of the services required.

(2) Every locality should have a multi-professional core team as the focus of care provision for mentally disordered offenders. This should cover the whole range of the professions concerned in the health and social services (and some others such as education staff and probation officers) including both general mental health staff and forensic specialists.

(3) The Care Programme Approach, which had been adopted in 1990 as the general basis for the care of severely mentally ill people (Department of Health 1990), should apply equally to mentally disordered offenders. The overall purpose of the approach was 'to focus the most resource-intensive assessment, care and treatment on the most severely mentally ill people, whilst ensuring that all patients in the care of the specialist psychiatric services receive the basic elements of the CPA' (Department of Health 1995). Its main elements were:

- systematic assessment of health and social care needs
- an agreed care plan
- allocation of a key worker
- regular review of the patient's progress.

Reed recommended that the Care Programme Approach should apply specifically to discharged prisoners with continuing mental health care needs, and to patients remitted to prison after mental health treatment in hospital.

(4) The over-representation of ethnic minority communities among those classified as mentally disordered offenders was an important issue. More should be done to establish the reasons for this, to ensure that ethnic minority members benefited fully from schemes for diversion from custody, and to make services more sensitive to their needs.

The basis of the Reed approach was, then, to place specialist forensic services firmly in the context of general mental health services. If mentally disordered offenders were fully accepted as part of the clientele of those services more specialist forms of care could be limited to those who really needed them rather than having to compensate for shortfalls in the general services. But even on this assumption Reed identified serious shortcomings in the specialist forensic services. The need for medium secure beds was reassessed and a new target of 1500 proposed. At the start of the review there had been only 70 consultant forensic psychiatrists nationally—nearly half of them working in the three special hospitals. The review calculated that this number would need to be more than doubled to meet the needs of the new medium secure units and provide an acceptable level of care in the special hospitals. Similar increases were needed in other professions such as forensic nursing and clinical psychology.

The level of 600 medium secure beds achieved by 1990 appeared even more inadequate when set against the new target. But the new emphasis on integrating forensic services with general mental health care also marked a decisive break with the basic assumptions of the old policy. Specialist forensic services were now seen as part of a spectrum of secure provision, with local secure services, working as an integral part of the local mental health service, at one end of it, and the special hospitals at the other. The local secure services were seen as including the formerly scorned 'locked wards'.

The problem with secure psychiatric provision was not simply that there were not enough beds. They were also in the wrong places. In particular, the shortfall in local medium secure beds had led to a substantial number of patients being left in the high security special hospitals whose condition did not justify that level of security. The Reed review identified divisions of responsibility between different agencies financed from different budgets as an important cause of this. Local health authorities had no financial incentive to make provision out of their own budgets for special hospital patients whose care was being paid for centrally by the Department of Health, through the Special Hospitals Service Authority.

The imbalance in the different levels of security was identified by Reed as a critical flaw in the forensic services. It worked against the central objective of a range of services which could be deployed flexibly to respond to patients' changing needs. The special hospitals were large and isolated. Those left stranded in them were effectively cut off from their local communities with poor prospects of long-term rehabilitation. Concern about this was compounded by periodic reports of ill treatment and improper care of patients in the hospitals. At Ashworth Hospital these were considered by a Committee of Inquiry which identified a large number of failings in the management of the hospital and its care of patients (Committee of Inquiry into Complaints about Ashworth Hospital 1992).

Implementation of Reed

The overall impact of the Reed proposals is not easy to assess. The review itself, and the wide publicity given to its extensive series of detailed reports, generated a great deal of discussion and debate. Its conclusions were endorsed by the then Government which in successive years identified mentally disordered offenders as a key priority for health and social services. It is certainly true that awareness of the problems and needs of mentally disordered offenders was greatly increased. A growing number of court diversion schemes were funded by the Home Office and the Department of Health provided 'pump-priming' funding for these and a variety of local multi-agency projects. But the impact of these initiatives on the care actually received by mentally disordered offenders, though undoubtedly significant, cannot readily be quantified.

The review did have a measurable effect on the provision of medium secure places. In 1992, following publication of the first series of consultation papers from the review, the Government announced that it was increasing the central capital allocation for this purpose from £3 million to £18 million. Funding continued at a similar level in subsequent years, and the original Glancy target of 1000 places (irrelevant as it now was) was finally reached in 1996. By 1998 the number had risen to 1600.

There was also a measurable, and large, increase in the number of prisoners transferred to hospital under the provisions of the Mental Health Act. The overall number rose more than three-fold between 1989 and 1993—after which it remained fairly stable at around 750 a year. Taking unsentenced and untried prisoners alone there was a more than five-fold increase between 1989 and 1994, from 98 to 536 (Home Office 1998).

High security services

Following the main Reed review a new working group (also chaired by Dr Reed) was formed specifically to seek solutions to the problems surrounding high security services. Its report, published in 1994 (Department of Health 1994), quoted findings by Maden and others from 1992 suggesting that as many as half of the 1700 patients then in special hospitals did not need care in high security conditions. The main reason for this was the inadequacy of medium and lower security facilities. The working party recommended that high security services should be dispersed among a larger number of units with no more than 200 high security patients each (these would include the existing special hospitals, operating on a reduced scale). It also made proposals for tackling the distortion of priorities caused by separate budgets through progressively greater involvement of NHS purchasers in high security services.

The then Government announced its decisions on the working party's proposals in 1995 (NHS Executive 1995). The proposal for dispersal of high security services was not accepted 'for the time being', but new funding arrangements were introduced on the lines recommended by the working party. These were co-ordinated by a new Commissioning Board on which NHS purchasers were represented (as were the Home Office and the Prison Service). The Special Hospitals Service Authority was abolished. These changes came into effect from April 1996.

The document setting out the Government's response also gave the results of the most detailed analysis yet undertaken of needs for secure mental health care. It covered 3580 patients who were then in the special hospitals, NHS and independent sector secure hospitals, or in prison. The analysis revealed a serious gap in the existing services, represented by the large group of 1360 patients needing longer-term care at medium or lower levels of security. Six hundred and forty of these were then in special hospitals, representing 42% of all special hospital patients. 'Longer-term' is defined in this context as a period of 24 months or more. Little or no specific provision had been made for this group. Its absence can be traced back to the view taken in 1974 by the Glancy working party which saw medium secure care as essentially a short-term requirement—stating in its report that: 'If no progress is being made after, say, 15 months, consideration should be given to an alternative placement such as return to prison, admission to a special hospital, or return to an ordinary psychiatric hospital'.

Better co-ordination of high and medium security services, and the removal of perverse financial incentives, remained an objective of the new Government elected in 1997. The Government announced in 'Modernizing mental health services' (see below) that regionally based specialized commissioning groups were being formed to commission both high and medium security services from April 2000. There was also to be legislation to enable high security hospitals to be constituted as NHS Trusts (subsequently enacted in the 1999 Health Act). But the Government still stopped short of endorsing the 1994 Reed proposal for dispersal of high security services. The three special hospitals would 'continue to be the main providers'.

At the beginning of 1999 the shortcomings of the special hospital system were again highlighted in the report of another inquiry (the Fallon Inquiry) into Ashworth Hospital (Committee of Inquiry into the Personality Disorder Unit, Ashworth Special Hospital 1999). This was specifically concerned with the personality disorder unit at the hospital. It was prompted by allegations made by a former patient in the unit about misuse of drugs and alcohol, financial irregularities and the availability of pornographic material. The report largely endorsed the account which had been presented of a ward 'where staff had lost control and where patients manipulated staff and systems more or less at will'. More generally, it summed up the picture painted by the series of earlier reports on the special hospitals of 'insular, closed institutions whose predominantly custodial and therapeutically pessimistic culture had isolated them from the main stream of forensic psychiatry'. The report concluded that Ashworth Hospital was not retrievable and should be closed once alternative regional services were in place. This was rejected by the Government (though it largely accepted the report's detailed recommendations for strengthening management and improving security at the hospital). The Government's response to the report (Department of Health 1999a) reaffirmed its view of the importance of Ashworth, Broadmoor and Rampton in providing high security psychiatric care and asserted that the changes introduced by the 1999 Health Act (to allow them to be managed by NHS Trusts) would bring them 'back into the NHS fold'.

Wider context

Any assessment of the impact of policy changes affecting mentally disordered offenders is complicated by the scale of the problems which the mental health services as a whole found themselves facing in the 1990s. The difficulties presented by dangerous or violent patients were an important factor in these. This made the shortage of secure facilities, and the relationship between forensic and general mental health services, a central issue.

Failings in the mental health services were highlighted by a series of homicides committed by psychiatric patients or former patients. These cases attracted wide publicity and so did the reports of the inquiries which were set up to establish what had gone wrong. The first of these was the 1988 report on the inquiry into the case of Sharon Campbell (Spokes 1988). The report highlighted the lack of effective co-ordination between the many different professionals involved in Miss Campbell's care. It made a series of recommendations directed at ensuring that each patient had a proper care plan and did not lose contact with the services. The care plan should be prepared before a patient was discharged and should be the subject of regular multidisciplinary review by all those concerned in the patient's care from both health and social services. These ideas formed the basis of the Care Programme Approach mentioned above.

In 1993 the report of the inquiry chaired by Miss Jean Ritchie into the care of Christopher Clunis (Ritchie 1994) highlighted the shortage of medium secure places in the then South East Thames region. The report also referred to the impression formed by the inquiry team that there was a shortage of such places serving the whole of central London. Because of this, 'sometimes patients who require to be admitted to a medium secure unit bed have to be contained within general psychiatric wards, which are not properly equipped to care for patients who are disturbed or violent'. Another consequence was that patients who were ready to leave medium secure units sometimes had to be discharged directly into the community, without having been involved in any local rehabilitation programme. There were also not enough forensic psychiatrists to care for mentally ill offenders and other disturbed or violent patients.

The Ritchie report also commented more generally on the insufficiency of general psychiatric beds in London hospitals to care for all the patients who should properly be admitted for treatment. It quoted bed occupancy figures of between 100% and 120% for the Hither Green, Horton and South Western Hospitals and of 130% for the Central Middlesex Hospital. Evidence of such a shortage can be found in many other sources. The Mental Health Act Commission (1997) recorded that, across the country, there were 98 patients for every 100 beds (though this fell to 86 per 100 beds if patients on leave were excluded). Eight per cent of wards had more patients than beds designated for them. The pressure was greatest in Inner London where the proportion of detained patients was three times that of other inner cities and four times the level for England as a whole.

These findings raise an obvious question about resources for mental health. Government had always denied that the closure of mental illness hospitals was meant to save money. The declared intention in 1975 (in 'Better services for the mentally ill'—see above) was that savings from the reduction in the number of in-patients should be redeployed to develop the health and social services needed by mentally ill people in the community. It is often argued that in reality the savings were used to develop acute medical and surgical services. There are no readily accessible statistics to prove or disprove this, but it is certainly the case that the number of NHS hospital beds for mental illness fell sharply. A survey undertaken in 1994 for the Mental Health Task Force showed that the number of such beds had fallen from 83 700 in 1982–83 to 47 296 in 1992–93—a reduction of 46% over the 10 years (Davidge *et al.* 1994). The 1982–83 figure—dating as it does from a period when the principle of community-based care for mentally ill people was firmly established—itself reflects a steep decline from the peak of 149 696 reached in 1955. The fall in NHS bed numbers over the 10 years to 1992–93 was offset to some extent by an increase in the number of local authority, voluntary sector and private sector beds and residential places. If these are added to the NHS beds the combined total shows a fall of only 5%, from 92 234 to 87 568. It cannot be assumed, though, that the new beds and places represented an equivalent level of service. The evidence, quoted above, of pressure on acute psychiatric beds suggests clearly that this resource was unequal to the demands being placed on it.

Cumulatively the series of failures contributed to the growing sense of cynicism about community care described at the start of this chapter, and the growing concern about risks to the public and to mentally ill people themselves. The Conservative Government did not go as far as its Labour successor in concluding that 'care in the community has failed' but it did take a series of steps directed at reducing the perceived risks—in particular, the introduction of supervision registers in 1994 and of the new 'supervised discharge' powers in 1996.

Labour Government policy

The new Government's vision for the future of mental health care was set out in 1998 in the policy document 'Modernising mental health services' (Department of Health 1998). This made a clear break with earlier approaches by acknowledging at the outset that there was a relationship between active mental illness and violence, and by including the protection of the public among the central aims of the new policy. The change proposed to the actual structure of services, which were to be 'safe, sound and supportive', was less radical. The main elements were to be 'extra beds of all kinds, better outreach services, better access to new anti-psychotic drugs, 24 hour crisis teams, more and better trained staff, regional commissioning teams for secure services, and development teams'. As mentioned above, the development of secure hospital services and the integration of forensic and general mental health services was given some prominence.

Where the new approach departed most sharply from the past was in abandoning the long held assumption that care and treatment outside hospital should rely on the patient's voluntary participation and that only those who were ill enough to be in hospital should be subject to compulsory treatment. 'Modernising mental health services' recorded the Government's judgement that 'the existing laws on mental health are now out of date', highlighting the absence of powers to enforce compliance with treatment outside hospital. It announced that there was to be a comprehensive review of the 1983 act. The proposals put forward by the Government following this review are discussed below.

The approach was further developed with the publication in September 1999 of the National Service Framework for Mental Health (Department of Health 1999b). This is likely to have a significant impact on all branches of psychiatry. For the first time, it sets out a comprehensive central strategy for adult mental health services. It places a strong emphasis—both explicit and implicit—on public safety, and more specifically on ensuring adequate risk assessment and management. This can be expected to fuel both direct and indirect pressures on forensic psychiatry by encouraging yet more conservative management of individuals who offend, or who are at risk of offending, and by increasing the significance of the sub-specialty as a source of advice and 'consultancy' as well as direct service provision.

Specific measures within the National Service Framework include:

- plans to provide a further 300 secure beds (subsequently modified to 471) by April 2002
- a requirement to set local milestones on access to assessment and services through the criminal justice system
- a national requirement to reduce the number of prisoners awaiting transfer to hospital
- enhanced training on risk assessment for staff working with severely mentally ill people

- a requirement to work towards reducing suicide rates in prison and in hospital
- a requirement to develop in-reach services to work with mentally ill people in prisons.

As financial underpinning of the strategy the Government committed itself to investing an extra £700 million over the three years 1999/2000–2001/02 in improving mental health services. The NHS Plan (Department of Health 2000) made new pledges to provide 200 additional long-term secure beds by 2004 and to move 400 patients from high security hospitals to more suitable settings. It also promised new places for people with severe personality disorder (see below).

New legislation

Following the publication of 'Modernising mental health services' in September 1998 the Government announced the appointment of an expert committee to carry out a fundamental review of the 1983 Mental Health Act. The committee submitted its advice in July 1999. The Government put forward its own detailed proposals for consultation in November 1999 (Department of Health 1999c). These took account of the expert committee's advice but did not follow it in all respects.

The new proposals were wide ranging, covering a large number of issues which had arisen during the 17 years of the 1983 act's operation. But in setting out the case for change the document again emphasized the Government's concern about the limited nature of the powers to compel patients to undergo treatment. The proposals were 'designed to provide greater flexibility in this area by breaking the automatic link between compulsory care and treatment and detention in hospital'. A further key objective was to ensure that the provisions of a new act were fairly and consistently implemented. To this end the Government proposed that some of the key principles underlying the legislation should be expressly stated in the act itself. It also envisaged greater clarity in the assessment procedures for patients subject to compulsory powers, and a process for independent decision making in all cases where this was to continue for longer than 28 days. This contrasts with the 1983 act under which decisions to apply compulsory powers are essentially taken by the professionals concerned. These elements, designed to provide more explicit protection of the rights of patients, can be seen as offsetting to some extent the increased restriction of patients' liberty implied by the creation of new compulsory powers. They also reflect the need to comply with the provisions of the European Convention on Human Rights, incorporated into UK law by the 1998 Human Rights Act.

Under the Government's proposals, decisions to impose compulsory care and treatment beyond an initial 28 day period would be taken by a new kind of tribunal. If it was satisfied that compulsory care and treatment were justified, and that a properly constituted care plan was in place, the tribunal would issue a 'compulsory order' reflecting the content of the care plan and specifying whether treatment was to be provided in hospital or in a community setting. In the latter case the order could state where the patient was to live and require him or her to comply with the specified arrangements for care and treatment. The health and social services would also be under a duty to deliver these arrangements. If the patient did not comply, the care team would be have powers to enter premises where he or she was and to convey the patient to a stipulated place for care and treatment, or to hospital. If necessary help could be sought from the police, though it was envisaged that this would be done only as a last resort.

In relation to offender patients the consultation document stated that 'the provisions of the 1983 act in respect of offenders have proved fundamentally sound'. The new arrangements for compulsory care and treatment would also be available for mentally disordered offenders, the compulsory order in these cases being made by the court instead of the new tribunal. The court would decide this in the light of a formal assessment in hospital. As for non-offender patients the order could specify care and treatment in a community setting, though the court would need to consider whether the risk to public safety required the offender to be detained in hospital. The court would retain the power to make a restriction order in cases where the offender presented a risk of serious harm to others.

The consultation document also proposed some detailed changes to meet problems which had arisen in operating the mentally disordered offenders provisions of the 1983 Mental Health Act.

Psychopathic disorder

Some of the most contentious issues raised by the 1983 act concern the way in which it deals with people with psychopathic disorder (or anti-social personality disorder). The new Government did not include this in its main review of the 1983 act but made it the subject of a separate, but linked, policy initiative. While the main review of the act was led by the Department of Health, the initiative on personality disorder was managed by the Home Office, reflecting its responsibility for the criminal justice system.

The legal, policy and management problems presented by this group of people have greatly troubled successive governments. The 1983 act defines psychopathic disorder as 'a persistent disorder or disability of mind (whether or not including significant impairment of intelligence) which results in abnormally aggressive or seriously irresponsible conduct on the part of the person concerned'. Thus, the disorder is defined by the behaviour it is said to produce, and this raises the question of the basis for distinguishing those with 'psychopathic disorder' from others who commit violent crimes.

Following an extensive review by the Butler Committee of the problem of psychopathic disorder, the 1983 act side-stepped the central question by stipulating that a person suffering from psychopathic disorder may only be admitted to hospital for treatment if it 'is likely to alleviate or prevent a deterioration of his condition'.

Whether or not this requirement is met is left to the judgement of the doctors who must recommend a person's admission to hospital under the act. In the absence of generally agreed criteria it may be a matter of chance whether an offender is sent to prison or admitted to hospital. A 1993 survey by Dolan and Coid of the existing research recorded that 'there is still no convincing evidence that psychopaths can or cannot be successfully treated (Dolan and Coid 1993).

The problems relating to psychopathic disorder were the subject of a further study undertaken in the wake of the Reed review, by a working group which was also chaired by Dr Reed. Its report, published in 1994 (Department of Health and Home Office 1994), included proposals for more research and evaluation and fuller use of facilities for assessment before decisions were taken on whether an offender should be imprisoned or made the subject of a hospital order.

The Reed working party also recommended the introduction of a new form of disposal which it termed a 'hybrid order'. This would be a combined prison sentence and hospital order imposed by a court, with the prison sentence set as an appropriate tariff for the offence. The offender would be sent initially to hospital; but if treatment proved ineffective he or she could be transferred to prison to complete his or her sentence there. The purpose was to obviate the problem described above when a psychopathically disordered hospital patient proves to be untreatable and there is no legal basis for continuing his or her detention. This proposal was subsequently adopted by the former Government in the shape of the 'hospital direction' introduced by the 1997 Crime (Sentences) Act.

The Labour Government's proposals, entitled 'Managing dangerous people with severe personality disorder', were published for consultation in July 1999 (Home Office 1999). Their intention was described, firstly, as ensuring that 'dangerous severely personality disordered (DSPD) people are kept in detention for as long as they pose a high risk', and secondly as 'managing them in a way that provides better opportunities to deal with the consequences of their disorder'. The law would be changed so that such people would not be released while they continued to present a risk to the public.

Under the Government's proposals the courts would no longer have the power to order the admission to hospital of offenders diagnosed as suffering from psychopathic disorder. The paper set out two options for the future legislative and service framework. The first would broadly maintain the existing framework with specific modifications to deal with the personality disorder group. In the case of those convicted of offences, the courts would be able to make greater use of discretionary life sentences and would have new powers to remand offenders for specialist assessment. For those not currently before the courts the new 'civil powers' (to be decided following the wider review of the 1983 act as described above) would be framed so as to allow DSPD individuals to be detained in hospital whether or not they were 'likely to benefit from hospital treatment'. These might include people approaching the end of a determinate prison sentence if they were still thought to present a risk to the public. Where a DSPD individual was placed would depend on whether he or she had been detained under criminal or civil legislation. Specialist facilities would be developed within both the prison and health services, possibly with joint funding and joint commissioning by a central agency.

Under the second option, a new legal framework would be introduced to provide for the indeterminate detention of DSPD individuals in both criminal and civil proceedings. In both cases this would have to follow a period of compulsory assessment in a specialist facility. There would also be powers for supervision and recall following a person's release from detention. A new specialist service would be set up for the management of DSPD individuals. This would be separate from, but closely linked to, the prison and hospital services.

A point which attracted much criticism when the Government's proposals were published was that they would allow indefinite detention of people who had not committed any offence and were not suffering from a treatable mental disorder. The document included provisions intended to ensure that the new arrangements complied with the European Convention on Human Rights—indeterminate detention would be authorized only on the basis of an intensive specialist assessment, there would be a process of appeal and the authority to detain would be subject to regular independent review.

Conclusion

The new direction signalled by the Labour Government can be seen as a watershed for both general and forensic mental health policies. The catchphrase 'safe, sound and supportive' (adopted as the subtitle of 'Modernising mental health services') reflects a determination to set the Government's own distinctive stamp on policy development. The point has been made in this chapter that this does not, in reality, represent an entirely clean break with the past. Nevertheless, the new emphasis on public safety, the commitment to legislation allowing compulsory treatment in the community, and the extra resources designated for mental health services add up to an important shift of approach. The measures set out in the National Service Framework (described above) and the NHS plan have started to give this some tangible shape.

All this suggests an enhanced future role for forensic services, which will be further extended if new specialist services are developed for people with severe personality disorder. Achieving it will present some formidable challenges. More forensic psychiatrists, psychologists, nurses, occupational therapists and others will be needed to work in secure settings. Moreover it cannot be assumed that the additional secure beds planned will be enough to meet continuing pressures from acute mental health services, the community and the criminal justice system. These will be intensified if (as many commentators have suggested) the increasing preoccupation with public safety leads to greater conservatism in practice. Concerns about safety and risk may also create more demands on forensic psychiatry for advice, training and research and development.

This chapter has described some other long standing difficulties affecting the work of forensic services. One of the most troublesome has been the position of the three special hospitals. The Government has followed its predecessors in insisting that these remain as the providers of high security services, in the face of unequivocal (and repeated) advice about the extreme difficulty of making them effective in a therapeutic role. High security care is clearly a key element of any forensic mental health service, and putting right the often identified shortcomings of the high security hospitals must therefore be a critical task.

In the past one of the key problems in getting the right balance between different levels of security has been the division of responsibility for funding. While the new Government has sought to address this by introducing regional commissioning of both high and medium security services, it remains to be seen whether the division between these regionally commissioned services and the general services commissioned by primary care groups or patient care teams will prove a source of new problems. A related issue is the stigma associated with secure psychiatric services which is likely to present continuing difficulties in relation to the siting of new units and the placement of patients who are ready to leave.

The over-representation of ethnic minorities among those identified as mentally disordered offenders has so far received only limited attention. Perceived injustice (whether apparent or real) in the way different groups are dealt with must work against the acceptability and effectiveness of forensic services. Ensuring that this is properly tackled will be another important challenge.

Finally, the Government's strategy places some weight on the proposed new powers to allow compulsory treatment to be imposed on patients living outside hospital. How effective these will be in improving the safety of the public and patients themselves remains to be seen. A recent study concluded that there was no clear evidence that new compulsory powers would have averted incidents of homicide committed by psychiatric patients or former patients (National Association for the Care and Resettlement of Offenders 1998). It will be important to guard against unreal expectations about this, leading in turn to a false sense of security. The introduction of the new powers will require very careful handling. Achieving the goals which the Government has set itself will call for imagination, flexibility and persistence—and a realistic appreciation of the resources needed for the task.

References

Committee of Inquiry into Complaints about Ashworth Hospital (1992) Report, Cm 2028. London: HMSO.

Committee of Inquiry into the Personality Disorder Unit, Ashworth Special Hospital (1999) Report, Cm 4194. London: Department of Health.

Davidge, M., Elias, S., Jayes, B. *et al.* (1994) Survey of English mental illness hospitals, March 1994. Birmingham: University of Birmingham.

Department of Health (1990) The Care Programme Approach for people with a severe mental illness referred to the specialist psychiatric services. London: Department of Health.

Department of Health (1994) Report of the working group on high security and related psychiatric provision. London: Department of Health.

Department of Health (1995) Building Bridges: A guide to arrangements for inter-agency working for the care and protection of severely mentally ill people. London: Department of Health.

Department of Health (1998) Modernising mental health services. London: Department of Health.

Department of Health (1999*a*) Government response to Fallon inquiry (press release 1999/0461). London: Department of Health.

Department of Health (1999*b*) National service framework for mental health. London: Department of Health.

Department of Health (1999*c*) Reform of the Mental Health Act 1983: proposals for consultation, Cm 4480. London: Department of Health.

Department of Health (2000) The NHS Plan, Cm 4818. London: Department of Health.

Department of Health and Home Office (1992) Review of health and social services for mentally disordered offenders and others requiring similar services: final summary report, London: HMSO (detailed reports on specific aspects of the services considered in the review were published in six further volumes in 1993 and 1994).

Department of Health and Home Office (1994). Report of the Department of Health and Home Office working group on psychopathic disorder. London: Department of Health and Home Office.

DHSS (1974) Revised report of the working party on security in NHS psychiatric hospitals. London: Department of Health and Social Security.

DHSS (1975) *Better services for the mentally ill.* London: HMSO.

Dolan, B. and Coid, J. (1993) *Psychopathic and antisocial personality disorders: treatment and research issues.* London: Gaskell.

Gunn, J., Maden, T. and Swinton, M. (1991) *Mentally disordered prisoners.* London: Home Office.

Home Office (1990) Provision for mentally disordered offenders, Circular No. 66/90. London: Home Office.

Home Office (1998) *Statistics of mentally disordered offenders in England and Wales 1997*, Issue 19/98. London: Home Office.

Home Office (1999) *Managing dangerous people with severe personality disorder: proposals for policy development.* London: Home Office.

Home Office/Department of Health and Social Security (1975) Report of the Committee on Mentally Abnormal Offenders. London: HMSO (an interim report by the committee was published in 1974).

National Association for the Care and Resettlement of Offenders (1998) *Risks and rights: mentally disturbed offenders and public protection* .London: NACRO.

NHS Executive (1995) High security psychiatric services: changes in funding and organisation. London: Department of Health.

Powell, J. E. (1961) Mental hospitals for the future. In *Emerging patterns for the mental health services and the public.* London: National Association for Mental Health.

Ritchie, J. (Chair) (1994) Inquiry into the care and treatment of Christopher Clunis. London: Department of Health.

Royal Commission on the Law relating to Mental Illness and Mental Deficiency (1954–57) Report. London: HMSO.

Spokes, J. (Chair) (1988) Report of the committee of inquiry into the care and after-care of Miss Sharon Campbell. London: HMSO.

Taylor, P., Mullen, P. and Wessely, S. (1993) Psychosis, violence and crime. In *Forensic psychiatry, clinical, legal and ethical issues.* Oxford: Butterworth-Heinemann.

The Mental Health Act Commission (1997) Seventh biennial report 1995–97. London: HMSO.

Chapter 4

Psychiatric disorder and individual violence: imagined death, risk and mental health policy

Joan Busfield

Introduction

The media show considerable fascination with deaths and violence that result from the actions of individuals with a psychiatric history. In the UK, the death of Jonathan Zito at the hands of Christopher Clunis in 1992 attracted considerable attention, as did the action of Ben Silcock who climbed into the lion's den at London Zoo. Similarly the death in 1994 of Christopher Edwards at the hands of Richard Linford when they were put in the same cell in Chelmsford prison was reported in the national as well as local press, as was that of the social worker, Jenny Morrison, killed by a psychiatric patient, Anthony Joseph, when she visited him in the community as part of her duties.

These homicidal or violent actions may result from delusions of persecution and the person who kills may have a diagnosis of schizophrenia. Alternatively the focus throughout their psychiatric history may have been on criminal activity and wrong-doing, or on alcoholism or drug dependence, and the individual may have received a diagnosis of conduct or anti-social personality disorder, or some other personality, behaviour or substance use disorder. Some of the individuals involved may have a criminal record; frequently, they will have had one or more spells in a psychiatric bed, either on a compulsory or informal basis, and have been discharged into the community, often under the care of a community psychiatric nurse (CPN). The CPN may see them once a month, perhaps giving them their injections, or they may refuse medication or disappear from contact with any form of community mental health service. Usually close examination of their psychiatric records in the aftermath of the violent incident produces evidence of earlier events or statements which can, retrospectively, be read as warnings of the dangers they posed: threats that they wanted to kill someone or a previous incident involving physical violence.[1]

---

[1] Joseph had, for instance, threatened to kill his mother some six months earlier. However, the problem with such retrospective readings is that it is usually possible to identify some significant event which, with the hindsight, can be read as predictive. The difficulties of prediction are discussed further below.

It is now common in the UK for deaths like these to be attributed to failures in the implementation of the policy of community care, or even to fundamental flaws in the policy itself. The detention of lunatics considered dangerous was one important justification for the establishment of asylums in the nineteenth century, along with optimistic assumptions about the therapeutic potential of asylum care, and issues of dangerousness still feature strongly in the rationales for the use of compulsory powers to detain individuals within the framework of mental health legislation. It is not surprising, therefore, to find that the introduction of policies of community care in the second half of the twentieth century, along with the closure of the old asylums, is often blamed for acts of violence by mentally disturbed individuals. On the one hand, it is suggested that community provision for those with a psychiatric history of severe mental disorder is in practice frequently inadequate—that too few resources are provided to support such individuals in the community, or that there are inadequate controls to ensure that they comply with treatment, usually in the form of medication. On the other hand, it is suggested that disturbed individuals with propensities to dangerousness need to be held in secure or semi-secure accommodation on a compulsory basis, and that the policy of community care has been taken too far, at least in relation to this group of people, and needs to be reversed. Here the argument is that whereas in the past the dangerous lunatic was locked up now she, or more usually he, is free to roam the streets and kill or attack at random.[2] Underpinning such analyses is the assumption that the move to community care has increased the risks of violence by those suffering from a psychiatric disorder, and that what we now need to do is to find ways of reducing those risks.

The official response in the UK to public concerns about violence by those with psychiatric problems has been two-fold. In the first place, individual deaths and the events that lead up to them have been the subject of a series of expensive and elaborate individual inquiries (see, for instance, Ritchie *et al.* 1994; Coonan *et al.* 1998; Herbert *et al.* 1999), inquiries that were made mandatory in 1994. These have generated a plethora of recommendations, many strikingly similar, intended to reduce the likelihood of reoccurrence of such events. Frequently mentioned is the need for better inter-agency co-operation, with individuals apparently falling between the cracks of health and social services, for more consistency of care over time, as well as for better communication between different types of worker, such as psychiatrists and CPNs.

Second, there have been a number of policy initiatives, particularly prompted by the adverse publicity surrounding Jonathan Zito's death, in an effort to allay public disquiet and to reduce violence by those with a psychiatric history living in the community. These include: the greater use of risk assessment of individual patients, often

---

[2] Analyses of such deaths indicate that men make up around two-thirds of assailants (Royal College of Psychiatrists 1996).

as part of the care programme approach (CPA) in which a plan of care is devised for those discharged into the community; the introduction in 1994 of a requirement for registers of persons with severe mental illness discharged into the community 'who are, or are liable to be at risk of committing serious violence or suicide, or of serious self neglect' (Department of Health, 1994); and, following legislation in 1995, the intro-duction of supervised discharge orders, which require those discharged under such orders to comply with a care plan developed for them.[3]

The most recent proposal is to rectify what is now considered by some to be a 'loop-hole' within the provisions of the 1983 Mental Health Act. This is that persons with a diagnosis of 'psychopathic disorder', unlike those with severe mental illness, cannot be compulsorily detained for any length of time under the provisions of the 1983 Mental Health Act if they are considered untreatable, a judgement commonly made of those identified as having this disorder. The term psychopathic disorder (see Ramon 1987), which is defined in the Act as 'a persistent disorder ... which results in abnormally aggressive or seriously irresponsible conduct' (paragraph 1), and is not a term widely usedin psychiatric classifications, is close to the *Diagnostic and Statistical Manual*'s (American Psychiatric Association 1994) 'antisocial personality disorder' and to the *International Classification of Diseases*' (World Health Organization 1992) 'dissocial personality disorder' and its 'conduct disorder', the latter referring to 'a repetitive and persistent pattern of dissocial, aggressive or defiant conduct' (ibid: 266).[4] Individuals with a severe mental illness, who are considered a threat to others or themselves and are unwilling to be admitted to hospital on a voluntary basis can be compulsorily detained. Depending on the circumstances this is either for observation (for 28 days under section 2 of the act) or treatment (initially for six months under section 3), or in emergencies for 72 hours (section 4). In contrast, persons with a psychopathic disor-der cannot be held under section 3 for treatment if that treatment is not likely to allevi-ate their disorder or prevent a deterioration in their condition. There is a clear logic to this (not holding for treatment those who will not benefit from it) which fits liberal concerns to protect the rights of the individual.[5] However, more recently politicians and policy makers, responding to public concerns about dangerousness, have argued that the law should be changed since some of the most difficult and potentially danger-

---

[3] If they refused to comply a mental health worker could take them to the place where the care plan had designated that they should reside. However, supervised discharge orders have not been widely used.

[4] These characterisations suggest conduct that might be viewed as closer to 'badness' than 'madness'. An alternative argument is that these individuals have a long-standing personality or behavioural 'problem'.

[5] The then legal director of MIND, Larry Gostin, spearheaded a successful campaign to reform the 1959 Mental Health Act, emphasizing the need for changes that strengthened the civil rights of individual pateints (see Gostin 1975).

ous individuals, if considered untreatable, cannot be held for longer periods in psychiatric facilities even if they are considered dangerous.[6]

It is vital, however, when considering the risk reduction strategies prompted by these widely publicized cases, cases which seem to confirm the stereotype of those with mental disorder as potentially dangerous individuals who need to be controlled, to put them into a broader social context. Sociological ideas and approaches, as well as those of other theorists, can cast light both on the extent of public attention that is given to deaths and violence at the hands of disturbed, and on efforts at risk reduction. In what follows I first seek to understand the public attention to deaths and violence by psychiatric patients. I then turn to examine the empirical evidence on the connection between psychiatric disorder and individual violence, focusing on violence against others rather than the self in order to keep the scope of the analysis within manageable boundaries.[7] I next examine the sociological literature on risk, exploring its potential contribution to understanding strategies of risk reduction in relation to individuals with psychiatric disorder. Finally, I assess the implications of this theoretical and empirical work for mental health policies in relation to dangerousness.

The media and imagined deaths

That deaths caused by individuals with a psychiatric history generate considerable attention in the media is not surprising. Violent deaths in general appear to exert a particular fascination on the human consciousness, or at least fin de siecle western consciousness. Death, especially unexpected death—death that should not have happened—provides the media with endless copy. On the one hand, there is the obsessive fascination with the death of public figures when it is unexpected and premature, as the deaths of Diana, Princess of Wales in 1997 and of John F. Kennedy in 1963 (and even the more recent death of his son) attest, or for that matter of the lesser known but nonetheless public figures of Gianni Versace or Jill Dando. All were killed in the prime of their lives, either as a result of accident or murder. Such deaths fill the newspapers and television screens, and generate books and films. They often, too, lead to detailed public inquiries of the causes of the accident, or to detailed investigations in the search for the killer and their motives. This obsession with the unexpected, premature deaths of individuals is paralleled by a popular, new, and rather different genre of narratives of death and dying, usually written by journalists and other media figures. These

---

[6] This includes the small number of individuals in England and Wales found not guilty by reason of insanity. They are usually sent to one of the special hospitals such as Broadmoor, but can be transferred to another psychiatric facility and then discharged when appropriate (though in practice their detention may be longer than it would be if they had been dealt with solely through the criminal justice system).

[7] I use the term individual violence to indicate that there is no attempt to encompass forms of collective violence such as war.

graphically and movingly describe their experiences and their struggle against death (frequently from cancer), often vividly portraying their feelings and emotions and those of their families and friends (the narratives of Liz Tilberis (1998), Ruth Picardie (1998) and John Diamond (1998) are recent examples). Here subjective experience and the inner world are brought into the picture very explicitly.

On the other hand, there is the endless media exploration of large-scale tragedies— of collective deaths—such as the sinking of the Herald of Free Enterprise, the crushing of spectators at the Heysel football stadium, the Lockerbie bomb that brought down an aeroplane, the King's Cross underground fire, the Dunblane shootings, or for a new generation, tragedies such as the sinking of the Titanic, recently recounted in both book (Bainbridge 1996) and film. These larger scale disasters often, too, lead to public inquiries in an effort to attribute blame, and can serve as a potent lever for policy change in relation to safety measures, depending on the interpretation of events and the current political climate. Both individual and collective deaths have now also spawned a generation of TV documentaries. One could also note the popularity of TV programmes about medical work involving death and threatened death.

In this context of a public obsession with unexpected, extraordinary death, the media attention to the deaths that result at the hands of a person with a psychiatric history is to be expected. Such deaths, especially those involving attacks on a stranger, not only belong to the category of the unexpected, unpredictable death, they also involve direct attacks by one person on another. Moreover, unlike many other unexpected deaths, they involve actions by people whose thoughts, feelings and behaviour are viewed, almost by definition, as irrational and uncontrollable (see Busfield 1996, Chapter 3). There is therefore a double unpredictability: not only is the death unpredictable, but so too is the killer. Indeed, where death involves the killing of one person by another, there is usually a tendency to view the killer as somehow disturbed, even if there is no formal psychiatric history—a tendency in part based on the difficulty of understanding how an individual could behave in such a way and on the ready elision between the apparent unintelligibility of the behaviour and mental disorder.[8] For instance, the Dunblane killer (who took his own life after the shooting) was described in the media as a 'loner', a standard media signifier for someone who is not quite normal or properly adjusted. The same applies to many of the frequent shootings in the USA, where the lives and psychological pathologies of killers are used to explain her, or more usually his, actions and to bring them back into the category of the explicable. In such cases the focus on the killer's pathology (which may well be clear cut), is part of a widespread tendency to individualize and personalize events, so drawing attention away from the social factors that have played their part, such as the USA's extremely liberal gun legislation, or the failure in the UK fully to use the tighter gun

---

[8] This linkage is emphasized by a diverse range of writers (see, for instance Laing 1967; Jaspers 1963).

control powers that are available, or indeed, in both cases, any examination of the character of contemporary society and community which may encourage such behaviour.

We can seek to understand this obsession with unexpected, extraordinary death in a number of different ways. Sociologists and historians have pointed to the different ways in which death is understood and given meaning across time and place. A common argument is that there has been a 'sequestration of death' in advanced western societies (Aries 1976; Mellor 1993)—that death has been increasingly hidden from public view. In the light of the discussion so far about the media fascination with death, such claims might seem surprising, or indeed patently false. However, the argument about the sequestration of death is that personal death, that is the death of those whom we know personally, now tends to be dealt with, and experienced, in private rather than public ways, including in particular our own feelings about it. Most visible here is the narrowing of the rituals of public mourning—the disappearance of the wearing of black armbands by mourners, of the slow funeral cortege with the mourners walking behind the coffin, of the public and open display of the body—rituals which were often sustained through religious institutions. In addition, there is the marked change in the location of death away from the home to the hospital where death is arguably much more hidden from view.[9]

Whilst some have seen the media obsession with death as calling into question theorists' claims about the sequestration of death, others have suggested that the media obsession is a product of that sequestration: that as personal deaths become more private and hidden away, and as our feelings about these deaths are not publicly expressed, so the public obsession with the unexpected deaths of others has increased. Our fears and anxieties about our own death and of the deaths of those to whom we are close find their outlet in the form of 'imagined deaths', relivings of the experiences of others, a process that involves some identification with the horrors of these extraordinary deaths, described so vividly in the media. We imagine what it would feel like to lose someone for whom we care. We imagine what it would have been like to die in the Herald of Free Enterprise or the Titanic as the ship went down, as well as trying to work though the significance of what it means to have one's life ended so abruptly.

The argument here is that our underlying anxieties and fears about death, including the knowledge that we ourselves will die, can be handled in different ways, and that in societies where personal death is less familiar (partly because of increased longevity), where the rituals surrounding death are more restricted, and where our belief in the afterlife has virtually disappeared, then interest in the unexpected death of others

---

[9] Although much is made by some theorists of the move from home to hospital as the place of death, and it is frequently seen as part of the sequestration of death (see Giddens 1991), the hospital is a public space, the home a private one, and the key issue is the social relations surrounding death—how visible the death is to the wider public.

increases.[10] Put in this way the argument tends to suggest some universality in fears and anxieties about death alongside varying culturally accepted ways of responding to death. However, a number of writers have argued that the degree of our underlying fear of death is itself variable between individuals and over time, as well as the way in which it is manifested. R.D. Laing used the notion of ontological security, a concept grounded in existential ideas, to characterize the psychologically healthy individual. Such a person, he contends has:

> a sense of his presence in the world as a real, alive, whole, and, in a temporal sense, a continuous person. As such, he can live out into the world and meet others: a world and others experienced as equally real, alive, whole, and continuous.
>
> Such a basically *ontologically* secure person will encounter all the hazards of life, social, ethical, spiritual, biological, from a centrally firm sense of his own and other people's reality and identity (Laing 1965:39)

Ontological security is contrasted with the condition of ontological insecurity, where the individual is less able to cope with the hazards of life, Laing viewing the latter as one of the defining characteristics of schizophrenia (though not restricted to it, and by implication the condition extends to those who are especially anxious and fearful but not schizophrenic).

More recently, Giddens (1991) has used the concept of ontological security in a similar fashion to characterize the sense of security and self-identity of individuals which allows society to function, but has added an historical dimension to the analysis. He argues that in late modern societies, where individuals have to construct their own sense of identity reflexively (that is, consciously and with self-awareness), the awareness of one's own potential death—fear of non-being—is one of the key threats to ontological security. Consequently, drawing on his ideas, we can see the portrayal of unexpected deaths in the media as reflecting fears and anxieties about death which are characteristic of the age and are not constant across time and place.[11] At the same time these fears and anxieties are enhanced and amplified by the media, since the media permit 'the *intrusion of distant events into everyday consciousness*' (Giddens 1991:27, author's italics).

Extended to deaths caused by individuals with a psychiatric history, sociological discussions therefore help us to understand the psychological grounding and social shaping of the powerful fears and anxieties, as well as fascination, that surround such deaths, fears which are tied to the character of contemporary society.[12] Significantly, such an analysis also suggests that the public's fears of death and violence may be exaggerated. We need therefore to determine how extensive the risks of violence are

---

[10] Public executions, which served to emphasize the importance of adherence to social norms, may in the past have exercised some of the same fascination.

[11] The eighteenth century is particularly notable for the public interest in, and attention to, death.

[12] A rather similar analysis could be developed of the fear of violent crime more generally which is out of proportion to the actual level of crime.

from those with mental disorder. Are the fears of violence out of proportion to the real dangers? What are the precise nature and extent of the links between psychiatric disorder and individual violence?

Psychiatric disorder and individual violence

The links between psychiatric disorder, as currently defined and measured, and individual violence are highly contested and have been explored in a range of empirical research.[13] A key point of contention is the extent to which those with psychiatric problems are more prone to violence than those without, violence here meaning attacks on other people using physical force, including physical fights, the use of weapons to intimidate or injure, rape and homicide. A number of mental health advocates have argued that the public stereotypes are false and that persons with a psychiatric disturbance are no more likely than those without psychiatric problems to engage in acts of violence. However, as a broad generalization, this claim is not supported by the evidence. An influential review by John Monahan in the early 1990s convincingly argued that certain forms of mental disorder do increase the chances of violent actions. However, and this is a very important qualification, the increased risks of violence do not apply to the majority of psychiatric disorders (Monahan 1992). One consequence is, and this is common in the field of psychiatric epidemiology, that precisely where you set the boundaries of psychiatric disorder affects the strength of the association.

An important source for Monahan's conclusions was the Epidemiological Catchment Area (ECA) study, carried out in the USA between 1980 and 1983, which Swanson and his colleagues used to explore the nature and extent of the association between psychiatric disorder and reported violence (Swanson *et al.* 1990; Swanson and Holzer, 1991). The ECA study involved a series of community surveys of psychiatric disorder assessed on the basis of the individual's symptom reports.[14] It was not therefore prone to the biases that contaminate many studies of the links between psychiatric disorder and violence which are based on psychiatric in-patient populations, where the occurrence or likely occurrence of violence is itself one of the reasons for admission to a psychiatric bed.[15] However, the measure of violence probably underestimated the level of violence amongst those surveyed, not only because of the restricted range of questions on violence, but also because of a common reluctance to admit to violence.[16]

---

[13] The boundaries of what constitutes mental disorder change and vary across time and place.

[14] Psychiatric disorder was measured using the 'diagnostic interview schedule'.

[15] However, there are issues about the reliability and validity of the measures of mental health used in these studies (see Busfield 1996).

[16] The measure of violence used by Swanson and his colleagues (1990) depended on the response to five separate questions on violence in relation to: spouse/partner; children; fights involving blows; use of weapons in fights; and physical fights while drinking. There was no specific question about rape.

Swanson and his colleagues' analysis showed that reported violence in the previous year was significantly raised amongst three groups with psychiatric problems: those with a 'major' psychiatric disorder (a psychosis, such as schizophrenia or manic depression) where the prevalence of violence was more than five times as high as amongst non-patients; and those with either alcohol or drug dependence where the prevalence was even higher (the former having rates 12 times as high, the latter 16 times as high as non-patients). The study also showed that those with multiple diagnoses (co-morbidity) were generally more prone to violence. However this increase in reported violence did not apply to other 'milder', more common mental disorders, such as anxiety and depression, where rates of violence were no higher than amongst the non-disordered group. It is important to note that Swanson and his colleagues did not examine the association between anti-social personality disorder and violence. This is because it is not possible to measure the two independently of one another since tendencies to violence are one symptom of this disorder.[17] This means that there is a fourth group of patients to add to the list of psychosis and alcohol and drug disorders that are associated with raised level of violence: those with certain types of personality or conduct disorders.

Swanson and his colleagues did not discuss the reasons for the associations they observed, but those with psychotic symptoms may engage in violence because of the precise character of their delusions (for instance, feeling themselves to be persecuted by someone, or particularly under threat). In fact Monahan (1990) contends, on the basis of other research (see Link et al.1992), that it is only in the 'active' phase of psychosis, when the person is experiencing symptoms like delusions and hallucinations, that the rates of violence are higher than those of non-patients. In the case of those with problems of alcohol or drug dependence, the impact of the drug or alcohol may well act as a stimulant and remove inhibitions, undermining some of the constraints that deter people from violence. However, other mechanisms may also be at work, as when drug users engage in violent crime to fund their drug taking (see Goldstein 1985).

The finding that alcohol and drug disorders are more strongly associated with violence than psychotic disorders is important. This is because, though included in some psychiatric classifications as behavioural rather than mental disorders, they are by no means always included in definitions and measures of psychiatric disorder, including those that explore the links with individual violence.[18] Nor do individuals with substance use or conduct disorders fit the stereotype of the 'mad' person driven to kill and destroy by disturbed thoughts and perceptions. In general the ECA data

---

[17] Four of the five violence questions used by Swanson and his colleagues were derived from the questions initially intended to measure anti-social personality disorder.

[18] The present state examination (Wing et al. 1974), for instance, does not include questions specifically designed to measure alcohol and drug disorders.

indicate that it would be more appropriate to talk of the links between behavioural disorders and violence than between 'mental' disorders and violence.[19]

One further limitation of the ECA study that needs to be noted is that no data were collected about the use of psychotropic medication, yet psychotropic drugs can reduce the danger of violence (indeed, as noted earlier, failure to continue with medication can be a factor precipitating violence). The issue is complex since certain prescribed drugs may actually increase violence in some individuals. However, overall the use of psychotropic medication is likely to reduce any correlations between psychiatric disorder and violence.[20]

An equally important issue is the size of the contribution of those with mental and behavioural disorders to the overall level of individual violence in a given society. This has been explored in a range of studies. For instance, Taylor and Gunn (1999) examined cases of homicide and argued that those with a severe mental disorder do not make a very significant contribution to the homicide level. Their focus was on the contribution of major psychosis to the incidence of homicide and, based on a number of studies, they estimated that in England and Wales around 10% of those convicted of homicide (or found not guilty by reason of insanity) suffer from a psychotic disorder. This amounts to only some 40–50 persons out of a total of around 450–500 homicide convictions per year, which they suggest is a relatively low proportion. They also argue that there is little evidence of any change over time in the contribution of psychosis to cases of homicide, despite increasing moves towards community care.

However, Taylor and Gunn's conclusion about the contribution of psychiatric disorder to cases of homicide needs to be treated with caution. Their focus, as I have noted, was on estimating the contribution of persons with psychosis to homicide. According to the data they present, rather higher proportions over the period 1986–95 had a verdict of 'diminished responsibility' or 'not guilty by reason of insanity', the annual figure varying between 11.5 and 18% (though this is still less than one in five of homicides).[21] In addition, over the same period a further 30–58 murder suspects annually committed suicide before they could be brought to trial, an action which might be taken to be indicative of some mental disorder, yet these cases are not included in the percentages.[22] Moreover, measuring psychiatric disorder in terms of these legal outcomes may often exclude persons with behavioural disorders—for instance, those with alcohol or drug problems or personality disorders. If these were included

---

[19] This is why I have largely used the term psychiatric disorder as the generic category rather than mental disorder or mental illness.

[20] There are recent reports that drugs such as Prozac can increase violence in a small proportion of individuals (see *The Guardian,* June 11 2001).

[21] There is of course a major problem about the interpretation of data on diminished responsibility since it is subject to the vagaries of decision making in the judicial process.

[22] Suicides are excluded from both the numerator and the denominator.

the contribution of all psychiatric disorders would be higher. A further important point to note here, which Taylor and Gunn also emphasize, is that the contribution which those with psychiatric problems make to the overall levels of violence in a society depends on how common violence is in the society. In the USA, for instance, where homicide rates are far higher than in the UK, the proportion of homicides attributable to severe mental disorder is lower than in the UK (Coid 1983).

Again the ECA data give us a rather fuller picture, but one, as with other research in the field, that differs according to the starting point. Approaching the data by focusing on reported incidents of violence (which parallels the Taylor and Gunn starting point for the study of homicide) indicates that psychiatric disorder does make a very significant contribution to acts of violence. In so doing it supports the view that Taylor and Gunn's interpretation of the data tends to underestimate the contribution of psychiatric disorder to violence. The ECA study shows that only 3.7% of the overall sample (368 persons out of a sample of 10059, a very small proportion) reported violent behaviour in the previous year. However, of these 368 individuals some 56% met the criteria for psychiatric disorder, compared with only 20% of the non-violent respondents.[23] Put another way over half of the people who reported violent behaviour in the previous year were also judged to have a psychiatric disorder. As we would expect, given the ECA findings on the significance of certain diagnostic groups in relation to violence, the most common diagnosis amongst those who reported violent behaviour was an alcohol or drug abuse disorder (42% of the violent group compared with only 9% of the non-violent group). But other diagnoses were also more prevalent in this group than in the non-violent group, including affective disorders (9% against 3%) and schizophrenia (4% of the violent group against 1% in the non-violent) (Swanson *et al.* 1990). Such data indicate that if the boundaries of psychiatric disorder are not restricted to severe psychosis and include, in particular, the substance use disorders, then the contribution of psychiatric disorder to violence is very considerable (and we need to remember that their analysis excluded those with anti-social personality disorder).

However, it is very important to look at the data on psychiatric disorder and violence from a rather different perspective, a perspective which starts with all those who are identified as having a psychiatric disorder. Such an analysis reveals that the apparently tight association between violence and psychiatric disorder manifest when we start with those who are violent is in fact much looser. If we take not violent people but all those with a psychiatric disorder as our starting point (significantly this was as many as 22% of the ECA sample—quite a high figure and one that indicates that the boundaries of psychiatric disorder were drawn rather widely) then the picture looks very different and gives strong grounds for challenging stereotypes of those with a psy-

---

[23] If more people had admitted to violence it might well be that a rather lower proportion of the violent would have also fallen into the group of those with psychiatric problems.

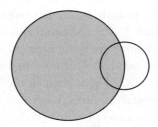

Fig. 4.1 Psychiatric disorder and individual violence.   ⬤ = psychiatric disorder ◯ = violence

chiatric disorder as usually prone to violence.[24] What we find is that almost all of the individuals with a psychiatric disorder did *not* fall into the group of those who were violent. Swanson and Holzer note, for instance, that 'more than 90 percent of persons with serious mental disorder (excluding substance abuse) were not violent by their own report' (Swanson and Holzer 1991), and even amongst those with drug and alcohol disorders some 65 and 75% respectively were not violent. Clearly if the rates of reported violence are underestimates then these percentages might well be reduced a little. Nonetheless it is reasonable to conclude that even though many who are violent do have a psychiatric disorder, a very large majority of those with a psychiatric disorder are not violent. This can be seen in Fig. 4.1, which portrays the association between psychiatric disorder and individual violence using a Venn diagram. To predict that an individual will be violent on the basis that he or she has a psychiatric disorder would usually be incorrect, and the ECA study suggests it will lead to errors in at least nine out of every 10 cases.[25]

A further point, often emphasized in studies of psychiatric disorder and violence, is that the majority of violence by those with a psychiatric history is not a matter of 'random' attacks on strangers as public stereotypes tend to suggest. In most cases the victim is known to the assailant and is frequently a family member. This is true of many incidents of violence, particularly of homicide. Whilst deaths of those known to the assailant constitute no less a tragedy, this does mean that random deaths as a result of attacks by a person with a psychiatric history on a stranger are exceptionally rare.

One implication of the analysis of the data on psychiatric disorder and violence is

[24] High prevalence rates of psychiatric disorder are common in community surveys of psychiatric morbidity.

[25] Swanson and colleagues do not provide a simple percentage of those who were disordered who also reported acts of violence. However, using their data it is possible to calculate such a figure. 2189 out of 10 059 were identified as having a psychiatric disorder and these persons contributed 55.5% of the 368 identified as violent—i.e. 204 individuals. This means that only 9.3% of the disordered were violent.

that in itself psychiatric disorder is a poor predictor of violence (though violence is a rather better predictor of psychiatric disorder). Moreover, even knowledge of the diagnosis does not increase the capacity to predict violence very greatly. The difficulty of predicting violence in those with a psychiatric disorder with any degree of accuracy was emphasized very forcefully by Gostin (1975) in MIND's campaign for the reform of the 1959 Mental Health Act. After reviewing the relevant research he concluded that the best, and only adequate predictor of dangerousness is a previous violent act—a point that has been frequently reiterated.[26] However, Gostin's claims about the difficulty of predicting dangerousness now need to be qualified. One of the findings of Swanson and colleagues' work is that, as other studies of violence also indicate, a number of socio-demographic factors are associated with increased levels of violence amongst those with a psychiatric disorder. Taking the ECA sample as a whole, violence was more common amongst lower class than upper class individuals, amongst the young than the old, and amongst men than women, and this applied as much to those with a psychiatric disorder as to those without one. Such observations, along with the predictive importance of past violence, have now been incorporated into some of the measuring instruments which have been developed in recent years to predict the likelihood of particular individuals being violent (see Borum 1996), such as the HCR-20 (Webster *et al.* 1997). As yet the instruments have not been well validated, but recent studies suggest that the capacity to predict violence in those with a psychiatric history can be somewhat improved.

However, even though there has been some improvement in the capacity to predict violence, and even though we may expect further improvement in future, there are strong grounds for considerable caution about the prospects for great improvement in the capacity to predict individual violence (Buchanan 1999). In the first place, it is more difficult to predict rare events, such as violence by a person with a psychiatric history, than more common ones. Second, even where more formal measures of risk assessment are used, these still depend on clinical judgements as to whether say an individual does have delusions, is angry or whatever—judgements that are likely to play a greater part as measures become more sophisticated. Third, the factors that predict one type of violence are not the same as those that predict others. Consequently, it is very difficult to develop measures of risk assessment that are sufficiently flexible to encompass the prediction of the diverse types of violence that can occur. And fourth, and related to this, violence is frequently circumstantial: the capacity to predict violence is likely to be limited by the fact that whether an individual is violent or not will depend on a range of circumstances and contingencies, on a particular constellation of events that are themselves hard to predict. A final point also needs to be noted: that in clinical contexts there are pressures to over-predict violence mainly because of the

---

[26] MIND's campaign helped to shape the subsequent 1983 Mental Health Act, which increased individual rights to contest the use of compulsory powers of detention (see also footnote 7).

more severe consequences for the clinician of failing to predict violence that then occurs than of predicting violence that does not.[27]

I consider the policy implications of this analysis in the final section. Before doing so, I want to explore the ways in which sociological ideas and approaches about risk can contribute to an understanding of the strategies deployed by professionals and policy makers for dealing with dangerousness in those with psychiatric problems.

Risk and dangerousness

Risk has become a key concept in sociological analyses of 'late modern' society and the ideas that have been developed help to illuminate the focus on risk in mental health policies. A number of theorists have argued that risk is a central feature of contemporary society, some terming it a 'risk society'. For example, Beck (1992) argues that late modern society, which has entered a period he calls 'reflexive modernization', is a risk society. Risk, he recognizes, is not a new phenomenon; however, as wealth replaces scarcity in western societies, new sources of risk emerge. These are the risks associated with new ways of producing wealth, such as the unknown risks associated with environmental degradation from chemical pollutants, the overuse of antibiotics, or the use of genetically modified organisms. These risks, he argues, tend to have a different character from earlier ones: they are more globalized, less predictable and less personal.

At first sight, Beck's analysis might appear to have little relevance for an understanding of the response to the violence of those with psychiatric problems since, though unpredictability is a key feature of this type of risk, it does not really belong to the group of new risks with which he is concerned, which relate mainly to global, environmental developments. Nonetheless his analysis is pertinent. In the first place, his characterization of contemporary society in terms of reflexive modernization is relevant to understanding the present-day desire to control risks. Beck contends that historically there has been a shift from the processes of modernization that characterized the move from a traditional, feudal society to an industrial one, to processes of modernization which transform industrial society to one that is characterized by 'modernity'. And a key feature of modernity is that science and technology, which made possible the processes of modernization leading to industrial society, are themselves called into question and are viewed with increasing scepticism. Risk is bound up with this reflexive modernization for attention to risk provides a way of trying to deal with the uncertainties of this new type of society: 'Risk may be defined as a *systematic way of dealing with the hazards and insecurities induced and introduced by modernization itself*' (Beck 1992:21, author's italics). And, whilst new risks undermine the standard bases of calculation, such as insurance, that were developed in industrial societies so that they cannot be adequately dealt with by the same means, nonetheless continuing to try to deal with

---

[27] This tendency has been identified in a number of studies (see Pfohl 1978).

new risks by these means is a 'very effective means of legitimizing them' (Beck 1992). Consequently we renew our efforts to control risk through rational, calculative means even though, he asserts, these efforts cannot succeed since the risks cannot be adequately predicted or controlled.[28] Although Beck suggests that old risks are more amenable to calculation than new ones, applied to the potential and unpredictable dangerousness of those with a psychiatric history the analysis helps to explain the increasing attention to risk and risk assessment in mental health policies, seeing the focus on risk as a widespread feature of late modern societies. It also help us to understand the difficulty of predicting violence by those with a psychiatric disorder, which though not one of the new environmental risks, nonetheless shares the characteristic of being highly unpredictable since it requires prediction of the individual event, not merely a statistical calculation of aggregate risks.[29]

Second, Beck's concept of reflexive modernization, with its emphasis on reflexivity, also draws attention to the increasing importance of our *awareness* of risk, with the implication that, whilst it is not necessarily the case that society (or those with psychiatric disorder) generates more risks than formerly, we are nonetheless more aware of them. This is a point developed by Giddens who talks of the rise of a 'risk culture':

> Modernity is a risk culture. I do not mean by this that social life is inherently more risky than it used to be; for most people in developed societies that is not the case. Rather, the concept of risk becomes fundamental to the way both lay actors and technical specialists organise the social world. Under the conditions of modernity, the future is continually drawn into the present by means of the reflexive organisation of knowledge environments (Giddens 1991:3)

Like Beck, he believes that as old risks are controlled, new risks are emerging, particularly high consequence global risks. What is crucial, however, is the changing consciousness of risk, with the measurement of risk itself further heightening that consciousness:

> Living in a 'risk society' means living with a calculative attitude to the open possibilities of action, positive and negative, with which, as individuals and globally, we are confronted in a continuous way in our contemporary social existence (Giddens 1991:28)

From this point of view, risk studies of those with severe mental health problems at one and the same time seek to control risk yet increase our awareness of it, and in so doing heighten anxiety.

Theoretical ideas about risk have been specifically deployed by Castel (1991) to examine the issue of dangerousness and mental disorder. He argues that risk has dis-

---

[28] Drafting this initially on the day after a major earthquake in Turkey, it is interesting to note that scientists are now accepting the impossibility of predicting earthquakes and arguing that the policy should be to try and minimize their impact through, for instance, the design of buildings (*The Guardian*, 18 August 1999).

[29] Insurance is a form of spreading or sharing of risks, though for those who sell insurance it may involve attempting to predict individual risk. However the success or failure of insurance does not depend on being correct in each case.

placed dangerousness in our ways of thinking about individuals with mental illness. His argument, like that of Beck and Giddens, is not so much that risk is a new concept, but rather, and here his emphasis differs from these authors (and draws heavily on Foucault's (1991) ideas about 'governmentality'), that we think about risk in a new and distinctive way. In the past, he suggests, within psychiatry risk meant 'essentially the danger embodied in the mentally ill person capable of violent and unpredictable action' (Castel 1991:283). It was an imputation, something that was imminent, and the proof of danger could only be provided after the act. The solution to this threat was confinement to prevent the threat being carried out. The new conception of risk does not see risk as embodied in individuals but as the product of a combination of 'risk factors' which 'render more or less probable the occurrence of undesirable modes of behaviour' (Castel 1991:287). This involves a different approach. Instead of starting from 'a conflictual situation observable in experience, rather one *deduces* it from a general definition of the dangers one wishes to prevent' (Castel 1991:289, author's italics). The approach is more probabilistic and more abstract and it focuses, as in Foucault's notion of governmentality, far more on populations than on individuals. But, like Beck, Castel argues that this attempt to control risk is doomed to failure: it is 'a grandiose technocratic rationalizing dream of absolute control of the accidental' (Castel 1991).

One way of reading Castel's analysis is to see it as an examination of the development of the technologies of risk assessment, and certainly there can be no doubt of the interest within medicine, including psychiatry, on quantifying risk through the assessment of risk factors. However I would argue, contra Castel, that, though grounded in epidemiological studies, risk assessment in psychiatry still focuses more on individuals than populations and is difficult precisely because, as I noted earlier, the aim is to predict the chances of a specific individual being violent, not just to aggregate risks.[30] Moreover, what is significant is the way in which, measured in terms of efforts at prevention, we seem to have a far greater fear of death at the hands of a violent individual than of death as a result of our own actions through say smoking or driving. Part of this links to issues of control—we fear most what we cannot seem to control—but it also indicates the way in which we still attribute dangerousness and risk to individuals, holding individuals responsible rather than looking at the social context in which that behaviour is generated.

We can see, nonetheless, how sociological discussions of risk help us to understand the contemporary character of the response to the threat of dangerousness in individuals with a psychiatric history. First, the work helps to explain the focus on risk and the belief in rational, technocratic solutions to the risks from individuals with a psychiatric history. Second, it calls into question how far it is possible to control risks by accurately

---

[30] Castel talks of the emergence of the 'epidemiological clinic', which he defines as 'a system of multifarious but exactly localized expertise which supplants the old doctor–patient relationship' (Castel 1991:282). His vision is highly dystopian.

identifying those who will commit a highly dangerous act. And third, it suggests that the focus on risk may actually increase anxiety about the dangers of violence from those with a psychiatric history.

Policy and practice

What are the policy implications of this analysis? First, let us consider the implications of sociological understandings of cultural attitudes to death and the public and media fascination with death. The analysis here suggests that the public and media fascination with the deaths caused by those with psychiatric problems, particularly psychotic disorders, is likely to continue at present, since these are precisely the type of unpredictable deaths that attract most attention, involving as they do human violence by an irrational assailant. It also suggests one reason why public campaigns that try to argue the case that psychiatric disorder does not heighten the likelihood of violence are not likely to be successful. Such campaigns have to contend with the ongoing media attention to, and public fascination with, the deaths that do result from the violence of the disturbed individual. In that respect politicians and policy makers will not be able to avoid the media attention generated by these deaths unless they can prevent them, which the examination of the difficulty of predicting individual violence by those with a psychiatric disorder suggests is unlikely.

However, the sociological analysis of death also suggests that we need to explore ways of giving expression to our fears and anxieties about death, so that imagined deaths become less important, and we feel less threatened by the risks of death and violence at the hands of a person with a psychiatric disorder and do not exaggerate the chances of such events. Whilst the sociological theorists suggest our sense of ontological security is linked to the character of late modern society and is not easily amenable to change, they also suggest that the fear of death is affected by social practices which could be changed more readily, such as the rituals (or lack of them) surrounding death and the openness with which we communicate our fears about it.

What, however, are the policy implications that can be drawn from an examination of the data on the relationship between psychiatric disorder and violence? The two over-riding empirical conclusions here are: first, that psychiatric disorder is in itself very poor predictor of violence; and, second, that even focusing on groups with a higher chance of violence, and bringing in a far broader range of information, the capacity to predict violence with any degree of accuracy is limited. These two conclusions have several important policy implications. First, they suggest that a return to more extensive preventive detention whether in small- or large-scale facilities is an inappropriate response to the issue of reducing the potential violence of those with a psychiatric history. In order to be effective the numbers who would need to be confined would be far higher than the numbers who, if allowed to remain in the community, would at some point be violent. And, allowing for the tendency of clinicians to overpredict violence, the actual numbers who would in practice be detained on grounds of safety would almost certainly end up being even higher. Moreover, the periods of detention would need to be lengthy, precisely the conditions for the accumulation of unwanted, marginal individuals which led to campaigns against the asylums both in this century and the last. And even then, given the problems of prediction, some individuals with a psychiatric history, who had not been detained, would prove to be violent. The civil liberties implications of such a strategy are enormous, particularly if the provision is made within the framework of health care arrangements, where principle of voluntarism are strong.[31] To put forward such arguments is not to deny that there are some people with a history of violence who are also psychiatrically disturbed, who need to be detained for longer periods of time. However, the numbers need to be kept to a minimum and the possibility of discharge kept under regular review.

Second, the difficulties of predicting dangerousness suggest that the focus within psychiatric services should be far less on risk assessment than on 'violence containment': that is on how to deal with individuals who start to show signs of becoming violent and difficult. Here the target groups are those who have most contact with those with the relevant types of psychiatric problem: mental health professionals, the police and social workers on the one hand, and families and close friends on the other. Teaching such groups how to deal with potential violence is likely to be a far better use of resources than general public education campaigns. Those who have most contact with those with a relevant psychiatric history need not only to be provided with information about the chances of violence, but also training in how to respond in situations when someone starts to become violent.[32]

Finally, what are the policy implications of the sociological analysis of risk? Are the efforts to predict and assess the risks of violence from psychiatric patients, as writers like Castel suggest, products of a mistaken conviction in our capacity to control the world—a product of the power of Enlightenment scientific rationality—that is doomed to failure. In my view such efforts are, indeed, a product of our belief in the power of reason and science. But it is not the belief in science that is misguided. Rather, it is the procedures and practices of reasoned argument and science that show us the limits to our capacities to predict violence.

However, the sociological analysis of risk, by suggesting that late modern societies have come to think about and organize the world in terms of risk, calls into question the priority that is being given to risk reduction and raises serious questions about the time and resources being devoted to the analysis of risk. There are two main grounds for questioning the concentration on risk reduction. First, the concentration on risk distorts policy priorities and diverts resources away from individuals with psychiatric

---

[31] Szasz (1970) made this point in his classic paper on involuntary mental hospitalization.

[32] There is some overlap between risk assessment and training in dealing with violence since part of the training will mean looking for the first signs of violence, but the overall approach is different.

problems who are not potentially dangerous, at the same time as narrowing the vision of those who are considered potentially violent to the risks they may pose and away from a wider understanding of their problems.[33] I have already argued that preventive detention would be very resource intensive because of the numbers who would be need to be detained in order to reduce significantly the violence of those with a psychiatric disorder. A major investment in such provision would be unlikely to represent the best use of resources, and would take resources away from other groups with psychiatric problems. Moreover, concentration on risk assessment and risk reduction is almost certainly increasing rather than reducing the public's and professionals' fear of violence. Of course, as I have indicated, the media play an important part in this, but so too do the professionals who concentrate on risk assessment, understandable though this tendency may be.[34]

Second, the concentration on risk reduction in relation to those with psychiatric disorders draws attention from the wider causes of violence in society. If the objective is the reduction of violence by those with psychiatric problems, there needs to be a far greater focus on wider strategies for violence reduction, including the reduction of sexual violence, which do not focus exclusively on this particular group. In the case of a society like the UK, the immediate policy solutions such as far tighter gun control do not present themselves in the way they do in the USA, where, as noted earlier, libertarian views on the right to carry guns underpin the high level of violent crime, particularly the mass murders resulting from armed assailants that are not uncommon. But this does not mean that there is no scope for more stringent implementation of the legislation concerning gun ownership in the UK. More importantly however, are general issues surrounding the acceptability and normative character of certain types of violence amongst certain groups. Here the ways in which masculinity is constructed in different groups in society and the way in which violence is embedded in some conceptions of masculinity are crucial, particularly those conceptions espoused by young, working-class men. So, too, is the way in which violence, including sexual violence, is often seen as a way for individuals (like states when they go to war) to achieve status and maintain power and control. What is important, too, is that the use of alcohol and drugs are also linked to these particular conceptions of masculinity thereby making their enactment in violent behaviour more likely. Consequently reducing the male abuse of drugs and alcohol, and the greater acceptability of 'tough', 'macho' behaviour, would have an impact on the tendencies to violence of those with psychiatric problems, who generally reflect the overall male bias in violence identified in so many other studies.

---

[33] The government is now proposing special facilities for those with "severe" personality disorders who are considered dangerous and admits this would require considerable resources. If such facilities are provided they are likely to divert resources from other mental health services.

[34] One reason for this is the fear of litigation.

Public fascination with unexpected deaths and violence regularly draws attention to the dangers posed by some individuals with psychiatric problems which become part of the landscape of imagined deaths. Our response to public concerns about these dangers should be careful and cautious. Above all it is vital to accept that dangerousness is difficult to predict with any great degree of precision and is likely to continue to be so. Risk assessments, now widely introduced in the mental health services, have some value but they do not and will not allow the accurate prediction of risks. Rather, all those engaged in dealing with persons with psychiatric problems, including friends and relatives, need to be given help and support in dealing with potential violence. This, of course, requires resources, but it should not mean a return to policies of locking up large numbers of people to prevent unpredictable violence—policies which are highly resource intensive and threaten civil liberties. Nor should it mean a concentration on the potentially dangerous at the expense of all others with psychiatric problems or at the expense of seeking to understand the behaviour of those who might be violent. Risk should not the dominant lens through which we view the realm of psychiatric problems.

Acknowledgements

I would like to thank Colin Samson and Nigel South for their constructive comments on an earlier version of this chapter and Paul Godin for his contribution to our discussions of risk and mental health services.

References

American Psychiatric Association (1994) *Diagnostic and statistical manual* (4th edn) (DSM-IV). Washington: American Psychiatric Association.

Aries, P. (1976) *Western attitudes to death*. London: Marion Boyars.

Bainbridge, B. (1996) *Every man for himself*. London: Duckworth.

Beck, U. (1992) Risk society: towards a new modernity. London: Sage.

Buchanan, A. (1999) Risk and dangerousness. *Psychological Medicine*, **29**, 465–73.

Busfield, J. (1996) *Men, women and madness: understanding gender and mental disorder*. London: Macmillan.

Borum, R. (1996) Improving the clinical practice of violence risk assessment: technology, guidelines and training. *American Psychologist*, 945–56.

Castel, R. (1991) From dangerousness to risk. In *The Foucault effect: studies in governmentality*, (ed. G. Burchell, C. Gordon and P. Miller). Hemel Hempstead: Harvester Wheatsheaf.

Coid, J. (1983) The epidemiology of abnormal homicide and murder followed by suicide. *Psychological Medicine*, **13**, 855–60.

Coonan, K., Bluglass, R., Halliday, G. *et al.* (1998) Executive summary of the report of the inquiry into the care and treatment of Christopher Edwards and Richard Linford. North Essex Health Authority.

Department of Health (1994) *Guidelines on Supervised Discharge*. HSG (94) 27. London: Department of Health.

Diamond, J. (1998) *Because cowards get cancer too*. London: Vermilion.

Foucault, M. (1991) Governmentality. In *The Foucault effect: studies in governmentality* (ed. G. Burchell, C. Gordon and P. Miller). Hemel Hempstead: Harvester Wheatsheaf.

Giddens, A. (1991) *Modernity and self-identity*. Cambridge: Polity.

Goldstein, P. J. (1985) The drugs/violence nexus: a tripartite conceptual framework. *Journal of Drug Issues* **15**, 493–506.

Gostin, L. (1975) A human condition: a review of the Mental Health Act from 1959 to 1975. Vol. I and II. London: MIND.

Herbert, P., Walters, J. and Ghosh, C. (1999) Report of the inquiry into the care and treatment of Micheal Donnelly. North Essex Health Authority.

Jaspers, K. (1963) *General psychopathology*. London: Manchester University Press.

Laing, R. D. (1965) *The divided self*. Harmondsworth: Penguin.

Laing, R. D. (1967) The politics of experience and the bird of paradise. Harmondsworth: Penguin.

Link, B. G., Andrews, H. and Cullen, F. T. (1992) The violent and illegal behavior of mental patients reconsidered. *American Sociological Review*, **57**, 275–92.

Mellor, P. (1993) Death in high modernity: the contemporary presence and absence of death. In *The sociology of death* (ed. D. Clark). Oxford: Blackwell.

Monahan, J. (1992) Mental disorder and violent behavior: perceptions and evidence. *American Psychologist*, 511–21

Pfohl, S. J. (1978) Predicting dangerousness: the social construction of psychiatric reality. Massachusetts: Lexington.

Picardie, R. (1998) *Before I say goodbye*. Harmondsworth: Penguin.

Ramon, S. (1987) The category of psychopathy: its professional and social context in Britain. In *The power of psychiatry* (ed. N. Rose and P.Miller). Cambridge: Polity.

Ritchie, J. H, Dick, D. and Lingham, R.(1994) The report of the inquiry into the care and treatment of Christopher Clunis. London: HMSO.

Royal College of Psychiatrists (1996) Report of the confidential inquiry into homicides and suicides by mentally ill people. London: Royal College of Psychiatrists.

Swanson, J.W. amd Holzer, C.E. (1991) Violence and ECA data. *Hospital and Community Psychiatry*, **42**, 954–5.

Swanson, J. W., Holzer, C. E., Ganju, V. K. *et al.* (1990) *Hospital and Community Psychiatry*, **41**, 761–70.

Szasz, T. S. (1970) Involuntary mental hospitalization: a crime against humanity. In *Ideology and insanity*. Harmondsworth: Penguin.

Taylor, P. J. and Gunn, J. (1999) Homicides by people with mental illness: myth and reality. *British Journal of Psychiatry*, **174**, 9–14.

Tilberis, L. (1998) *No time to die*. London: Weidenfeld & Nicholson.

Webster, C., Douglas, K., Eaves, D. *et al.* (1997) HCR-20. *Assessing Risk of Violence. Version 2*. Burnaby, British Columbia: Mental Health Law and Policy Institute.

Wing, J., Cooper, J. and Sartorius, N. (1974) *Measurement and Classsification of Psychiatric Symptoms*. Cambridge: Cambridge University Press.

World Health Organization (1992) *The ICD-10 classification of mental and behavioural disorders*. Geneva: World Health Organization.

Part 2

Clinical aspects of care of the mentally disordered offender in the community

Chapter 5

Mentally disordered offenders and models of community care provision

James Tighe, Claire Henderson and
Graham Thornicroft

Introduction

This chapter examines models of community care for mentally disordered offenders (MDOs). Any model has to balance the needs of the MDO, the wider community, carers and staff. Central to the operation of any model is the way that the risk of violent offending is managed. The service developments described in the chapter have co-incided with a cultural shift in preoccupations with sources of risk. Threats of war or epidemics dominated until the middle of the twentieth century; the extensive media coverage now given to homicides committed by mentally disordered people suggests a shift in perception of major threats. We review perceptions of risk, and how these are translated into clinical practice and public policy. A typology of possible service interfaces between general and forensic psychiatry is discussed; its merits and demerits are delineated. A volume and quality argument applies at the more severe end of the spectrum of MDOs, in that forensic psychiatry enables concentration of skills in dealing with those who need high or medium secure care. The central question of this chapter is: To what extent does the volume and quality argument apply to those classed as MDOs who are not currently (and may never have been) admitted to secure facilities and who are living in community settings?

Risk: perception

Both forensic and general psychiatrists take decisions about risk on a daily basis, for example whether to discharge or compulsorily detain a patient. How a psychiatrist assesses the probability that a patient may commit a serious offence may make the difference between community or institutional care.

Taylor and Gunn (1999), using Home Office statistics, estimate that in 1995 11.5% of prosecutions for homicide resulted in the accused being found to have a mental disorder. In the late 1950s and early 1960s this figure was as high as 48% for some years. Of the fewer than 20 homicides per year committed by people with schizophrenia, only 10 have had contact with the mental health services (Department of Health 1999*a*). Mental illnesses such as psychoses are less associated with violence than the misuse of alcohol and drugs (National Association for the Care and Resettlement of Offenders 1998). Nonetheless, instances of homicide by psychiatric patients receive high levels of press attention. This has resulted in significant political pressure for public protection from the minority of mentally ill people who pose a risk of violence. While the policy is high on the government agenda (Home Office/Department of Health 1999) there has been criticism from mental health professionals. They argue that it would be more effective to improve care for all patients (Eastman 1997; Taylor and Gunn 1999), reflecting recognition that this issue does not provide the justification for specialized services for those targeted.

When either homicide or suicide in England or Wales involves a known psychiatric patient, the National Confidential Inquiry into Suicide and Homicide by People with a Mental Illness (Appleby *et al.* 1999) is informed. There can also be internal inquiries, coroner's hearings, civil litigation for negligence (Harrison 1997) and for homicides, criminal proceedings. Meanwhile, mental health services are expected to manage risk effectively within tight budgetary constraints, while adhering to the principle of using the least restrictive alternative for their patients. A substantial legislative framework and a network of non-statutory organizations advocating for service users is in place to ensure least restrictive practice.

(a) Clinical versus actuarial risk

The clinical approach to risk focuses on the individual; other approaches focus on risks for organizations (corporate risk). Individual risk is also the focus of insurers who use statistical models to make inferences about individuals from populations. This actuarial methodology has some application to clinical risk, but clinical risk assessment has ultimately to be more than the uniform application of a statistical model to each patient. Any assessment of risk has to take account of which outcomes are of concern and what events or factors are indicative of those outcomes. It is on this point that the difference between clinical and actuarial risk resides. Buchanan (1999) points out:

> A table providing estimates of the risk of interpersonal violence over a 5-year period, which uses as one of its predictors the number of convictions for violence, is of little use to a clinician who wishes to predict the risk of his patient committing arson before his next appointment and who does not have access to the patient's criminal record.

Let us say that a table of risk for violence is available to the clinician along with this patient's notes. The clinician can now count up the number of convictions for violence in the past five years, and make a risk assessment based on the table. Let us also say that the patient had a two-year period of non-compliance with anti-psychotic medication during which he drank alcohol in excess, and had several convictions for violent offences. Since then he has complied with medication, ceased drinking alcohol and had no further incidents of aggression. According to the table this patient is still a high risk for aggression. However there are a number of extra factors not taken into account in the table that may be considered better predictors. Can a table ever be constructed that could take into account all the possible relevant factors in assessing risk of violence or self harm? Buchanan comments: 'Because people often do what they intend, the clinician who discusses intentions may be able to predict events that have not happened before. This, a table cannot do.'

There are a number of tools to assess the risk of violence. Some, such as the HCR-20 (Webster *et al.* 1995) include both clinical and actuarial elements. Both unaided clinical judgement and several risk assessment tools have been shown to have some effectiveness at predicting violence in the short term (Mossman, 1994).

(b) Public perception of risk

The influence of scientific research and how it is presented in the press needs to be viewed in the context of an increasingly risk-averse society. Furedi (1998) points out that the prominence and coverage of a risk is not necessarily an indicator of the likelihood or severity of the negative outcome concerned. Rates of child murder, as distressing as they are, have remained steady over the last 20 years at about 85 per year (one child in a city or large town), the majority of these committed by parents (Prins 1999). Yet fear of what is labelled 'stranger danger' appears to have an increasing impact on child rearing in the UK. In 1971 80% of seven- and eight-year-olds took themselves to school everyday; in 1996 it was estimated that fewer than 10% did so (*The Independent* 22 July 1996). Jackie Lang, president of the Girls' School Association, voiced concern (*Daily Telegraph* 27 November 1997):

> The fears of parents are perfectly understandable but we may be exaggerating the likelihood of these frightful things. If we teach children in a blanket way that all strangers are evil, they must never smile at an unknown adult and that they must be ferried from door to door, you are creating an unhealthy climate when it is not true by far and away for the majority of children . . . . If drink and drugs and dodgy sex and driving too fast are the only ways left to satisfy a natural urge to be daring, we shall have done young people a disservice.

Hence psychiatrists operate in a milieu of reportage of risk that seems to have an increasingly invidious impact on public perceptions. It is not difficult to find examples of reportage about mental health service users that contribute to a generally distorted view of the risk that these persons pose to society. Such material has been reviewed and its impact upon attitudes analysed (Philo 1997). It is worth noting that in the UK, the risk of being killed by a stranger with psychosis is about one in 10 million (Szmukler 2000), one person in a province or country. This risk is minor compared to that, for example, of being killed in a road accident, which is about one in 15 000 (one person in a large or small town).

When optimal placements are hindered by public perception of *all* those with psychosis as threatening, it can result in resistance to the use of residential properties for supportive housing. The result may be a paradoxical increase in the risk of adverse events due to lack of community support.

Risk: society and psychiatry

Society has two expectations of mental health services: first, to manage the risk that patients may represent to themselves and to society, and second, to curtail the freedoms of their patients by the absolute minimum amount. Given the problems of risk management and perception there is an inevitable tension between these two.

(a) Defensive practice

Wall *et al.* (1999) reviewed admissions to acute psychiatric beds in the UK between 1984 and 1997. They found that total numbers had increased from 13 488 to 24 639; the percentage of admissions that were compulsory increased from 7 to 12%. They pointed out two possible reasons. The first is the increase in drug and alcohol use by psychiatric patients. It is important to bear in mind that co-occurring substance abuse is one of the few reliable indicators of risk of violence or self harm (Marshall 1998). The second is that during the period 1982–1992 there was a drop of 43 000 in the number of psychiatric beds available. They suggest that public fear of violence by mentally ill patients have led to pressures to keep patients in hospital longer than necessary and so have put further strain on the availability of beds. This in turn leads to delays in admission and treatment and may mean that patients' illnesses are becoming more severe and that compulsory treatment is being initiated in cases in which informal admissions would previously have been possible. An alternative to allowing a patient to deteriorate to the point where compulsory admission is necessary is to use some form of compulsion in the community. One commentator has suggested that defensive practice could lead to a new form of institutionalization, with intrusive surveillance by over cautious mental health teams (Harrison 1997).

(b) Society and the profession of psychiatry

It is usual for professions to have a code of practice laid down, stipulating amongst other things that no practitioner should attempt any task beyond their abilities. Applying this to risk assessment raises questions about the routine practice of psychiatry. Given the daily burden on the psychiatrist to assess risk, and the vagaries of predicting all but the most immediate risks, it could be argued that many psychiatrists are routinely having to practice beyond their ability. At the same time concern has been expressed that the imprecise nature of risk assessment will inevitably lead to some patients being wrongly assessed and being subject to unnecessary restrictions (Grisso and Appelbaum 1992).

Risk: policy on management

(a) Legal requirements—legislation

Since 1714 there have been 14 acts of Parliament affecting the treatment of MDOs (Vaughn and Badger 1995). The 1959 Mental Health Act is seen as a watershed in the development of mental health legislation. It allowed wider use of voluntary admission, and was part of the foundation for the development of community care. At that time there was movement towards open door policies in psychiatric institutions. The 1959 Mental Health Act carried forward the values that underpinned the open door policy into community care. The optimism of 1959 was tempered by the realism of the 1983 Mental Health Act (1983 MHA) which introduced stricter control of treatment against consent and a Mental Health Act Commission (MHAC) to ensure that hospitals treat patients in accordance with their rights. Nonetheless the 1983 MHA is still seen as offering an alternative to dangerousness as a criterion for civil commitment (Appelbaum 1997). Yet even this paradigm includes risk of harm to self and others in its criteria, though the 1983 MHA includes the requirement that the patient 'be suffering from a mental disorder' requiring treatment and that detention may be authorised 'in the interests' of the patient's health. There is also the criterion that admission be in the interests of the patient's, 'safety or with a view to the safety of others'. Table 5.1 shows the powers accorded to professional groups under 1983 MHA.

The 1983 MHA is currently under review. The Expert Committee (Richardson, 1999) and the Green Paper (Department of Health 1999b) state that it should be possible to assess and treat patients compulsorily in either hospital or the community. Two crucial issues in determining models of forensic community care are encapsulated here. Firstly again there is a statement of the importance of risk assessment without specific guidance on what constitutes risk. Secondly there is the possibility of compulsion in the community, leading to the question of under which circumstances and how such compulsion should be applied.

In addition to the 1983 MHA, MDOs can fall within the remit of:

(1) *National Health Service (NHS) and Community Care Act 1990.* This was a broad ranging re-organization of mental health care in the UK. It places responsibility for co-ordinating care of community psychiatric patients in the hands of the local authority. Each patient has a care manager who co-ordinates the different agencies involved with the patient, monitors progress and adjusts the care package accordingly, involving new agencies where appropriate. This ushered in the care programme approach (CPA) covered later in this chapter.

(2) *Criminal Procedure (Insanity and Unfitness to Plead) Act 1991.* Allows for those found unfit for trial or not guilty by reason of insanity to be subject to procedures similar to those which follow the making of a restriction order under Section 41 of the 1983 MHA.

Table 5.1 Powers of professions under the Mental Health Act 1983, to detain and treat

Section	Recommendation by	Powers
2	Two doctors and one social worker	Detain patient for 28 days for assessment, and possibly treatment
3	Two doctors and one social worker	Detain patient for up to six months for treatment
4	One social worker or the patient's nearest relative	Detain patient for three days in case of urgent necessity
5(2)	One doctor	Detain patient for three days if already voluntarily admitted and attempting to leave the ward
5(4)	One nurse	Detain patient for six hours if already admitted and attempting to leave the ward
7	Two doctors and one social worker	Guardianship—to require the patient to reside at a specified address and attend a specified place for treatment. Also the guardian, or their representative, has access to the patient at their residence
25	Two doctors and one social worker	Supervised discharge—to require the patient to reside at a specified address and attend a specified place for treatment. Also the guardian, or their representative, has access to the patient at their residence *and* the power to convey the patient to out-patient treatment
35	Crown and Magistrates Courts	Prisoners held on remand, sent to specified hospital for reports
36	Crown Court	Prisoners held on remand, sent to specified hospital for treatment
37	Crown and Magistrates Courts	Convicted prisoner admitted for treatment or made subject of Guardianship (MHA Section 7, see Table 5.2)
38	Crown and Magistrates Courts	Convicted prisoner admitted for assessment
41	Crown Court or Court of Appeal	Convicted prisoner held under Section 37 (above), special restrictions imposed to protect the public
47	Home Secretary	Convicted prisoner transferred from prison to a hospital for treatment
48	Home Secretary	Prisoners held on remand transferred from prison to a hospital for treatment
135	Magistrates Court	Entry to premises and removal to a place of safety, with a view to further detaining the patient, up to three days
136	Police	Removal from public place to a place of safety, up to three days

(3) *Criminal Justice Act 1991.* Allows a court to make a Guardianship order under 1983 MHA Section 37, with the agreement of the appropriate health authority or trust, who must state the form that the guardianship will take. In addition under this act, a Crown Court judge can make a direction for psychiatric treatment as part of a probation order.

(4) *Police and Criminal Evidence Act (PACE) 1984.* Provides for the provision of an 'appropriate adult' to advise and advocate on behalf of anyone in police custody who is believed to be mentally ill or mentally handicapped.

(5) *Sex Offenders Act 1997.* Requires sex offenders to inform local police of where they are living. In cases where an offender is judged to present a serious risk this information can be passed on to third parties. There is no guidance on what constitutes a serious risk.

(6) *Crime and Disorder Act 1998.* This introduced Sex Offender Orders. These allow for civil action to restrict convicted sex offenders from accessing designated public areas or applying for designated jobs. This can be done whatever the year of conviction. The act also requires health authorities and trusts to co-operate with local authorities and the police in joint crime prevention initiatives. The exact implications of this for health authorities and trusts are not yet clear. It seems possible that the collecting of anonymized data on victims of unreported crimes could be one requirement.

(b) Legal requirements—common law

Clearly this legislative framework imposes responsibilities on treatment services, yet most of it is couched in terms of what the various agencies can do to, or require of, the MDO. Responsibility for the safety of the MDO and the public is specifically mentioned in the sections of the 1983 MHA, but these statements are not elaborated. Hence the gap between risk management, as discussed in the first part of this chapter, and possible action under legislation are considerable.

The 'Tarasoff' decision, handed down by the California Supreme Court in 1976, concerned a patient who told a therapist that they intended to murder a specified third party. The therapist offered no warning to this person, who was eventually murdered by the patient. The court held the therapist to have been wrong not to warn the victim. Thus in the USA there is at least one clear criterion for risk assessment laid down in law, this is the statement of intention with regard to a specified third party. This principle seems to have been followed in a recent UK case, though Tarasoff was not directly cited. In Palmer versus Tees Health Authority and Another (*The Times Law Report* 6 July 1999), the health authority was not found to be liable for the sexual assault and homicide of a child committed by a patient who had ceased to attend for out-patient appointments. The patient had admitted a sexual attraction to children and stated a homicidal intent while an in-patient. However there was no threat expressed to any specific child. The judgement stated:

> In cases where it is alleged that a defendant by his negligence is responsible for the actions of a third party it must be shown that the victim or injured person was one who came into a special or exceptional or distinctive category of risk from the activities of the third party. It was not sufficient to show that the victim or injured party was one of a wide category of members of the general public.

W versus Egdell (1990) primarily concerns confidentiality but is relevant also to the management of risk. Dr Egdell was an independent psychiatrist retained by W to prepare a report for a Mental Health Review Tribunal (MHRT). He formed the view that W constituted a serious danger to the community. In the light of this W withdrew his application to the MHRT. Concerned that W, who had previously committed a multiple homicide using a firearm, might be in need of further treatment Dr Egdell gave a copy of his unfavourable report to the hospital authorities. W was unsuccessful in his attempt to sue Dr Egdell for breach of confidentiality. The evidence on which Dr Egdell based his view was not a specific threat to any individual but W's ongoing interest in firearms and explosives, in the context of his previous behaviour. Here risk to the broadest possible category, the general public, was the issue. This is the kind of balancing of alternatives that is necessary for effective risk management.

Whether and how actuarial criteria could be established in either statute or common law is a difficult question. The use of such criteria would inevitably and rightly raise a number of human rights issues. Actuarial criteria would by definition be identifying a population. This population having been identified as being potentially dangerous to the community could be subject to restrictions. In jurisprudence (Raz 1975; Collett 1977) a distinction is made between regulative and constitutive rules. The regulative determine what should be done, while the constitutive determine under what circumstances the regulative rules can be applied. The issue here is not so much the regulative rules; it is uncontroversial that a dangerous person should be detained. The issue is the constitutive rule: under what circumstances do we feel that dangerousness is clearly enough identified to allow the regulative rules regarding detention to be used? Restricting an individual's freedom on the basis of membership of a population could be a breach of their human rights, dependent on how the population is defined. Even if being male and a heavy drinker raises the probability of a person committing a violent act, to detain all male heavy drinkers might justifiably lead to comparisons being drawn with totalitarian regimes.

(c) Policy and risk management

In addition to statue and case law there have been two major policy initiatives during the 1990s which aim to establish systems which will allow better management of care generally and risk particularly.

(1) *Care Programme Approach.* This was introduced in 1991 as part of the NHS and Community Care Act, with the aim of reducing the number of psychiatric patients who fall out of contact with services due to breakdowns in communication

between health and social services. Each patient has a care plan jointly agreed by health and social services staff which is regularly reviewed. Key workers are responsible for co-ordinating the process by maintaining contact with the patient, reviewing the care plan and calling meetings for review. Dependent on the level of the patient's need and their potential for harm to self and others they can be placed on one of two levels of CPA. The lowest level usually equates to stable patients in need of only minimal contact and the middle to patients requiring the kind of case management standardly available in most sector psychiatric services. The enhanced level of CPA is reserved for patients seen as being at high risk.

(2) *Supervision Register.* This was introduced in 1994 (NHS Management Executive 1994) following recommendations in the Report of the Inquiry into the Care and Treatment of Christopher Clunis (1994). Mental health services are required to maintain a register of patients who are considered to be at significant risk of self harm or neglect, or of violence to others. The decision to place a person on this usually follows discussion with the care team but rests with their consultant psychiatrist. Patients have to be informed orally and in writing that they are on the register and why. The main point of the register is to provide a central reference of individuals at high risk and to ensure proper allocation of resources to them, though no new resources are made available as a result of being on the register. Nonetheless having a patient on the supervision register should encourage a key worker to be more cautious with that patient than they might be with others. In future, the supervision register will be absorbed into the enhanced level of the CPA.

Current service structures

Central to an understanding of the development of community services for MDOs is an understanding of their relationship with in-patient forensic services and with community general psychiatry services.

(a) Levels of security for in-patient settings

More than one commentator has pointed out that the development of open door policies in old psychiatric hospitals led to the development of a new culture which was less able to cope with patients in need of a secure environment (Vaughn and Badger 1995). A need developed for facilities which, while secure, are not as restrictive as those in the special hospitals: Broadmoor, Rampton and Ashworth. In 1974 the Glancy Report (Department of Health and Social Security (DHSS) 1974) recommended that there should be about 1000 medium secure beds in the UK. The Butler Committee (Home Office and DHSS 1975) the following year stated that the number of secure beds needed might be as many as 2000 (see also Chapter 3). In 1992 the Reed Report (Department of Health and The Home Office 1992) found that there had been disappointing

Table 5.2 Formal detentions under the Mental Health Act 1983 Part III by: Section and National Health Service (NHS) or Private (P) Facility, with ratio of change[1]

Sections under which admitted	1986	1991/92	1992/93	1993/94	1994/95	1995/96	1996/97
37(NHS)	1026	986	904	963	924	791	703
Ratio of change		0.96	0.88	0.94	0.90	0.77	0.69
37(P)	31	57	72	64	54	66	46
Ratio of change		1.84	2.32	2.06	1.74	2.13	1.48
% Private	2.9	5.5	7.4	6.2	5.5	7.7	6.1
35, 36, 47 and 48 (NHS)	411	893	882	1059	953	924	891
Ratio of change		2.17	2.15	2.58	2.32	2.25	2.17
35, 36, 47 and 48 (P)	6	45	45	58	60	37	39
Ratio of change		7.50	7.50	9.67	10.00	6.17	6.50
% Private	1.5	5.0	5.1	5.5	6.3	4.0	4.4

Source: Department of Health (1998); in-patients formally detained in hospitals under the Mental Health Act 1983 and other legislation. Prepared by Government Statistical Service.

[1] 1986 base year.

progress towards these goals. Where extra beds were needed the private sector was quick to establish provision. Table 5.2 shows the extent and development of private bed use for MDOs nationally between 1986 and 1997.

Differing approaches to the problem in different regions as well as differing special needs amongst the populations complicates the relationship between the different levels of security.

The low frequency of transfer of patients between general and medium secure units and the pressure for long term medium and low secure local forensic units suggests that increasing numbers of patients will be cared for by forensic services for the foreseeable future. Many see forensic services as already a separate but parallel system of care (Beck 1995). However, viewed as a separate system it has gaps in care settings, levels of security and possible lengths of stay. Based on recent government proposals (Home Office/Department of Health 1999; Department of Health 1998), an expanded portfolio of places with differing levels of security, admission time and care may include:

(1) Separate facilities for those deemed untreatable but in need of detention.

(2) For those deemed treatable
   • high secure (most likely in special hospitals)
   • long-term medium secure for stays over two years

- short-term medium secure for stays under two years
- long-term low secure
- short-term low secure, i.e. intensive care units
- forensic hostels
- bail and probation hostels
- community forensic mental health teams
- prison services run by NHS forensic mental health services.

It is possible that the difference between patients in medium and low secure wards is one of duration of risk. Many in-patients in low secure environments will have short episodes of risk, following which they can be referred back to an open acute admission ward, whereas the average length of stay is between 18 and 24 months on medium secure units, and 8 years at Broadmoor. MIND states that 'Secure beds are likely to be used as an easy option unless alternatives are available—and so demand may continue to outstrip provision'. This statement suggests the need to consider forensic provision in the context of the whole service, as opposed to a segmental approach, where a local difficulty may be fixed but the problem displaced to another part of the service (Thornicroft and Tansella 1999). Murray (1996) draws attention to this phenomenon, citing the negative correlation between provision for the mentally ill and for criminals first described by Penrose in 1939. He stresses that forensic services must not be provided at the expense of general services, which provide care at an earlier stage in a patient's illness that may help prevent later offending and the need for secure care. Evidence of subsidization of forensic services by general mental health exists. The index of need for psychiatric services included in the York resource allocation formula implies a three-fold difference in spending between areas (Peacock and Smith 1995). In inner city areas (other than London) with high need, many health authorities are spending under the predicted level for general mental health services (Bindman 1999), but are spending more than the formula predicts on secure care. In inner London, four health authorities spend higher amounts on both general mental health services and MDOs than predicted by the York formula. It is not clear whether the budget for general mental health services or other health budgets are being used to pay for these higher levels of spend for MDO services.

A recent study (McCrone et al. in press) found that four-fifths of variation in high and medium secure service use could be explained by a model including Black ethnicity, Asian ethnicity, population density, number of people aged over 65, number of people single/widowed/divorced, number of people registered as permanently sick, and the number of new registrations of drug use. The fit of the model was particularly good in inner London and other urban areas, but poorer in rural areas. The addition of supported housing significantly increased the variation explained. The use by different health authorities of medium secure unit beds varies by around ten-fold (Thake 1997) in England and Wales. The studies suggest that a separate assertive outreach service for those discharged from MSUs might suit some areas more than others.

There is thus a clear view that other interventions should be used to reduce this demand, although it is not known how effective they are in doing so. Until the evidence is clearer on this it is hard to know whether more in-patient services are needed (in line with the Butler report) and, if so, to what extent.

(b) Models for community forensic services

Six papers on the subject of community-based forensic psychiatry treatment have been published in UK-based peer-reviewed journals since 1977 (Gunn 1977; Higgins 1981; Snowden 1985; Gallwey 1990; Whittle and Scally 1998; Snowden et al. 1999). Much of the debate turns on whether community forensic services should run parallel to community mental health teams, or be integrated with them. In the USA, Heilbrun and Griffin (1998) reviewed 21 papers from eight states, written since 1977. Here, the terms of the debate are slightly different; the authors identify a tension between three possible models; centralized, community mental health centre (CMHC) embedded and private. The first two of these appear to equate with the two identified UK models. The third option has not been seriously considered as an alternative for community care in the UK.

General/forensic psychiatry relationship; parallel and integrated models

Snowden et al. (1999) argued that the definitions of the terms 'integrated' and 'parallel' are problematic. They identified three different uses of the terms (see Table 5.3):

- organizational
- descriptions of patient care model
- directions for development of practice.

Thus under the taxonomy of Snowden et al. (1999) it is possible for a service to be managed by the local mental health service (organizationally integrated) but with a staff of specialist clinicians seeing MDOs (patient care parallel). However the taxonomy then seems to allow that some MDOs with more local contacts and lower risk might be treated by local general psychiatric services (integrated patients), while others with fewer local contacts and higher risk are treated by a specialist forensic team (parallel patients). It seems that in this taxonomy the 'organizational' and 'patient care aspects' are independent of one another, while the 'practice development' part is simply one operationalization of the 'patient care aspect'. We argue that this is the at the root of the confusion that Snowden et al. (1999) feel that these terms cause. Whatever the intention of services, Henderson et al. (1998) estimate that up to 70% of

Table 5.3 Snowden's (1999) taxonomy of terms 'integrated' and 'parallel' in describing community forensic mental health teams

	Integrated	Parallel
Organizational	Responsibility for planning and supervising services lies within existing mental health service structures	Responsibility for planning and supervising services lies with dedicated specialist teams
Patient care model	MDO seen by local general adult team	MDO seen by specialist forensic mental health team
Practice development	MDOs with local social networks, having offended during an exacerbation of a psychosis and having had minimal contact with the criminal justice system, remain integrated into general psychiatric services	MDOs without local social networks, having come from prison or a high secure hospital, and are assessed as carrying a higher risk to others or themselves

MDOs are treated within general psychiatry. Even when a service has a clear parallel patient care model, the issue of what criteria define an appropriate referral to community forensic psychiatry team remains problematic.

Parry (1991) described a parallel model with clear boundaries as to what constitutes a forensic patient: one discharged under Section 37 (and possibly Section 41) of 1983 MHA, or one with a serious conviction which could result in a prison sentence. Parry describes his service in Merseyside as providing community psychiatric nurses (CPNs), crisis intervention, day and drop-in centres, all closely linked to the local regional secure unit (RSU) to which re-admissions are quickly arranged. He acknowledges that an integrated model is preferable but points to the high level of input that is required to maintain some forensic patients in the community, especially those on 'enhanced' levels of the CPA. In his service only 20% of patients discharged from the RSU were followed-up by his service. The rest went either to higher security units or straight back to general psychiatric services. Unfortunately he does not give the percentages in these last two groups. Nonetheless there does seem to be some form of integrated service operating if patients can be discharged direct from RSU to general services.

Daly and Lord (1998) offered several criteria for a patient to be taken on by their forensic team:

(1) Those with an 'active forensic history'.

(2) Patients on Section 37 (and possibly 41) of the MHA who had been referred back to locality teams.

(3) 'Private sector' patients who would return home to locality teams.

(4) Patients discharged from prison with known psychiatric history.

(5) Dual diagnosis/personality disorder/challenging behaviour group with forensic concerns.

(6) Known patients on the 'enhanced' CPA supervision register who generate ongoing concerns although may not have offended.

These criteria are considerably broader than those of Parry in that any patient with a petty criminal conviction could be fitted into one of the categories. Having said this, the team clearly refers most of their referrals onwards or back to the general team. Perhaps a more relevant set of criteria would be those for keeping a patient under the care of the community forensic mental health team. Out of 137 referrals over an 8 month period about 24% were taken on by the team and 29% were referred back to sector services with management advice following assessment. The remaining 46% patients were referred on to a variety of services. It seems from these that whatever the intention the actual operation of most community forensic mental health teams fits into the 'practice development' definition of Snowden *et al.* (1999) of the integrated/parallel taxonomy. Any service is a mixture of both models, with some direct care of forensic patients going on alongside assessment and consultation with general services.

From discussion with key informants, it seems clear that rather than being actual models to choose between, the concepts of parallel versus integrated services represent two extremes at the end of a continuum of possible types of service interface. Both would be undesirable to both general and forensic psychiatrists. It is more useful to consider what possible forms intermediate types of interface could take (see Chapter 11).

Snowden *et al.* (1999) propose a practical taxonomy to characterize the relationship of forensic and general psychiatry teams in the community. Their four-level model (see Table 5.4) does much to resolve the confusion about integrated/parallel services by allowing for the existence of both approaches with graded levels of shared care in between. The framework provides a strategic approach to how general and forensic services should share the care of MDOs. There remains the practicality of how team members communicate and refer, and who the MDO sees and where. Three options are discussed.

(a) Forensic community psychiatric nurses in general teams

Community psychiatric nurses with a special interest in the care of MDOs could be allotted a small caseload of patients resident within the catchment area of a sector team and provide specialist interventions, such as anger management, while liaising with agencies such as bail hostel staff and probation officers. This might introduce greater patient level effectiveness than general adult care alone, without the loss of service level effectiveness entailed by separate services. But who would provide supervision to such a CPN, and which consultant would be responsible for their caseload? If the psychiatrist were to be the sector consultant, the CPN would need forensic advice from another source outside the team. To locate supervision and responsibility in the same

Table 5.4 Snowden's (1999) levels of community care for forensic psychiatry

Level of care	Description
Level 4: All care by forensic community mental health team	Equates to parallel model of 'patient care'
Level 3: Shared care—led by forensic community mental health team	Patient key worked by forensic psychiatrist or CPN in association with social worker or probation officer
Level 2: Shared care—led by local community mental health or probation service	Patient key worked by general psychiatrist with a forensic CPN and a social worker or probation officer
Level 1: All care by local community mental health or probation service	Equates to integrated model of 'patient care'

consultant would require that the forensic CPN belonged to a forensic community mental health team (CMHT) with staff shared among several sectors. This would address the problems created by the large catchment area size needed for a forensic CMHT.

(b) Consultation–liaison model

In this model members of a CMHT meet with a visiting forensic consultant to discuss cases rather than referring them for a forensic out-patient appointment. Only after agreement at such a discussion can a case be referred to forensic services. In this model, the population served by the forensic community teams outlined above would instead be served by intensive general adult services. The problems of liaising with other agencies are reduced by the less stigmatizing nature of the service. Integration with sector teams may facilitate more comprehensive care and make team members more geographically accessible to patients. The consultation–liaison model involves changing resources and incentives in order to influence what generalists are prepared to do. Currently many general services are unable to provide intensive management of any form, nor do they have the ease of access to forensic advice described. Without such changes generalists will continue to be unwilling to accept some referrals from forensic psychiatrists and to provide mental health services for people released from prison.

(c) Shared care by general and forensic keyworkers

This model allows for education of general adult staff by forensic staff, reducing problems of deskilling. The latter could provide specific interventions for referred patients while responsibility remained clearly that of the general CMHT. Supervision for the forensic keyworker and screening of referrals for shared care would be required from a forensic consultant outside the CMHT, who may or may not provide a consultation–

liaison service as described above. These last two models represent the furthest degree of integration of forensic and general community services, representing ways in which recommendations in the Reed report (Home Office and DHSS 1992) might be implemented. Both service and patient level effectiveness may improve as a result, while lines of accountability remain clear.

Style of care

What follows in this section is drawn from the literature on schizophrenia. Mueser *et al.* (1998), identify three models of community care each with two varieties of sub-model (see Table 5.5). Our descriptions of these models have come from several sources. It is clear that the rehabilitation-oriented models seem to be practised within either case management or intensive comprehensive models, hence such terms as 'strengths case management' (Solomon 1992).

Both case management and assertive community treatment (ACT) have been the subject of Cochrane reviews (Marshall *et al.* 2000; Marshall and Lockwood 2000). In the review of ACT (Marshall and Lockwood 2000) four varieties are included. The results compare ACT to standard community care, hospital-based rehabilitation services and intensive case management. Those receiving ACT were less likely to drop out of contact or to be admitted to hospital than those receiving standard community care; less likely to be admitted to hospital than those receiving hospital-based rehabilitation; and spent fewer days in hospital than those receiving intensive case management. Those receiving ACT were more likely to be living independently than those receiving hospital-based rehabilitation, however there were no other clear advantages for ACT on measures of social functioning for any of the other conditions.

The criteria for inclusion in the case management were those studies that failed to fulfil the criteria for the review of ACT. It includes studies of interventions described as; 'home-treatment', 'brokerage', 'intensive', 'clinical' or 'strengths', with no distinctions made between them. Ccase management appears to reduce drop-out but increase rates of hospital admission.

This raises the question of how should CMHTs, whether general or forensic, engage with MDOs who are directly under their care? Given the level of social expectations to monitor the risk an MDO represents to others, it is not unreasonable to expect the model to be of the intensive comprehensive variety. However, this does raise ethical issues about the role of psychiatry within the criminal justice system. Firstly, the advantages of the brokerage model have to be maintained and no patient should be denied a service simply on the basis of being an MDO. Secondly, if the function of mental health services is simply one of monitoring and observation then it simply becomes another form of policing. To justify what can be an intrusive style of intervention the content has also to be therapeutic. This would suggest that the inclusion of rehabilitation-oriented models is essential. It is worth noting that one of the principles

Table 5.5 Models of patient community care

Model	Sub-model	Content
Case management	Clinical case management	One assigned key worker who (1) maintains contact with the patient (2) monitors their mental state and treatment compliance (3) delivers a limited amount of therapeutic intervention (4) involves other members of the CMHT as necessary
	Brokerage of care (Holloway 1991)	One assigned key worker who (1) assesses and identifies patient need at regular intervals (2) identifies deliverers of care who can meet the needs, and then negotiates and monitors the delivery of packages of care
Intensive comprehensive	Intensive case management	One assigned key worker who (1) provides most of the care and therapeutic intervention themselves (2) has a small caseload (3) maintains intensive contact with their patients
	Assertive community treatment	A team which (1) works with small caseloads (2) delivers care and therapeutic intervention as necessary (3) matches the presenting need to the skills of team members (4) provides 24 h emergency cover
Rehabilitation-oriented	Rehabilitation	Emphasizes addressing skills deficits (1) social skills (2) self-care skills (3) work skills (4) learning skills
	Strengths (Rapp 1993)	Six principles (1) focus on individual strengths, not pathology (2) key worker/client relationship is 'primary and essential' (3) interventions based on client self-determination (4) community is an oasis of resource, not an obstacle (5) aggressive outreach preferred mode of intervention (6) sufferers of mental illness can learn, grow and change.

of the strengths model is that interventions should be based on client self-determination. Where this conflicts with clinical and social values overt coercion follows.

Risk as a criterion for community forensic mental health care

If a general CMHT is already using an intensive case management or ACT model what will be the rationale for involving extra community forensic psychiatrists or CPNs? We could use risk as a criterion. If this were to happen, would it be ethical to only take risk to others as the criterion, or would these teams have an expanded role in working with those at risk of suicide or serious self-harm? If so they would become *de facto* the ACT branch of CMHTs but run the risk of stigmatizing their patients, as described above. And could this role be integrated with that of providing long term support and input into MDOs who have been discharged from secure accommodation? For such patients the level of need is as crucial in determining care as the level of risk. How these two aspects of care planning can be resolved is another discussion.

Conclusions

The argument for specialist care is based on the relationship between volume and quality. Clinicians caring for a particular group develop more experience and expertise, providing higher quality care, than clinicians for with a broader caseload. Other psychiatric specialities (old age, learning disabilities etc.) are based on common developmental characteristics of patients. By contrast the speciality of forensic psychiatry is based on a social category for which there is no consensual definition. The case for separate forensic CMHTs is based on their ability to provide continuity of care for MDOs leaving secure care, given the volume and quality argument (Snowden *et al.* 1999). While this may be the case for some individual level treatments, the associated stigma and larger catchment area might hamper service level effectiveness for community rehabilitation and have negative impacts on autonomy, accessibility, comprehensiveness, equity, accountability, co-ordination and efficiency.

From the review presented here and our own discussions with professionals, we conclude: while some forensic psychiatrists advocate greater provision of local forensic services (such as long-term low secure beds and community forensic teams), many general psychiatrists and advocacy groups would prefer more comprehensive community care with assertive outreach teams and access to forensic consultation. Arguments about who should be responsible for patients admitted to low secure units reflects the absence of consensus about the nature of the interface between the two services. The research question arising from this is what impact would the provision of more comprehensive community care versus long-term low secure units have on demand for each other and on other system components, such as acute local units or MSUs? While the provision of each would clearly affect resources available for provision of the other, it is not clear to what extent these services can be substituted one for another. Establishing the extent to which general adult psychiatric care can prevent offending behaviour and the resultant need for forensic services will necessitate local agreements about the shape of the forensic–general psychiatry interface. This process, and the greater contact that may result in between the two specialities, may facilitate some resolution of more fundamental differences.

Two service administration models have been identified, the parallel and the integrated. We argue that these approaches are not in reality mutually exclusive, rather two ends of a continuum. The views of key informants support models toward the integrated end of the continuum, but the point was made that different models might suit areas with different demographics. The model of care chosen for MDOs will be influenced by the model of care used for patients who are not considered to be MDOs. This latter group may include people with mental illness who have had contact with the courts but who are not considered to represent a significant risk to the public.

Given the current problems of transferring patients between general and forensic services, creation of parallel local services might create an additional boundary where teams could refuse to accept referrals from each other. The need to keep forensic service caseloads relatively small could reduce their ability to take on new cases, particularly if referrals the other way were few. Meanwhile the possible diversion of money from general to local forensic services could leave general psychiatry teams less able to care safely for difficult patients. Further, general services could experience staffing problems if nurses were attracted by the higher pay and smaller caseloads of forensic work.

Finally we propose the following criteria for care by community forensic psychiatry teams:

(1) A pre-determined cut-off score on a well-evaluated risk management tool that uses both clinical and actuarial items.

(2) Being placed under Section 37 (with or without a Section 41 restriction) of the MHA.

We are aware that these can only be tentative criteria, and welcome the comments that they will provoke. It is also true that different teams may use different instruments, and so there might be inequity in the use of restrictions and supervision. However, if all community forensic teams were using such instruments and their performance were to be regularly audited the differences between such instruments would soon become clear, and improvements could be developed amongst those instruments that continued to be used.

References

Appelbaum, P. S. (1997) Almost a revolution: an international perspective on the law of involuntary commitment. *Journal of the American Academy of Psychiatry and Law*, **25**(2).

Appleby, L., Shaw J., Amos, T. *et al.* (1999) Safer services. Report of the national confidential inquiry into suicide and homicide by people with mental illness. London: Stationery Office.

Beck, J. (1995) Forensic psychiatry in Britain. *Bulletin of the American Academy of Psychiatry and Law*, **23**, 249–60.

Bindman, J. (1999) Allocation and expenditure on mental health services in England: Implications for equity. MSc thesis, London School of Hygiene and Tropical Medicine.

Buchanan, A. (1999) Risk and dangerousness. *Psychological Medicine*, **29**, 465–73.

Calman, K. and Royston, G. (1997) Risk language and dialects. *British Medical Journal*, **315**, 939–42

Collet, P. (1977) The rules of conduct. In *Social rules and social behaviour* (ed. P. Collett). Oxford: Basil Blackwell.

The Daily Telegraph—www.the-telegraph.co.uk/

Daly, R. and Lord, A. (1998) An overview of the early developing stages of Community Forensic Team. Poster Presentation at Royal College of Psychiatrists Forensic Section Annual Conference.

Department of Health (1998) Modernising mental health services. London: Department of Health.

Department of Health (1999*a*) National confidential enquiry into suicide and homicide by people with mental illness: Safer services. Leeds: Department of Health.

Department of Health (1999*b*) Reform of the Mental Health Act 1983: Proposals for consultation. London: HMSO.

Department of Health and The Home Office (1992) Review of health and social services for mentally disordered offenders and others requiring similar services, final summary report. London: HMSO.

DHSS (1974) Revised report of the working party on security in NHS psychiatric hospitals (Glancy report). London: HMSO.

Eastman, N. (1997) The Mental Health (Patients in the Community) Act, 1995. *British Journal of Psychiatry*, **170**, 492–6.

Furedi, F. (1998) Culture of fear: risk taking and the morality of low expectation. London: Cassell.

Gallwey, P. (1990) The development of a district-based psychiatric service for difficult and offender patients. *Journal of Forensic Psychiatry*, **1**(1), 52–71.

Grisso, T. and Appelbaum, P.S. (1992) Is it unethical to offer predictions of future violence? *Law and Human Behaviour*, **16**, 621–33.

Gunn, J. (1977) Management of the mentally abnormal offender. *Proceedings of the Royal Society of Medicine*, **70**, 877–80.

Harrison, G. (1997) Risk assessment in a climate of litigation. *British Journal of Psychiatry*, **170**, 37–9.

Heilbrun, K. and Griffin, P.A. (1998) Community-based forensic treatment. In *Treatment of offenders with mental disorders* (ed. R. M. Wettstein). New York: The Guilford Press.

Henderson, C., Bindman, J. and Thornicroft, G. (1998) Can deinstitutionalised care be provided for those at risk of violent offending? *Epidemiologia E Psichiatria Sociale*, **7**, 1.

Higgins, J. (1981) Four years experience of an interim secure unit. *British Medical Journal*, **282**, 889–93.

HMSO (1983) Mental Health Act 1983.

HMSO (1984) Police and Criminal Evidence Act (PACE) 1984.

HMSO (1990) National Health Service and Community Care Act 1990.

HMSO (1991) Criminal Procedure (Insanity and Unfitness to Plead) Act 1991.

HMSO (1991) Criminal Justice Act 1991.

HMSO (1998) Crime and Disorder Act 1998.

Home Office and Department of Health (1999) Managing dangerous people with severe personality disorder: Proposals for policy development. London: HMSO.

Home Office and DHSS (1975) Report of the committee on mentally abnormal offenders (Butler Report). London: HMSO.

Home Office and DHSS (1992) Interim report of the committee on mentally abnormal offenders (Reed Report). HMSO: London.

The Independent—www.independent.co.uk/

McCrone, P., Leese, M., Glover G. and Thornicroft G. (submitted for publication) Social deprivation and the use of secure psychiatric beds.

Marshall, J. (1998) Dual diagnosis: Co-morbidity of severe mental illness and substance misuse. *Journal of Forensic Psychiatry*, **9**, 9–15.

Marshall, M and Lockwood, A. (2000) Assertive community treatment for people with severe mental disorders (Cochrane Review). In *The Cochrane Library*, Issue 4. Oxford: Update Software.

Marshall, M., Gray, A., Lockwood, A. and Green R. (2000) Case management for people with severe mental disorders (Cochrane Review). In *The Cochrane Library*, Issue 4. Oxford: Update Software.

Mueser, K. T., Bond G. R., Drake, R. E. and Resnick, S G. (1998) Models of community care for severe mental illness: a review of research on case management. *Schizophrenia Bulletin*, **24**(1), 37–74.

Miller, R. (1991) The ethics of involuntary commitment to mental health treatment. In *Psychiatric ethics* (ed. S. Bloch P. and Chodoff). Oxford: Oxford Medical Publications.

MIND Mind's policy on people with mental health problems and the criminal justice system. MINDfile, MIND.

Mossman, D. (1994) Assessing predictions of violence: being accurate about accuracy. *Journal of Consulting and Clinical Psychology*, **62**(4), 783–92.

Murray, K. (1996) The use of beds in NHS medium secure units in England. *Journal of Forensic Psychiatry*, **7**, 504–24.

NACRO (1998) *Risks and rights: Mentally disturbed offenders and public protection*. London: NACRO.

NHS Management Executive (1993) Executive letter, EL(93)68.

NHS Management Executive (1994) Introduction of supervision registers for mentally ill people from 1st April 1994, Health Service Guidelines HSG (94) 5.

Parry, J. (1991) Community care for mentally ill offenders. *Nursing Standard*, **5**(23), 29–33.

Peacock, S. and Smith, P. (1995) The resource allocation consequences of the new NHS needs formula, Discussion Paper 134. York: Centre for Health Economics, University of York.

Penrose, L. (1939) Mental disease and crime: outline of a comparative study of European statistics. *British Journal of Medical Psychology*, **18**, 1–13.

Philo, G. (1997) Changing media representations of mental health. *Psychiatric Bulletin*, **21**, 171–2.

Prins, H. (1995) *Offenders, deviants or patients?* London: Routledge.

Prins, H. (1999) But will they do it again? Risk assessment and management in criminal justice and psychiatry. London: Routledge.

Raz, J. (1975) Practical reason and norms. London: Hutchinson.

Report of the inquiry into the care and treatment of Christopher Clunis (1994) HMSO.

Richardson, G. (1999) Draft outline proposals by scoping study committee April 1999 review of the Mental Health Act 1983. London: Department of Health.

Snowden, P. (1985) A survey of the regional secure unit program. *British Journal of Psychiatry*, **147**, 499–507.

Snowden, P., McKenna, J. and Jasper, A. (1999) Management of conditionally discharged patients and others who present similar risks in the community: integrated or parallel? *Journal of Forensic Psychiatry*, **10**(3), 583–96.

Solomon, P. (1992) The efficacy of case management services for severely mentally disabled clients. *Community Mental Health Journal*, **28**, 163–80.

Szmukler, G. (2000) Homicide inquiries: What sense do they make? *Psychiatric Bulletin*, **24**, 6–10.

Szmukler, G., Thornicroft, G., Holloway, F and Bowden, P. (1999) Homicides and community care: the evidence. *British Journal of Psychiatry*, **174**, 565–5.

Thake, T. (1997) Information to assist with population based needs assessment in secure psychiatric services. London: High Security Psychiatric Services Commissioning Board.

Thornicroft, G. and Tansella, M. (1999) *The mental health matrix: A manual to improve services.* Cambridge: Cambridge University Press.

Tarasoff versus Regents of the University of California (1976) 131 California Reporter 14 (California Supreme Court). In Kennedy, I. and Grubb, A. (1994) *Medical law: text with materials.* London: Butterworths.

Taylor, P. J. and Gunn, J. (1999) Homicides by people with mental illness: myth and reality. *British Journal of Psychiatry*, **174**, 9–14.

The Times—www.the-times.co.uk/

Vaughn, P.J. and Badger, D. (1995) Working with the mentally disordered offender in the community. London: Chapman and Hall.

W versus Egdell (1990) 1 All England reports (1989) 4 Butterworths medical law review 96 (Court of Appeal). In Kennedy, I. and Grubb, A. (1994) *Medical law: text with materials.* London: Butterworths.

Wall, S., Hotopf, M., Wessely, S. *et al.* (1999) Trends in the use of the Mental Health Act: England, 1984–96. *British Medical Journal*, **318**(7197), 1520.

Webster, C. D., Douglas, K. S., Eaves, D. *et al.* (1995) HCR-20: Assessing risk for violence (version 2). Vancouver: Mental Health, Law and Policy Institute, Simon Fraser University.

Whittle, M. C. and Scally, M. D. (1998) Model of forensic psychiatric community care. *Psychiatric Bulletin*, **22**, 748–50.

Chapter 6

Assessing the risk of violence posed by mentally disordered offenders being treated in the community

Jennifer L. Skeem and Edward P. Mulvey

Introduction

People with mental illnesses often come into contact with the criminal justice system, and a substantial proportion of individuals in the criminal justice system have significant mental health problems (Monahan 1992*b*). The prevalence of individuals with both legal and mental health problems, or mentally disordered offenders (MDOs), seems to be on the rise because of a 'psychiatrization of criminal behaviour' associated with establishing dangerousness as a criterion for civil commitment (Cocozza *et al.* 1978), or a 'criminalization of the mentally ill' related to inadequate community-based treatment resources and restrictive civil commitment criteria (Teplin 1984; for a review, see Rice and Harris 1997). Regardless of the policy causes, this growing group of patients presents clinicians with complex assessment, treatment and service coordination needs.

Addressing these needs is particularly challenging when MDOs have previously engaged in serious violent or anti-social conduct and are being treated in a community-based setting. Once a rare event for practising clinicians, this set of circumstances is becoming more common (Dvoskin and Steadman 1994; Slobogin 1994; see also Chapter 9), in part because community-based care, even for previously violent or anti-social individuals, may be more therapeutic than institutional care (Andrews *et al.* 1990; Rice and Harris, 1997). In this situation, clinicians are responsible for providing cost-effective services in the least restrictive setting possible while optimizing public safety (Petrila 1995; Rice and Harris 1997; Tarasoff versus Regents of the University of California 1976; Shelton versus Tucker 1960). Achieving this delicate balance requires ongoing risk assessment that focuses intervention efforts on factors related to violence potential.

This chapter provides limited, specific support for clinicians engaged in this task by presenting a strategy and structure to apply when conducting ongoing assessment of the MDO's risk for future violence. The chapter does not dwell on the content of risk assessments (e.g. specific risk factors to weigh in assessing risk), nor does it review therapeutic approaches designed to prevent violence. The best form of risk management takes a broad array of factors into account, including the strength of the therapeutic alliance and the levels of care available, and is addressed elsewhere (see Chapters 5 and 8; Rice and Harris 1997; Truscott *et al.* 1995). This chapter is written under the assumption that high quality risk assessment requires not only a consideration of risk factors relevant to each patient (Bonta *et al.* 1998; Eronen *et al.* 1998; Melton *et al.* 1997) in light of jurisdictional definitions of dangerousness (e.g. Parry 1994), but also a clear and consistent *process* for analyzing these factors (see also Litwack and Schlesinger 1999; Monahan 1981; Poythress 1990; Webster 1997). This chapter describes ways in which clinicians can make more systematic and reasoned decisions about when and how to intervene with MDOs.

Research on clinicians' predictive accuracy: its relevance to risk assessment with mentally disordered offenders

Research on clinicians' risk assessments has focused mainly on predictive accuracy, rather than on the information gathering and decisional processes associated with this task. This focus on accuracy stems from researchers' efforts to address a policy concern about the wisdom of legal standards that predicated long periods of institutionalization and deprivation of patients' constitutional rights upon clinicians' predictions of future patient violence (Monahan 1996; Mulvey and Lidz 1995). Early studies painted a bleak picture of clinicians' predictive accuracy (see Litwack and Schlesinger 1999; Mulvey and Lidz 1993; Monahan and Steadman 1994). More sophisticated research conducted over the past decade, however, suggests that clinicians have a modest ability to assess risk, with levels of predictive accuracy significantly better than chance (see Lidz *et al.* 1993; Otto 1992, 1994; Mossman 1994). The extent to which these newer findings apply to assessments of MDOs is unclear. On the one hand, clinicians may be less accurate in identifying potentially violent MDOs because, unlike general psychiatric patients, all MDOs have offence histories. Mentally disordered offenders' lack of variability with respect to this predictive variable may increase the difficulty of the violence prediction task. On the other hand, the higher base rate of violence among MDOs, relative to general psychiatric patients, should *decrease* the difficulty of the prediction task (see Otto 1992, 1994).

Unfortunately, very few studies of clinical risk assessment target MDOs. The results of those that do, however, are not encouraging. For example, in a six-year follow-up of community residents who had been evaluated in a forensic clinic, Menzies and Webster (1995) found that even the most accurate clinicians' predictions of which MDOs would be violent were 'neither powerful nor pragmatically of any value'. Although such findings may indicate reduced clinical accuracy in predicting MDOs' future violence, there are two reasons to reserve judgement. First, like most other studies of MDOs, the criterion measure of violence used in this study was based upon record reviews, which often fail to identify violent incidents detected when researchers interview patients and collateral sources (Mulvey et al. 1996). Second, and more importantly, the judgement task studied in this and most other prior research may differ markedly from the one faced by a clinician monitoring the MDO in a community setting.

The context of, and the information considered in, assessments of MDOs differ from those associated with assessments tested in most prior research on clinical accuracy. Over recent years, hospital stays have been drastically shortened, with (a) the adoption of policies of deinstitutionalization and treatment in the least restrictive setting, and (b) the rising dominance of managed care over the mental health care market, and its restrictions on reimbursable services (Lerman 1981; Regier et al. 1993; Kiesler and Simkins 1993). Given this shift, clinical predictions of future violence are less commonly used as gateways to institutionalization, and are more commonly associated with the ongoing responsibility to protect third parties while working with potentially violent patients in the community (Monahan 1996).[1] A clinician assessing the MDO in this environment is less concerned with whether the patient may be justly deprived of liberty than with when and under what controllable conditions he may commit a violent act (Heilbrun 1997; Monahan and Steadman 1994; Rice and Harris 1997). Relatively few studies of predictive accuracy account for these dramatic changes that have occurred in the general context and purpose of assessing violence risk over recent years.

The ongoing nature of risk assessment with MDOs also yields different information for predicting violence. The community clinician has repeated contact with the MDO, should be intimately familiar with his current symptoms, problems and life circumstances, and should develop a relatively well-articulated narrative for his[2] patterns of violence. Theoretically, this permits the clinician to make short-term evaluations of risk that are grounded in a frequent, recursive, experience-based assessment of the patients' current state and capacity for adaptive coping with particular environments and stressors. Almost 20 years ago, Monahan (1981) observed that clinicians' risk assessments may be relatively accurate under these types of circumstances (i.e. short-term predictions in community-based settings). Although Mossman (1994) found that clinicians' short-term predictions of violence were no more accurate than their

---

[1] There are context-specific exceptions to this statement. For mentally disordered offenders in the USA, these include predictions of dangerousness as (1) gateways to civil commitment for sex offenders who have fulfilled their criminal sentences (Kansas versus Hendrick, 1997), (2) requirements for the continued detention of insanity acquittees (Foucha versus Louisiana 1992), or (3) justification for increased levels of security with MDOs (Rice and Harris 1997). Given this chapter's focus on risk assessment as it pertains to treating MDOs in the community, however, the statement is appropriate.

[2] For reading ease only, the pronoun 'he' is used in this chapter to reference mentally disordered offenders, based on the predominance of males in this population.

long-term predictions, predictive accuracy in the treatment context described above has not been systematically tested.

Finally, the likely courses of action for a community clinician working with the MDO differ from those studied in prior research. If a community clinician believes that a patient is at risk for violence, he or she may attempt to reduce violence potential by intensifying treatment efforts, attempting to manage critical aspects of the patient's environment, using the therapeutic alliance to develop a safety plan with the patient, increasing the patient's level of care (e.g. to partial or brief hospitalization), or warning or arranging to protect the potential victim (Beck 1987; Monahan 1993; Truscott et al. 1995). Most prior research studies only clinicians' decisions about whether or not to hospitalize a patient. Given the reduced availability of hospitalization, contemporary clinicians are under more pressure to consider other risk management options. Thus, violence potential may more often be managed without forcibly and indefinitely depriving patients of their liberty.[3] In addition, contemporary clinicians' risk assessments are sensitive to the fact that violence potential is affected by the availability of particular treatment resources. A clinician's knowledge about available interventions and beliefs about their potential effectiveness could increase or decrease the MDO's real or perceived violence potential. For example, given a residential treatment unit in which only milieu- and pharmaco-therapy are available, a clinician might perceive the MDO with traits of psychopathy as more highly at risk for violent reoffence than the MDO with schizophrenia.

In summary, there are considerable differences in the situation facing a community clinician working with the MDO and those facing clinicians examined in prior studies, based both on differing clinical populations (MDOs versus general psychiatric patients) and judgement contexts (ongoing risk management in the context of a therapeutic relationship versus a one-time evaluation). As a result, the overall accuracy that might be expected from clinicians working with MDOs is difficult to gauge. The best hope for maximizing accuracy, however, clearly rests with performing the assessment task consistently and thoughtfully.

Research and practice: How do clinicians assess risk?

A logical approach to improving the assessment of violence potential is to develop an understanding of existing risk assessment practices and then to modify these practices. Unfortunately, current knowledge about how clinicians perform risk assessments is limited. Risk assessment research has largely 'sidestepped' the first, critical stage of describing clinicians' judgement processes (Mulvey and Lidz 1985).

....

[3] The range of less intrusive options available for managing risk renders clinicians' tendency to err on the conservative side by overpredicting potential violence (e.g. Mossman 1994; Otto1992) less costly or even desirable, given the serious consequences of failing to identify and intervene with a violent MDO in the community.

Descriptive research about clinical decision making is necessary, however, for conducting informed investigations of predictive accuracy. As noted by Jackson (1989), 'with more detailed knowledge about *how* clinicians work, it might well be possible to return later to the unsolved issue of validity of judgement' (emphasis added). Although a few authors have observed clinicians' risk assessments and have provided their interpretations of the decisional bases for individual cases (Litwack 1996) or biases across cases (Pfohl 1978; Pflafflin 1979; see Jackson 1989; Mulvey and Lidz 1985), there are very few systematic investigations of clinicians' risk assessments with respect to particular process or content variables.[4] Instead, most research on risk assessment has been *prescriptive*, that is, focused on how violence can best be predicted (see Borum 1996; Litwack and Schlesinger 1987; Ferris *et al.* 1997; Monahan 1996; Monahan and Steadman 1994; Otto 1992).

The currently dominant research agenda, which explicitly focuses on identifying specific risk factors for violence in order to better inform clinical assessment (e.g. Monahan and Steadman 1994; Webster *et al.* 1997), extends earlier research that assumed a more implicit, but nonetheless still prescriptive, approach. Many early studies assessed the accuracy of clinicians' decisions by examining how clinicians applied commitment criteria (e.g. Steadman and Cocozza 1974; Thornberry and Jacoby 1979), using involuntary hospitalization decisions as proxy variables for clinicians' judgements of dangerousness (see Litwack and Schlesinger 1999; Mulvey and Lidz 1985). These studies often adopted a 'black box' view of the judgement process, providing no data on the bases for the clinicians' conclusions (Buchanan 1997). More recent studies attempted to identify case variables that were maximally predictive of clinicians' decisions to hospitalize (e.g. McNiel *et al.* 1992; Yesavage *et al.* 1982) and/or judgements that a patient would be violent (e.g. Menzies *et al.* 1982; Segal *et al.* 1988). In addition, a few simulation studies presented clinicians with case vignettes in which particular cues are manipulated to assess their effect on assessments of dangerousness (e.g. Esses and Webster 1988; Jackson 1986, 1988; Slovic and Monahan 1995; Werner *et al.* 1983). Although these studies begin to describe clinical decision making, they are primarily prescriptive in that the universe of potential cues is defined by the researcher (cf. Sweetland 1972, as cited in Monahan 1981). Their results seem to provide more information about the researchers' insight regarding the variables that clinicians *may* or *should* consider in assessing risk than about the cues that clinicians actually perceive as salient in particular cases. Moreover, the statistical models produced in these studies typically explain little of the variance in clinicians' judgements, indicating that 'the

---

[4] Some investigators have surveyed clinicians about how they render decisions (see Jackson 1989; Mulvey and Lidz, 1985). However, the factors that clinicians describe as strongly related to dangerousness typically fail to powerfully predict their judgements about dangerousness. This may be because individuals often have difficulty describing the bases for their judgements and mental processes (Nisbett and Wilson 1977). For this reason, we recommend systematic observational strategies for describing how clinicians assess risk.

decisions rendered [by clinicians] ... are by no means purely mechanical' (Menzies *et al.* 1982).

Oftentimes this research is based on the cue utilization model (see Grisso 1981), a model of clinical judgement with limited capacity for capturing the nuances of human decision making and contemporary clinical practice. This model frames the task of predicting dangerousness as a clinical exercise in developing and applying a maximally predictive, context-free algorithm for combining individually based risk factors. However, a large body of research on clinical judgement indicates that clinicians are not 'consistent, cue-utilizing, rational problem solvers' (Mulvey and Lidz 1995; see also Meehl 1954; Turk and Salovy 1988). Instead, clinicians are likely to assess risk in a more insightful manner, guided by cognitive heuristics and experience-based knowledge structures, such as prototypes, schemas and scripts (see Borum *et al.* 1993; Garb 1998; Fiske 1993; Genero and Cantor 1987; Melton *et al.* 1997; Schneider 1991). Specifically, clinicians may be less likely to mechanistically gather data about a predetermined set of predictor variables (e.g. age, gender, violence history, substance dependence), then mathematically combine that data to arrive at a judgement about violence risk. They may be more likely to assess basic risk factors that they believe are critical in most cases (e.g. age, gender, violence history) and risk factors they believe are important to the specific case (e.g. compliance with treatment; command hallucinations). They might then, for example, intuitively compare the extent to which the MDO's characteristics matched those of their prototypes of violent offenders (see Litwack and Schlesinger 1987). As the number of features that the MDO shared with their prototype of a violent offender (e.g. an acutely psychotic violent offender) increased, so would the likelihood that the MDO would be deemed potentially violent. In order to be deemed potentially violent, the MDO would not have to share all of the prototype's characteristics, or even a predetermined subset thereof. Instead, his characteristics would be intuitively weighted and combined to arrive at a scaled judgement about his degree of fit with the violent prototype (for reviews, see Hampton 1993; MacLaury 1991; Rosch 1977; Way 1997).

These ideas are, of course, speculative, and would require systematic research to verify. To describe the nature of clinicians' decisional process, investigators might extrapolate methods from cognitive research for eliciting, coding and testing clinicians' violence prototypes, narratives, or 'vignettes' (see Ericsson and Simon 1984; Pennington and Hastie 1992; Smith 1991). The closest approximation to research of this nature was conducted by Mulvey and Lidz (1995), who assigned observers to record nearly verbatim transcripts of 410 interviews by clinicians of patients and their families in a psychiatric emergency room. These transcripts were coded and entered into a database, as were clinicians' judgements about the likelihood of patients' future violence. Qualitative analyses revealed that clinicians developed contextualized judgements about violence that were guided by implicit scripts about how a patient's violence would unfold and the conditions that would be present when it occurred:

Clinicians' predictions about the occurrence of violence are based upon an assessment of what particular type of violence the patient might commit and the circumstances under which it will be done. Clinicians do not generally view a patient as either being 'dangerous' or 'not dangerous', but instead see a patient as possibly doing some type of act (e.g. beating his mother) if certain situations either persist or present themselves (e.g. his mother keeps living with her present boyfriend) (Mulvey and Lidz 1995).

Subsequent research that elicited clinicians' judgements using this conditional model indicated that clinicians may be differentially effective in their assessments of future violence, depending on the conditions that they believe are related to violence (Mulvey and Lidz 1998; Skeem *et al.* 1999).

Further research is needed to determine the nature, variability and effect of clinicians' experience-based knowledge structures, including their narratives for violence and prototypes of violent offenders. Research of this nature may generate two critical payoffs. First, if the complexity and contextual nature of clinicians' decision-making processes can be fully 'built in' to tests of predictive accuracy, we may discover that clinicians are more accurate than traditionally assumed or more accurate with some types of cases than with others. Second, an understanding of clinical decision making may be a prerequisite for developing effective methods for improving practice in risk assessment. Because knowledge structures such as prototypes and stereotypes are resistant to change, specialized methods have been developed for modifying them to improve decision making and judgement. For example, Smith (1993) found that prototypes of crime categories (e.g. burglary) could be revised, but *only* when they were refuted point-by-point and replaced with the legal definitions for the crimes.[5] Thus, prototypes must be specifically described before they can be modified. Similarly, most methods designed to change stereotypes, including the development of sub-types to replace superordinate categories, assume that the original stereotype has been identified and targeted for change (see Hilton and Von Hippel 1996 for a review).

In summary, there are little existing data on *how* clinicians assess risk and these data only begin to capture the complex task facing clinicians who must monitor the risk of MDOs living in the community. In the absence of clear empirical guidance, a careful consideration of what this task entails seems to be the best strategy for refining both practice and future research.

---

[5] For example, subjects' prototype of burglary involved a person breaking into a dwelling to steal something of value. In order to revise this prototype, subjects had to be specifically informed that, contrary to their conceptions, the law did *not* require that a residence, forced entry, nor theft be involved in burglary. Instead, burglary was defined by statute as entering a building without authority with the intent to commit a felony.

Demands of assessing risk with mentally disordered offenders in the community

Emphasis on risk state

Most research on clinical prediction of future violence is squarely focused on *risk status*, or determining which individuals are at greatest risk for violence. When treating a mentally disordered offender in the community, however, information about risk status is of limited utility. It can help clinicians to identify patients on their caseload who are at higher 'baseline' level of risk, but it provides little guidance for their key task of monitoring and reducing each patient's violence potential. In order to be maximally effective in this latter task, clinicians must go beyond evaluating risk status, which focuses on inter-individual variability in risk, to assessing *risk state*, which focuses on intra-individual variability in violence potential.

Risk state is a patient's propensity to commit a violent act at a given time. It varies based on particular changes in biological, psychological and social variables in the patient's life. For example, individuals with severe mental illness may be more likely to commit violent acts when suffering from *acute* symptoms of psychosis, including delusions and hallucinations (e.g. Link and Stueve, 1994; McNiel 1994; Modestin and Ammann 1996), or perhaps during periods of heavy substance abuse and poor compliance with medication (Swartz *et al.* 1998).[6]

In assessing risk state, rather than risk status, an emphasis is placed on dynamic risk factors that might change over time or be modifiable with treatment. Risk factors may be conceptualized as ranging from static, fixed or unchangeable (e.g. gender, race, history of violence) to dynamic, variable or potentially changeable (e.g. weapon availability, social support) (Heilbrun 1997; see also Kazdin *et al.* 1997; Kraemer *et al.* 1997).[7] Static risk factors describe the MDO's risk *status*, while the combination of static and dynamic factors describes the MDO's risk *state*. For example, a young man

---

[6] This study presents cross-sectional data only. The authors are currently conducting longitudinal research to determine whether there are causal relationships among medication compliance, substance use and violence in civil hospital patients. This will determine whether medication compliance and substance abuse are components of risk status (e.g., patients who tend to be non-compliant with medication and abuse substances are at greater risk for violence), or risk state (e.g. individuals are more likely to become violent when they become non-compliant with medication or increase substance abuse).

[7] Most authors dichotomize static and dynamic, or fixed and variable risk factors. However, risk factors may be placed on a continuum based on the extent to which they are modifiable. For example, fixed risk markers such as race and gender are absolutely unchangeable. Relatively static, but not necessarily fixed risk factors include personality disorders and traits such as psychopathy, age (which changes slowly) and criminal history (which is fixed at a given point in time). Dynamic, or variable risk factors such as substance abuse, stage of mental illness and quality of interpersonal relationships change more quickly or dramatically over time. Conceptualizing the degree of malleability of risk factors may be crucial in planning risk assessment strategies.

with several traits of psychopathy and a history of domestic assault has a relatively high risk status. However, a clinician may intervene to manage risk only when the patient's risk state is acutely elevated, as indicated by increased alcohol consumption and his perception that his wife is attempting to gain more autonomy. Based on knowledge that similar dynamic factors precipitated past violent episodes, the clinician may attempt to reduce short-term risk of violence by intensifying treatment efforts focused on marital and substance abuse issues, warning the patient's wife or facilitating her temporary move to a safe setting, or initiating short-term hospitalization of the patient.

To assess risk state, clinicians must collect and analyze data on changes in a patient's violence potential over time. This process is likely to reveal patterns of causality that can inform treatment and risk management strategies. For example, a patient's primary treatment goals may assume a much different focus if (a) a deterioration in the quality of his interpersonal relationships is followed by an exacerbation of his psychotic symptoms, and then violence; than if (b) an exacerbation of his psychotic symptoms is followed by a deterioration in his relationships, which then leads to violence. Systematic attention to sequences of behaviours and events that precede violence during the course of a patient's treatment provides critical information about when and where to focus ongoing risk assessment and management efforts.

Unfortunately, very little research is available to determine the relative value of emphasizing state versus status in assessing and managing risk with MDOs, primarily because few studies focus on risk state. Two recent studies of risk assessment with civil psychiatric patients (Douglas et al. 1999) and mentally disordered offenders (Strand et al. 1999) suggest that dynamic, state-related risk factors (e.g. 'exposure to destabilizers') assessed by the 'risk management' scale of the 20-item historical/clinical/risk management scheme (HCR-20, Webster et al. 1995, 1997; see below), predict future violence at least as well as static, status-related risk factors assessed by its 'historical' scale (e.g. 'previous violence'). These results must, however, be considered in the light of research which indicates that historical, 'status', risk factors such as criminal history consistently predict violence moderately well (e.g. Bonta et al. 1998) but provides more mixed evidence about the predictive power of dynamic, 'state', risk factors such as symptoms of acute psychosis (see Buchanan 1999). Because there are compelling logical reasons for focusing on risk state in managing MDOs' risk, research is clearly needed to systematically compare the value of 'state' versus 'status' risk assessment approaches, especially with MDOs.

Utility of individualized data and anamnestic methods

Assessing the risk of MDOs in the community calls not only for a shift in focus to risk state and dynamic predictors of violence, but also for a change in the way that clinicians conceptualize the data gathering and interpretation process. Ongoing risk assessment of MDOs requires consideration of more individualized risk factors and more tailored methods of combining data.

In an oft-cited article, Miller and Morris (1988) list three types of risk assessment, including (a) the anamnestic approach, which involves evaluating the pattern of violence evident in the patient's case history and assuming that past aggression will be repeated under similar circumstances, (b) the actuarial approach, which, in practice,[8] involves using empirical data to determine how groups of people with characteristics similar to those of the patient tend to behave and (c) the clinical approach, which involves applying clinical experience, training and intuition about particular types of cases to interpret information and arrive at a professional judgement about the patient's level of risk (for alternative definitions, see Buchanan 1999).

The distinctions among these approaches are not as straightforward as they may seem at first blush. Though conceptually useful in a broad sense, the above typology confounds methods of data *collection* with methods of data *combination* and fails to clearly define different *types* of data. In a cogent analysis, Sawyer (1966) explains that most clinical judgement research, including Meehl's (1954) classic work, fails to distinguish well between these components of the decision-making process. According to Sawyer, methods of data *collection* may be classified as actuarial (i.e. 'mechanical') or clinical, based on whether or not a clinician is involved. Actuarial data are collected via self-report, clerical administration or record gathering. Clinical data range from the common clinical interview to standardized measures that clinicians use to rate symptoms or traits. Methods of data *combination* are classified as actuarial or clinical based on whether or not one applies a fixed set of rules to make a prediction. Data may be combined by applying an actuarial formula or equation that systematically weights variables, or by relying upon clinical knowledge and training to integrate information.

Distinguishing between methods of data collection and data combination reveals crucial shades of grey between Miller and Norris' (1988) and others' seemingly categorical distinctions between 'actuarial' and 'clinical'decision-making techniques. For example, a patient's score on the psychopathy checklist—revised (PCL—R; see below) is a clinical source of data because it is dependent upon a clinician's use of judgement in scoring the items and reflects information gleaned from an interview. Nevertheless, PCL—R scores are easily and effectively used in actuarial models to predict violence (e.g. Salekin *et al.* 1996). Failing to distinguish between methods of data collection and data combination in this example would neglect clinicians' valuable contributions to predictions of violence.

A refined conception of risk assessment involves distinguishing not only among methods of data collection and data combination, but also between data *types*. In the clinical judgement literature, the terms 'clinical' and 'actuarial' are often used interchangeably with 'anamnestic' and 'nomothetic', respectively. Although this practice

---

[8] A truly actuarial approach would involve systematically weighting a set of variables to generate a prediction about the likelihood that a patient would be violent. However, as noted by Melton *et al.* (1997), 'research has not delivered an actuarial equation suitable for clinical application in the area of violence prediction'.

reflects differences in the ways in which clinicians and statisticians typically predict behaviour (see Stouffer 1941), the terms are not truly synonymous. Learning to conduct flexible, individualized interviews in order to assemble a coherent case history is a staple of clinical training, but anamnestic data may also be collected mechanically or 'actuarially' (e.g. by obtaining case records or using computer programs to obtain historical information, see Farrel 1999). In a similar sense, actuarial techniques virtually always produce and rely upon nomothetic, or group-based data. Nevertheless, actuarial rules of data combination could theoretically be applied to anamnestic data (e.g. 'drug use' and 'living with brother' could be built into a prediction equation). Again, the overlap among Miller and Norris' anamnestic, clinical and actuarial approaches is more complex than it seems at first.

For the purposes of this chapter, our approach to this complexity is simply to distinguish between anamnestic (case-based) and nomothetic (group-based) data, mainly to highlight the importance of anamnestic data in assessing risk with MDOs. Mentally disordered offenders are likely to have a history of aggressive or violent behaviour that can be carefully analysed to yield crucial information about the nature and context of their violence, and carefully examining this anamnestic data can be the key to capitalizing on the oft-cited fact that repeated prior violent offences are the 'single most robust predictor of future violence' (Melton *et al.* 1997; Bonta *et al.* 1998).

A nomothetic approach has limited utility in these situations. Group-based data may not provide an adequately rich source for identifying *which* offenders are likely to become violent, and estimating when and how violence may unfold. Because MDOs are a heterogeneous population with varied offences, symptomatology, living situations and mental health and criminal histories (Rice and Harris 1997), the paths toward violent behaviour may differ substantially across individuals, and MDOs with equally serious violence potential may be characterized by markedly different risk factors. For example, a 35-year-old insanity acquittee with a history of assaulting his brother in what he mistakenly believed was a pre-emptive strike, who is suffering from paranoid delusions that are becoming increasingly focused on his room-mate, may be as much at risk for violence as a 13-year-old juvenile gangster with severe conduct disorder who has become increasingly reactive, hostile and threatening toward his mother since she began attempting to curb his truancy and firesetting. Clearly, clinicians must be prepared to identify, monitor, and, if necessary, intervene with both patients' violence potential. A consideration of a patient's risk factors based on nomothetic data (e.g. a history of assault; acute symptoms of psychosis), in conjunction with his individual offence pattern (e.g. past assault on his brother because he believed he was an impostor who intended to invade and use him for 'the organization') and current circumstances (e.g. developing doubts about his room-mate's true identity and motivation for renting with him), will aid clinicians in developing well-reasoned strategies for doing so. Thus, in keeping with Allport (1962), we recommend that the clinician 'come back to the individual' after applying nomothetic generalizations, 'not for the mechanical application of laws ... but for a fuller, supplementary, and more accurate assessment ...'.

Blending methods and data types to assess the mentally disordered offender's risk

As suggested above, our recommended approach to assessing MDOs' risk heavily emphasizes anamnestic *data*. The emphasis does not, however, mean that these data are the only relevant considerations in formulating a sound risk assessment. These data must be collected along with nomothetic data, and then systematically combined.

Clinical judgement is the primary method of data *combination* currently in use, and it will likely remain so in the foreseeable future (Monahan 1997). The challenge for new risk assessment technologies, therefore, is to aid, rather than to replace clinical judgement. Hopefully, any new actuarial tools will aid clinicians in systematizing assessments, thus addressing the well-founded critique that clinical judgements are difficult to challenge because the criteria upon which they are based are implicit (Melton *et al.* 1997; Miller and Morris 1988).[9] Guidelines and methods that help clinicians to 'stay close to the data' clearly articulate the reasoning that links these data to their predictions, and systematically integrated clinically and actuarially collected information will achieve this goal.

There are several ways that clinicians can use nomothetic data to promote an integrated form of clinical assessment. Clinicians may use published studies to identify variables that strongly predict violent behaviour in MDOs (e.g. Bonta *et al.* 1998), and determine the extent to which these variables match the characteristics of the patient being assessed. If available, they may also consider base rates of violence in groups of MDOs with characteristics similar to those of the patient (see Borum 1996 for a review of base rate data and risk assessment tools that provide additional information). They may administer risk assessment tools and risk-relevant measures of psychopathology and personality. As a group, however, these approaches heavily emphasize relatively static, dispositional predictors of violence such as age and psychopathy that aid little in assessing risk state and developing plans for risk management (Rice and Harris 1997). They also fail to incorporate potentially complex, case-specific information that may reduce or exacerbate a patient's violence potential (e.g. the MDO involved in a deteriorating relationship with a psychiatrist whose approach is particularly authoritarian is likely to become non-compliant with medication and, if he begins using alcohol, violently reoffend).

Because of these limitations, anamnestic data must also be gathered and considered.

---

[9] Although clinical judgements are also often criticized as inferior to actuarial formulas, Melton *et al.* (1997) and Litwack and Schlesinger (1999) review data that suggest that the research upon which this is based has underestimated the effectiveness of clinical judgement, which may often be as accurate as actuarial prediction.

A clinician should carefully evaluate the nature, extent, context and meaning of the MDO's past violent or aggressive behaviour. In doing so, the clinician may attempt to reconstruct past violent episodes in order to identify recurrent themes and to develop coherent narratives about violence that involve 'person or situational factors, or person–situation interactions, that inform judgements of risk-level or risk-management strategies' (Melton *et al.* 1997). Specific guidelines for applying this approach follow.

Guidelines for the process of risk assessment with mentally disordered offenders being treated in the community

As is evident from the literature interpreted above, there are unique demands associated with assessing the MDO's risk of violence in the community. This section translates the arguments presented above into more specific, practical points to aid the clinician engaged in this task. These points do not represent profound insights that form a recipe for success, but instead represent commonsensical guidelines that can be used to structure these risk assessments to better address the demands of a difficult clinical situation.

(1) Get the right information

Specifically assess for risk

When treating the MDO in the community, a clinician must *specifically* assess his risk for violence. Mental disorder is related to violence potential, but by poorly understood mechanisms (Mulvey 1994; Taylor 1997). Because violence potential cannot be equated with mental illness, traditional diagnostic assessments are merely the starting point in risk assessment.

Several authors have observed that clinicians may be reluctant to directly ask a patient about his past violence and present risk state because they fear that challenging the patient will risk their own safety (Borum *et al.* 1996; Litwack and Schlesinger 1999; Tardiff 1996) or damage the therapeutic relationship. To accommodate these concerns, initial interviews with MDOs should be carefully conducted in the safest setting available (Borum *et al.* 1996), and in a manner designed to preserve the therapeutic alliance (see Mills *et al.* 1987).[10] Moreover, if a clinician perceives a patient to be so vulnerable to stress that matter-of-fact questioning about violence in a structured setting will elicit aggressive behaviour, appropriate action should be taken to manage his risk state because he will undoubtedly encounter stressors and frustrations of at least equal severity in the community (for a discussion of 'stress interviews', see Borum *et al.* 1996; Litwack and Schlesinger 1999).

---

[10] See Mills *et al.* (1987) for data that indicate that clinicians' fears that fulfilling the Tarasoff 'duty to protect' will damage the therapeutic relationship are often misplaced.

Clearly, direct questioning is essential. As astutely observed by Prins (1988), 'the price that [clinicians] pay for ensuring the liberty of the [MDO] to live safely in the community is that of "eternal vigilance". [Clinicians] must therefore be willing to ask "unthinkable" and "unaskable" questions if they are to engage effectively in this work'. The initial risk assessment will require 'a very thorough probing of all forms of past violence', which may be initiated with specific questions such as 'What is the most violent thing you've ever done? What is the closest you've come to being violent?' (Monahan 1981), or with an exploration of the precipitants of past police visits, arrests or hospitalizations. After the initial assessment, clinicians must question the patient on an ongoing basis about anger, aggression, violence and the case-specific conditions that are most relevant to these issues (e.g. 'How are you getting along with X this week?', 'How tempted have you been to drink this week?'). Monitoring fluctuations in a patient's violence potential as they relate to his life circumstances (e.g. mental state, substance abuse, medication compliance, relationships, living conditions) may also enable a clinician to refine hypotheses about the causes of violence, thereby increasing the validity of risk assessments.

Use all available sources of information

Clinicians should make specific, and, if necessary, repeated efforts to obtain as much information as is reasonably possible regarding a patient's violence potential. The files should be reviewed immediately upon accepting the case to indicate the records that remain to be gathered (Webster and Polvi 1995). Although the process of obtaining and applying consent to release records may be time consuming and the records for particular cases may be voluminous, it is well worth the effort to scan the files for relevant information, check that information for accuracy, search for data to corroborate or refute that data, and attempt to resolve important inconsistencies (Litwack and Schlesinger 1999; Webster 1997; see below). As observed by Monahan (1993; see also Carstensen 1994):

> The only [*Tarasoff*, "duty to protect"] cases in which I have been involved that were, in the words of defense attorneys, "born dead" were those in which the patient had an extensive history of prior violence that was amply documented in reasonably available treatment records, but those records were never requested. In these cases, the clinician has been forced to acknowledge on the witness stand that if he or she had seen the records, preventive action would have been taken

Sometimes, despite diligent efforts to obtain information from several alternative sources during the course of an MDO's treatment, there are unavoidable gaps in a clinician's knowledge about potentially relevant risk factors. When confronted with this situation, clinicians should estimate the importance of the missing information and determine whether there are reasonable proxies for critical components. For example, if a formal assessment of psychopathy is unavailable, a clinician may search available information to analyse the frequency and type of the MDO's offences and any behaviour that suggests (or contradicts) traits of callousness, deceitfulness, impulsivity, lack of remorse, etc. If no reasonable proxies for important missing information exist, and a clinician believes that this seriously compromises his or her ability to assess the MDO's risk, this concern should be carefully documented. In general, clinicians should acknowledge doubts about their risk assessment based upon missing data, and record all efforts to address these by obtaining relevant records and making collateral contacts.

Critical sources of historical data to obtain to assess an MDO's violence potential include: arrest histories or 'rap sheets'; police reports on all prior offences, including victims' statements; psychological evaluations; trial transcripts; presentence investigation reports; and treatment records. These will aid in assessing the frequency, severity, nature and context of past episodes of violence, as well as describe compliance with treatment and the impact of any past interventions on risk state. Given the task of ongoing risk assessment and management, it is also critical to establish and maintain contact with a collateral source of information, preferably someone who has regular contact with the patient and is the most familiar with his behaviour in the community (e.g. a family member or friend). This contact can provide a first-hand account of fluctuations in variables relevant to risk state and information about aggressive episodes.

Patients may be surprisingly forthcoming about their involvement in violence (Monahan 1981). For example, Steadman et al. (1998; see also Mulvey et al. 1996) found that when agency records were used as the sole source of information about violence over a one-year period, 5% of patients in their study had apparently engaged in at least one violent act, compared with 24% when patient self-report was added, and 28% when a collateral informant who knew the patient was added. Although instructive, the conditions under which these data were obtained are not totally analogous to those associated with treating MDOs in the community. Mentally disordered offenders have greater motivation than research participants to minimize or distort their involvement in violence (e.g. to obtain reduced levels of supervision; to maintain a positive image with their therapist). Also, it is arguably easier for research participants to identify whether they have been violent over the past few months than it is for MDOs to recall and reconstruct past episodes of violence in a manner that is detailed, complete and accurate enough to pinpoint conditions for violence to inform effective treatment planning. Because human recall is imperfect and tends to be reconstructed in light of subsequent experience, clinicians should (1) obtain available records on past violent events to aid in reconstructing timelines between critical variables and piecing together violence narratives, and (2) assess risk on an ongoing basis, since information obtained prospectively is more accurate than that obtained retrospectively (see Kazdin et al. 1997; Kraemer et al. 1997).

Use risk-relevant assessment tools

As suggested above, risk for violence cannot be reduced to psychopathology, personality or intelligence. Traditional clinical assessments do not translate neatly into violence potential, in part because violence is the product of complex, reciprocal interactions between individual and situational–environmental variables (see Cervone 1991; Monahan 1981). As a unique construct, it requires specific evaluation.

Over recent years, a few groups of researchers have designed instruments to help structure the collection and the evaluation of relevant data as part of a comprehensive professional risk assessment (Borum 1996) as well as actuarial decision rules for specific populations. A review of these measures exceeds the scope of this chapter, and is available elsewhere (see Borum 1996; Litwack and Schlesinger 1997). In brief, the most thoroughly investigated risk assessment instruments include (1) the violence prediction scheme (Webster *et al.* 1994; see also Quinsey *et al.* 1998), which may be most appropriate for use with MDOs from secure forensic psychiatric settings with established histories of serious violence, given the samples used to develop the actuarial component of the instrument, the violence risk appraisal guide (VRAG), and (2) the 20-item HCR-20 (Webster *et al.* 1995, 1997), which is a more 'broad-band' instrument that explicitly provides for considering risk management issues. Because norms have yet to be developed for the HCR-20, it is most appropriately used as a semi-structured interview. Nevertheless, recent research indicates that, when compared to other risk assessment instruments including the VRAG, the HCR-20 adds incremental validity in predicting violence (Douglas and Webster 1999). Finally, the use of the psychopathy checklist (PCL-R, Hare 1991) should be considered. Although not a risk assessment tool *per se*, the PCL-R and other measures of psychopathy (see Lilienfeld 1998) are robust predictors of violent behaviour (Salekin *et al.* 1995; see also Hart *et al.* 1994) and, in many cases, may yield important data about violence potential (Serin and Amos 1995).

We recommend that clinicians include such measures in their assessments of violence potential for two reasons (see Monahan 1997). First, these measures may be used as semi-structured interviews or checklists to systematize essential areas of inquiry, thereby improving the reliability and validity of risk assessments. Although there are few data available on normative practices in risk assessment, analyses of clinicians' forensic evaluations indicate that their judgements are more reliable, and may be more valid, when they use issue-specific tools such as semi-structured interviews to organize their examinations (e.g. Nicholson and Kugler 1991; Skeem *et al.* 1998). Researchers and clinicians have long used similar tools to improve the reliability and validity of psychiatric diagnoses by structuring data collection and decisional processes (see Luria and Guziec 1981). Second, these measures are specifically tailored to address the correct issue. Normative research on assessments of other psycholegal issues such as competence to stand trial and criminal responsibility indicate that clinicians tend to rely on traditional clinical measures of personality and intelligence (e.g. the WAIS-R;

MMPI-2) much more often than issue-specific tools (Grisso 1987; Heilbrun and Collins 1995; Skeem *et al.* 1998). Instruments designed to measure such clinical constructs should be used to assess risk only when they generate information that is relevant to the patient's violence potential. For example, if a patient's offences appear to be based partially on paranoid delusions about governmental agencies, a clinician may administer a measure of delusions to aid her in specifically defining key dimensions and manifestations of the belief and determining how these change prior to violent episodes (Taylor *et al.* 1994).

(2) Distinguish between risk markers and risk factors

In the discussion above, a distinction was made between a patient's risk status (involving relatively static risk factors) and risk state (involving both static and dynamic risk factors) to demonstrate the utility of focusing on risk state in developing risk monitoring and treatment strategies. To refine these strategies, risk factors may be further distinguished based on the extent to which they are causally linked with violence. Developing and maintaining an intense, specific focus on likely *causal* risk factors for the MDO's violence will optimize the accuracy of risk assessment and the effectiveness of intervention, particularly if those risk factors are dynamic and potentially affected by therapeutic intervention.

Recently, a group of scholars developed a typology of risk factors that is useful for thinking about how a particular variable is related to an outcome (Kazdin *et al.* 1997; Kraemer *et al.* 1997). According to this typology, a *correlate* is a characteristic that is associated in an undefined manner with an outcome (e.g. when stressors are merely shown to co-occur with violent behaviour at a given point in time, inferences about whether stressors caused, or were caused by, violence cannot be drawn). A *risk factor* is a correlate that has been shown to precede an outcome, and comes in two varieties. A *risk marker* is a risk factor that is not known to be causally related to the outcome (e.g. a history of arrest is a risk marker for, but does not cause, subsequent violence). In contrast, a *causal risk factor* is a risk factor that, when modified, results in a change in the likelihood of the outcome (e.g. when an acute exacerbation of psychotic symptoms precedes violent behaviour, and aggression decreases when psychosis is under better control). Although the mechanisms or processes by which causal risk factors operate may be unclear, 'a plausible explanation of the mechanisms through which antecedent and outcome are related' (Kazdin *et al.* 1997) bolsters an argument that the relationship is causal.

Because causal risk factors have the greatest implications for effectively assessing and modifying the MDO's violence potential, developing an understanding of them is a crucial goal in contemporary risk assessment. To identify, understand and best utilize causal risk factors for the reduction of violence, clinicians could usefully address the following questions, adapted from Kazdin *et al.* (1997):

(1) *Is this characteristic, experience, or event a risk factor for violence?* Where does it occur in the timeline of events? Does it precede and increase the likelihood of the MDO's violence?

(2) *If so, do particular dimensions of the risk factor influence the likelihood of violence?* The relationship of risk factors to violence may depend on certain characteristics, including the timing, intensity, or 'dose' of the risk factor itself (e.g. for violence, psychosis may be a risk factor only during acute episodes; psychopathy may be a risk factor only when it exceeds a particular threshold; and alcohol use or poor medication compliance may be risk factors only when they occur in particular 'doses'). Moreover, some risk factors must be disaggregated to identify the facets that contribute most to violence potential (e.g. exposure to others' aggressive behaviour may be the dimension of poverty that best predicts a patient's violence).

(3) *Are there other conditions (e.g. individual characteristics, situations, additional risk factors), that influence the relationship between the risk factor and violence?* The relationship between the risk factor and violence may depend on conditions such as (a) individual characteristics including age (e.g. deviant peer relationships may strongly predict violence during early adolescence, but not adulthood), (b) situations or events such as treatment or institutionalization or (c) other risk factors (e.g. substance abuse may be more strongly related to violence during periods of medication non-compliance).

(4) *Does the risk factor play a causal role in relation to the outcome? If so, is the relationship direct, or might there be intervening steps? If indirect, what other variables or processes mediate or moderate the relationship (Baron and Kenny 1986)?* A clinician may, for example, believe that a patient's drug use is a causal risk factor for violence. After focusing her efforts on monitoring and reducing drug use, the patient's drug use may decline. His violence potential, however, will remain unchanged if drug use was merely a surrogate variable for his attachment to a deviant peer group that repeatedly engages in anti-social and aggressive behaviour.

(5) *If causal, is the risk factor capable of being modified?* As explained above, focusing on risk state and dynamic risk factors may yield the most effective ongoing risk assessment and management strategies. A belief that an offender is or is not amenable to treatment given available resources affects one's estimation of his degree of risk.

While answering these questions, it is important to bear in mind that a causal risk factor is rarely 'the cause' or the necessary and sufficient condition for violence. The risk factor approach presumes that there are multiple causal risk factors and multiple paths toward a given outcome like violence. This complexity must be considered and incorporated in risk assessment.

(3) **Consider history in detail**

As suggested by the nature of the questions posed in the previous section, the causal risk factors for the MDO's violence cannot be identified without carefully analysing his history. By applying the anamnestic approach introduced earlier, a clinician may attempt to identify the conditions under which an individual MDO is likely to react violently.

When there are past violent offences

When the MDO has a history of violence, it can be mined to provide rich information about which factors to focus on when monitoring violence potential. Broadly construed, a history of violence includes acts of battery (e.g. pushing, grabbing, slapping, hitting, kicking, biting, choking), sexual assault and using or threatening someone with a weapon (see Silver *et al.* 1999; Steadman *et al.* 1998). All forms of the MDO's prior violence should be analysed, using reasonably available sources of information, to answer the four questions below.

What happened?

At a basic level, one must determine the facts about what occurred during prior violent incidents (e.g. precipitants; time; location; victim(s); behaviour of MDO, victims and relevant others before, during and after the violence; and consequences, including extent of injury), in order to construct a timeline that specifically describes the sequence of events. It is also crucial to determine what thoughts, emotions and actions characterized the MDO before, during and after each violent event, much as one would for an evaluation of criminal responsibility or insanity (see Golding *et al.* 1999; Melton *et al.* 1997). For example, exploring how the MDO felt while conducting anti-social acts, and how he responded immediately after them (e.g. with remorse, relief, attempts to 'cover up') often yields critical data (Webster 1997). A specific emphasis should be placed on developing an understanding of the MDO's motivation for violence, based on consideration of issues such as victim–offender dynamics, the degree of injury intended, and the meaning attributed to the event (Melton *et al.* 1997; Tardiff 1996). The purpose of this inquiry is to form hypotheses about the individual, situational and interactive factors involved in the MDO's violence by identifying recurrent patterns that occur across events. Factors that repeatedly emerge in the descriptions of violence may then be specifically targeted to identify whether they are 'triggers' for violence that will aid in risk management.

What explains the event? What are the mentally disordered offender's causal risk factors?

Timelines and descriptions of violent events can be transformed into coherent violence narratives if the risk factors that cause them are correctly estimated. In order to do so, clinicians must specifically assess the link between particular risk factors and the MDO's violence. Because individuals may differ in the extent to which particular risk factors are related to violence (Melton *et al.* 1997), it is important to avoid automatically assuming that salient risk factors are causally linked to violence. For example, alcohol consumption is consistently identified in the literature as a risk factor for violence (e.g. Swanson 1993). A clinician familiar with this fact may attribute an alcoholic MDO's violence to drinking because (a) drinking is a highly visible risk factor in his case and (b) he is typically drunk when he becomes violent. This attribution may be in error, however, if the MDO is rarely sober. In this case, drinking may not be a risk factor for, or even a correlate of violence (see above).

In general, clinicians must guard against a range of biases, including 'illusory correlations' between certain variables and violence that stem from selectively attending to confirmatory cases or information (see Borum *et al.* 1993; Garb 1998; Melton *et al.* 1997). Errors in judgement can be reduced by systematically assessing the extent to which particular factors are causally related to violence, using the questions enumerated above. In addition, early impressions should not be reified: as with any case formulation, violence narratives must be open to revision based upon new information.

To refine assessments of violence potential, potentially causal risk factors should be defined as specifically as possible (see Monahan 1981). For example, if an irrational persecutory belief is related to violence, one should carefully analyze the specific content of the delusion and the feelings that it evokes (Juninger 1996; see also Golding *et al.* 1999; Link and Stueve 1994; Wessely *et al.* 1993). Because delusions are complex constructs, available instruments should be used to assess the belief with respect to key dimensions such as degree of conviction, preoccupation and systematization (Taylor *et al.* 1994; see also Appelbaum *et al.* in press; Garety and Hemsley 1994; Harrow et al. 1988; Kendler *et al.* 1983). If substance abuse or poor medication adherence appear related to violence, attempts should be made to specify the specific drugs and extent of (non)use required for violence (i.e. is there a 'dose–response' relationship?). If poor interpersonal relationships are linked with violence, an analysis of the typical victim, amount and quality of contact with him or her and types of long-standing and/or immediate interpersonal behaviour (or perceptions thereof) that precipitate conflict may be in order (see Estroff and Zimmer 1994; Estroff *et al.* 1998). If family, peer group or employment stressors appear related to violence, attempts should be made to determine what themes these stressors share, or how they were appraised by the patient (Monahan 1981).

Are there factors that protect against violence?

To balance one's assessment, protective factors against violence potential should also be identified, based on an analysis of the patient's history. A protective factor may be defined as an antecedent characteristic, event, or experience that substantially decreases the likelihood of violence for a high-risk individual (Kazdin *et al.* 1997). In essence, one should determine whether the MDO has been exposed to high-risk situations (e.g.

when dynamic causal risk factors were at a peak) without becoming violent. The factors that enable restraint in these situations (e.g. perceived social support; anger management techniques) have considerable implications for risk management. Protective factors should be carefully explored if the MDO has had considerable time at risk (e.g. with little supervision) since his last violent incident.

Important protective factors may be gleaned from analysing the MDO's response to treatment or institutionalization. Treatment records and other sources of information may provide relatively detailed information about the effect of specific interventions on the MDO's critical risk factors, and indicate the degree of structure and supervision required to reduce his violence potential. The impact of treatment may be further evaluated by assessing the patient's level of insight about his violence and its causes, and his capacity for using specific coping and preventive strategies or seeking increased treatment during times of stress (Litwack and Schlesinger 1999).

Which historical risk and protective factors are currently in effect?
After forming a coherent narrative of violence that incorporates risk and protective factors, a clinician can estimate the MDO's risk state by applying this knowledge to an assessment of his current and forseeable life circumstances (Monahan 1981). In essence, the clinician must determine which individual and situational risk and protective factors are, or will soon be, in effect. This will probably involve an assessment of the MDO's present symptomatology and mental state (e.g. fantasies about violence; perception of usual target), as well as his current living conditions (e.g. work, social and family circumstances; see below).

When there are no past violent offences

Not all MDOs will have committed violent acts. Although a lack of prior violent offences is a critical piece of data to weigh in assessing risk, it introduces a difficult level of uncertainty to the assessment process. Nevertheless, potential risk factors for violence may be identified in these cases by (a) applying the anamnestic approach outlined above, focusing on events in which the MDO came 'closest' to being violent and (b) using actuarial data on individuals with characteristics similar to those of the MDO to identify strong correlates of their violent acts.

An essential goal of assessment in these cases is to determine whether the MDO has experienced a risk state as high as his present one without incident. If a patient has weathered particular combinations of severe stressors, symptoms, substance abuse or other factors in the past without becoming violent, he may be capable of doing so in the future. When his symptoms, behaviour or circumstances have recently changed, however, it is critical to assess their impact on his coping capacity. If, for example, the MDO begins providing more focused, intense and heated descriptions of arguments with his wife, some reasoned preventive action should be taken, even if he has long endured marital conflict and abused substances without serious incident.

(4) Take context seriously

Clinicians are principally trained to identify, diagnose and treat psychopathology, and they spend the bulk of their professional careers doing so. In combination with the current zeitgeist in 'the decade of the brain' (Cacioppo and Berntson 1992; Gabbard 1992) this renders clinicians particularly likely to conceptualize and assess violence potential as a symptom or trait (Melton *et al.* 1997). However, as implied throughout this chapter, violence is a transactional process which, like most other forms of human behaviour, reflects reciprocal interaction between an individual and his environment (e.g. Cervone 1991; Monahan 1981). Because 'certain people may be dangerous in certain situations' (Mulvey and Lidz 1985), clinicians should be aware of their understandable tendencies to approach violence potential as a 'strictly diagnostic enterprise', and work diligently to determine how pathology, personality and intellect interact with contextual factors to create violence.

Systemic theories provide useful frameworks for organizing this task (see Altman and Rogoff 1987; Bronfenbrenner, 1977, 1999). A clinician may use one of these frameworks to consider reciprocal influences between the MDO and his partners, family members, peers, work environment, neighbourhoods, mental health and criminal justice system and other contexts. Researchers who have investigated some of these contextual influences have found them to be powerful predictors. For example, violent behaviour is more likely among patients who perceive that their significant others treat them in a hostile or aggressive manner (Estroff *et al.* 1994) and among patients who live in aggressive environments and/or impoverished neighbourhoods (Huesmann 1988; Silver *et al.* 1999). Considering such factors may add a valuable dimension to the clinical assessment process.

Considering contextual information not only reveals critical risk and protective factors for violence, but also permits an assessment of the MDO's general opportunity and means for aggression, including the availability of likely targets of violence and access to weapons. When the MDO with a history of assaulting his mother complains that his mother has been attacking and intrusive lately, a clinician's decision about whether and how to intervene may differ if the patient is 'stuck' at home alone with his mother in daily contact, or if he sees her only weekly, when she and her boyfriend visit him at a group home.

To obtain a richer and more accurate assessment of the nature and effect of contextual factors, clinicians may visit and observe the social environment in which the patient usually functions. Home visits can provide crucial first-hand information about the patient's level of functioning; the structure, organization, support and supervision available in the home; and the nature and quality of interactions with important others. This information cannot be meaningfully accessed in the far-removed, controlled setting of the clinician's office.

(5) **Be explicit**

Clinicians should *explicitly* describe their predictions and the data and reasoning that support them (Litwack and Schlesinger, 1999; Webster 1997). Using the processes described above for developing detailed, coherent violence narratives, a clinician should be able to clearly envision the general types of violence that are of greatest concern and the conditions under which they are most likely to occur. These narratives should be translated into specific, probabilistic, conditional predictions of violence because reducing them to 'either/or' judgements provides little or no guidance for monitoring and managing risk state (Litwack and Schlesinger 1999; Webster 1997). Clearly, explaining that 'this patient is moderately likely to become violent over the next month if his mother's health continues to deteriorate, she becomes unable to supervise him, and he discontinues taking olanzapine' is much more useful for disposition and planning than is stating that 'this patient is dangerous'.

The level of specificity with which a clinician should describe foreseen violent acts, however, is less clear, and there are no clear professional standards for communicating risk assessments to provide guidance (see Heilbrun *et al.* 1999; Slovic *et al.* in press). Available research on violence indicates that past violence predicts future violence, but has yet to determine whether specific types of violence predict the same type of violence (Buchanan 1999). When MDOs have clear, circumscribed patterns of prior violence, clinicians may reasonably estimate that one MDO is quite likely under particular circumstances to assault someone, while another is likely to commit a robbery. If clinicians can reasonably depict the violent act that they foresee (e.g. when an MDO has begun struggling with impulses to assault his brother, and has a history of repeatedly doing so), it seems reasonable to do so. It is often not possible to attain such clarity, however. For example, the first occurrence of violence (or of a particular *type* of violence) is much more difficult to predict, especially if the violent act is rare (e.g. bombing a school). In these situations, the clinician may have to settle for more general estimates of the likelihood that the MDO will become violent (e.g. low/medium/high) and the potential seriousness of that violence (e.g. mild/moderate/severe).

In describing predictions, the clinician should provide the data and reasoning that underlie them. Based on the patient's history, a clinician can describe particular risk and protective factors, the way in which they are linked to violence potential, and the extent to which they match the patient's current state and circumstances. This information should be carefully documented in the MDO's clinical record at the initial risk assessment, as should all ongoing efforts to evaluate, monitor and reduce violence potential. At a minimum, clearly documenting and supporting one's prediction reduces exposure to liability (Monahan 1993; Poythress 1990) and may raise consciousness about the factors that bias one's judgements (Mulvey and Lidz 1984; see Borum *et al.* 1993 for a review). Ideally, sequential records that detail the risk assessment and management process as data accrue allow the clinician to iteratively refine and improve the violence narrative.

Clear documentation and explicit reasoning may also promote ethical practice in challenging situations associated with monitoring MDOs in the community. For example, functioning as both therapist and risk assessor could be viewed as a dual role relationship capable of seriously impairing one's objectivity (American Psychological Association (APA) 1992, Sections 1.17, 7.03, 7.05; Committee on Ethical Guidelines for Forensic Psychologists (EGFP) 1992, Section IVD; see also Greenberg and Shuman 1997; Miller 1990). A clinician may underestimate the MDO's risk because they become invested in perceiving progress, attending carefully to data that suggest that the MDO is developing skills to cope with critical stressors, and thereby either fail to elicit or minimize the importance of data that indicate that his risk state remains high. Nevertheless, acting as both therapist and risk assessor is an unavoidable task for clinicians treating MDOs in the community. In such unavoidable situations, ethical codes mandate that psychologists 'be sensitive to' the likely influence that one role relationship will have on the other, and do everything possible to minimize harm (APA 1992; EGFP 1992). For example, according to the *Specialty Guidelines for Forensic Psychologists*:

> When it is necessary to provide both evaluation and treatment services to a party in a legal proceeding (as may be the case in ... small communities), the ... psychologist takes reasonable steps to minimize the potential negative effects of these circumstances on the rights of the party, confidentiality, and the process of treatment and evaluation.

The APA's ethical code recommends that harm be minimized by (a) disclosing the limits of confidentiality and clarifying role expectations with the patient at the initiation of treatment and as changes occur (APA 1992, Section 7.03) and (b) acting only as a fact witness in legal proceedings and refraining from providing opinion testimony (APA 1992, Section 7.05, 1994; Greenberg and Shuman 1997). More generally, to minimize errors in judgement, clinicians must make every effort to give balanced consideration to arguments that both support and legitimately contradict their opinions (Appelbaum and Gutheil 1991; Litwack and Schlesinger 1999; Monahan 1981). They should also periodically seek second opinions from colleagues who are not involved in the MDO's care, particularly when making decisions about changing his level of supervision. In fact, in settings where several clinicians have MDOs on their caseloads, it may be useful to establish regular mechanisms for reviewing cases (e.g. a risk management team that meets weekly for peer supervision). Even with help, however, violence prediction is a difficult task. Thus, when clinicians have reasonable doubts about a prediction, these should be directly acknowledged and addressed proactively in the documentation and handling of the case.

Conclusion

Effectively treating mentally disordered offenders in the community requires competent, ongoing risk assessment. However, an analysis of risk assessment research suggests that the research is limited in its ability to provide sound guidance for clinicians who treat MDOs in this setting. To aid clinicians, we presented a process for system-atically assessing risk that focuses on discerning the MDO's risk state based on the risk factors that explain his past violent behaviour. Because the research on clinical practice is very limited, the extent to which such processes and guidelines are incorporated in current risk assessment, and the areas most in need of improvement, are unknown.

Several years ago, Webster *et al.* (1995) observed that 'the greatest challenge in what remains of the 1990s is to integrate the almost separate worlds of research on the pre-diction of violence and the clinical practice of assessment. At present the two domains scarcely intersect'. Several recent advances suggest that this gap may be narrowing. Investigators are increasingly acknowledging the need to develop actuarial tools that can readily be integrated into practice (e.g. Borum 1996; Elbogen *et al.* 1999; Gardner *et al.* 1996; Webster *et al.* 1995).

Until the gap narrows appreciably, however, both researchers and clinicians face considerable challenges. Researchers must find innovative ways to capture and accom-modate to the realities of clinical practice. Clinicians, meanwhile, must work diligently to improve practice through thoughtful application of what is known, by using com-mon sense and attending to detail. Ultimately, however, improving practice will rest on better understanding existing clinical practices and applying that knowledge systematically.

Acknowledgements

We gratefully acknowledge the helpful comments of Stephen L. Golding PhD, on an earlier draft of this chapter.

References

Allport, G. (1962) The general and the unique in psychological science. *Journal of Personality*, **30**, 405–22.

Altman, I. and Rogoff, B. (1987) World views in psychology: Trait, interactional, organismic and transactional perspectives. In *Handbook of Environmental Psychology* (ed. D. Stokols and I. Altman), pp. 7–40. New York: John Wiley.

APA (1992) Ethical principles of psychologists and code of conduct. *American Psychologist*, **47**(12), 1597–1611.

Andrews, D. A., Bonta, J. and Hoge, R. D. (1990) Classification for effective rehabilitation: Rediscovering psychology. *Criminal Justice and Behavior*, **17**, 19–52.

Appelbaum, P. S. and Gutheil, T. G. (1991) *Clinical handbook of psychiatry and the law* (2nd edn) Baltimore, MD: Williams and Wilkins.

Appelbaum, P., Robbins, P. and Roth, L. (in press) A dimensional approach to delusions: Comparisons across delusion types and diagnoses. *American Journal of Psychiatry*.

Baron, R. M. and Kenny, D. A. (1986) The moderator/mediator variable distinction in social psychological research: Conceptual, strategic and statistical considerations. *Journal of Personality and Social Psychology*, **51**, 1173–82.

Beck, J. C. (1987) The psychotherapist's duty to protect third parties from harm. *Mental and Physical Disability Law Reporter*, **11**, 141–8.

Bonta, J., Law, M. and Hanson, K. (1998) The prediction of criminal and violent recidivism among mentally disordered offenders: A meta-analysis. *Psychological Bulletin*, **123**, 123–42.

Borum, R. (1996) Improving the clinical practice of violence risk assessment: Technology, guidelines and training. *American Psychologist*, **51**, 945–56.

Borum, R., Otto, R. and Golding, S. (1993) Improving clinical judgement and decision making in forensic evaluation. *Journal of Psychiatry and Law*, **21**, 35–76.

Borum, R., Swartz, M. and Swanson, J. (1996) Assessing and managing violence risk in clinical practice. *Journal of Practicing Psychiatry and Behavioral Health*, 205–15.

Bronfenbrenner, U. (1977) Toward an experimental ecology of human development. *American Psychologist*, 32(7), 513–31.

Bronfenbrenner, U. (1999) Environments in developmental perspective: Theoretical and operational models. In *Measuring environment across the life span: Emerging methods and concepts* (ed. S. Friedman and T. Wachs), pp. 3–28. Washington DC: American Psychological Association.

Buchanan, A. (1997) The investigation of acting on delusions as a tool for risk assessment in the mentally disordered. *British Journal of Psychiatry*, **170**, 12–16.

Buchanan, A. (1999) Risk and dangerousness. *Psychological Medicine*, **29**, 465–73.

Burgess, E. (1941) An experiment in the standardization of the case-study method. *Sociometry*, **4**, 329–48.

Cacioppo, J. T. and Berntson, G. G. (1992) Social psychological contributions to the decade of the brain: Doctrine of multilevel analysis. *American Psychologist*, **47**(8), 1019–28.

Cacioppo, J. T. and Berntson, G. G. (1992) The principles of multiple, nonadditive and reciprocal determinism: Implications for social psychological research and levels of analysis. In *The social psychology of mental health: Basic mechanisms and applications* (ed. D. Ruble and P. Costanzo), pp. 328–49. New York: Guilford Press.

Carstensen, P. C. (1994) The evolving duty of mental health professionals to third parties: A doctrinal and institutional examination. *International Journal of Law and Psychiatry*, **17**, 1–42.

Cervone, D. (1999) Bottom-up explanation in personality psychology: The case of cross-situational coherence. In D. Cervone & Y. Shoda (eds.), *The coherence of personality: Social-cognitive bases of consistency, variability, and organization*, pp. 303–41. New York: Guilford Press.

Cocozza, J, Melick, M and Steadman, H. (1978) Trends in violent crime among ex-mental patients. *Criminology*, **16**, 317–34.

EGFP (1992) Specialty guidelines for forensic psychologists. *Law and Human Behavior*, **15**(6), 655–65.

Douglas, D. and Webster, C. (1999). The HCR-20 violence risk assessment scheme: Concurrent validity in a sample of incarcerated offenders. *Criminal Justice and Behavior*, 3–19.

Dvoskin, J. A. and Steadman, H. J. (1994) Using intensive case management to reduce violence by mentally ill persons in the community. *Hospital and Community Psychiatry*, **45**, 679–84.

Elbogen, E., Calkins, C., Tomkins, A. and Scalora, M. (1999) Clinical judgements in violence risk assessment: Availability of the MacArthur risk cues in mental health settings. In *Predicting violence in mental health settings* (Chair S. Hart), Symposium conducted at the Psychology and Law International Conference, Dublin, Ireland.

Ericsson, K. A. and Simon, H. A. (1984) *Protocol analysis: Verbal reports as data.* Cambridge, MA: MIT Press.

Eronen, M., Angermeyer, M. C. and Schulze, B. (1998) The psychiatric epidemiology of violent behaviour. *Social Psychiatry and Psychiatric Epidemiology*, **33**, S13–23.

Esses, V. M. and Webster, C. D. (1988) Physical attractiveness, dangerousness and the Canadian Criminal Code. *Journal of Applied Social Psychology*, **18**, 1017–31.

Estroff, S. E. and Zimmer, C. (1994) Social networks, social support and violence among persons with severe, persistent mental illness. In *Violence and mental disorder: Developments in risk assessment* (ed. J. Monahan and H. J. Steadman), (pp. 259–95). Chicago: University of Chicago Press.

Estroff, S. E., Zimmer, C., Lachicotte, W. S. and Benoit, J. (1994) The influence of social networks and social support on violence by persons with serious mental illness. *Hospital and Community Psychiatry*, **45**(7), 669–79.

Estroff, S. E., Swanson, J. W., Lachicotte, W. S. *et al.* (1998) Risk reconsidered: Targets of violence in the social networks of people with serious psychiatric disorders. *Social Psychiatry and Psychiatric Epidemiology*, **33**(Suppl. 1), S95-S101

Farrel, A. (1999) Development and evaluation of problem frequency scales from Version 3 of the Computerized Assessment System for Psychotherapy Evaluation and Research (CASPER) *Journal of Clinical Psychology*, **55**, 447–64.

Ferris, L. E., Sandercock, J., Hoffman, B. *et al.* (1997) Risk assessments for acute violence to third parties: A review of the literature. *Canadian Journal of Psychiatry*, **42**, 1051–60.

Fiske, S. T. (1993) Social cognition and social perception. *Annual Review of Psychology*, **44**, 155–94.

Foucha versus Louisiana (1992) 504 U.S. 71.

Gabbard, G. O. (1992) Psychodynamic psychiatry in the "decade of the brain.". *American Journal of Psychiatry*, **149**(8), 991–8.

Garb, H. (1998) *Studying the clinician: Judgment research and psychological assessment*. Washington, DC: American Psychological Association.

Gardner, W., Lidz, C. W., Mulvey, E. P. *et al.* (1996) A comparison of actuarial methods for identifying repetitively violent patients with mental illnesses. *Law and Human Behavior*, **20**(1), 5–48.

Garety, P. and Hemsley, M. (1994) Delusions: Investigations into the psychology of delusional reasoning. New York: Oxford Press.

Genero, N. and Cantor, N. (1987) Exemplar prototypes and clinical diagnosis: Toward a cognitive economy. *Journal of Social and Clinical Psychology*, **5**, 59–86.

Golding, S. L., Skeem, J. L., Roesch, R. *et al.* (1998) The assessment of criminal responsibility: Current controversies. In *The handbook of forensic psychology* (ed. A. Hess and I. Weiner), pp. 519–47.

Greenberg, S. A. and Shuman, D. W. (1997) Irreconcilable conflict between therapeutic and forensic roles. *Professional Psychology: Research and Practice*, **28**(1), 50–7.

Grisso, T. (1981) Clinical assessment for legally-relevant decisions: Research recommendations. In *Law and mental health: Major developments and research needs* (ed. S. Shaw and B. Sales), pp. 49–81. Washington, DC: National Institute of Mental Health.

Grisso, T. (1987) The economic and scientific future of forensic psychological assessment. *American Psychologist*, **42**, 831–9.

Hampton, J. (1993) Prototype models of concept representation. In *Categories and concepts: Theoretical views and inductive data analysis* (ed. I. Van Mechelen, J. Hampton, R. Michalski and P. Theuns), pp. 67–95. London, England: Academic Press.

Hare, R. (1991) *The Hare Psychopathy Checklist—revised*. Ontario, Canada: Multi-Health Systems.

Harrow, M., Rattenbury, F. and Stoll, F. (1988) Schizophrenia delusions: An analysis of their persistence, of related premorbid ideas and of three major dimensions. In *Delusional beliefs.* (ed. T. Oltmanns and B. Mahrer), pp. 184–211. New York: John Wiley.

Hart, S., Hare, R., and Forth, A. (1994) Psychopathy as a risk marker for violence: Development and validation of a screening version of the revised Psychopathy Checklist. In J. Monahan and H. Steadman (eds.), *Violence and mental disorder: Developments in risk assessment*, pp. 81–98. Chicago: University of Chicago Press.

Heilbrun, K. (1997) Prediction versus management models relevant to risk assessment: The importance of legal decision-making context. *Law and Human Behavior*, **21**, 347–59.

Heilbrun, K. and Collins, S. (1995) Evaluations of trial competency and mental state at time of offense: Report characteristics. *Professional Psychology: Research and Practice*, **26**, 61–7.

Heilbrun, K., Dvoskin, J., Hart, S. et al. (1999) Violence risk communication: Implications for research, policy and practice. *Health, Risk and Society*, **1**, 91–106.

Heilbrun, K., Philipson, J., Berman, L. et al. (1999) Risk communication: Clinicians' reported approaches and perceived values. *Journal of the American Academy of Psychiatry and the Law*, **27**, 397–406.

Hilton, J. L. and Von Hippel, W. (1996) Stereotypes. *Annual Review of Psychology*, **47**, 237–71.

Huesmann, L. R. (1988) An information processing model for the development of aggression. *Aggressive Behavior*, **14**(1), 13–24.

Jackson, M. W. (1986) Psychiatric decision-making for the courts: Judges, psychiatrists, lay people? *International Journal of Law and Psychiatry*, **9**, 507–20.

Jackson, M. W. (1988) Lay and professional perceptions of dangerousness and other forensic issues. *Canadian Journal of Psychiatry*, **30**, 215–29.

Jackson, M. A. (1989) The clinical assessment and prediction of violent behavior: Toward a scientific analysis. *Criminal Justice and Behavior*, **16**, 114–31.

Juninger, J. (1996) Psychosis and violence: The case for a content analysis of psychotic experience. *Schizophrenia Bulletin*, **22**, 91–103.

Kansas versus Hendricks (1997) No. 95–1649/95–9076 65 U.S.L.W. 4564.

Kazdin, A. E., Kraemer, H. C., Kessler, R. C. et al. (1997) Contributions of risk-factor research to developmental psychopathology. *Clinical Psychology Review*, **17**, 375–406.

Kendler, K. S., Glazer, W. M. and Morgenstern, H. (1983) Dimensions of delusional experience. *American Journal of Psychiatry*, **140**(4), 466–9.

Kiesler, C. and Simkins, C. (1993) *The unnoticed majority in inpatient care*. New York: Plenum.

Kraemer, H. C., Kazdin, A. E., Offord, D. R. et al. (1997) Coming to terms with the terms of risk. *Archives of General Psychiatry*, **54**, 337–43.

Lerman, D. (1981) *Deinstitutionalization: A cross-problem analysis*. Rockville, MD: Department of Health and Human Services.

Lidz, C. W., Mulvey, E. P. and Gardner, W. (1993) The accuracy of predictions of violence to others. *Journal of the American Medical Association*, **269**(8), 1007–11.

Lilienfeld, S. (1998) Methodological advances and developments in the assessment of psychopathy. *Behaviour Research and Therapy*, **36**, 99–125.

Link, B. G. and Stueve, A. (1994) Psychotic symptoms and the violent/illegal behavior of mental patients compared to community controls. In *Violence and mental disorder: Developments in risk assessment* (ed. J. Monahan and H. J. Steadman), pp. 137–59. Chicago: University of Chicago Press.

Litwack, T. R. (1996) "Dangerous" patients: A survey of one forensic facility and review of the issue. *Aggression and Violent Behavior*, **1**(2), 97–122.

Litwack, T. R. and Schlesinger, L. B. (1987) Assessing and predicting violence: Research, law and applications. In *Handbook of forensic psychology* (ed. I. Weiner and A. Hess), pp. 205–57) New York: John Wiley.

Litwack, T. R. and Schlesinger, L. B. (1999) Dangerousness risk assessments: Research, legal and clinical considerations. In *Handbook of forensic psychology* (ed. A. Hess and I. Weiner), pp. 171–217. New York: John Wiley.

Luria, R. and Guziec, R. (1981) Comparative descriptions of the SADS and PSE. *Schizophrenia Bulletin*, **7**, 248–57.

MacLaury, R. (1991) Prototypes revisited. *Annual Review of Anthropology*, **20**, 55–74.

McNiel, D. E. (1994) Hallucinations and violence. In *Violence and mental disorder: developments in risk assessment* (ed. J. Monahan and H. J. Steadman), pp. 183–202. Chicago: University of Chicago Press.

McNiel, D. E., Myers, R. S., Zeiner, H. K. *et al.* (1992) The role of violence in decisions about hospitalization from the psychiatric emergency room. *American Journal of Psychiatry*, **149**, 207–12.

Meehl, P. E. (1954) *Clinical vs. statistical prediction: a theoretical analysis and a review of the evidence.* Minneapolis: University of Minnesota Press.

Melton, G. B., Petrila, J., Poythress, N. G. and Slobogin, C. (1997) *Psychological evaluations for the courts: A handbook for mental health professionals and lawyers* (2nd edn). New York: Guilford Press.

Menzies, R. and Webster, C. D. (1995) Construction and validation of risk assessments in a six-year follow-up of forensic patients: A tridimensional analysis. *Journal of Consulting and Clinical Psychology*, **63**, 766–78.

Menzies, R. J., Jackson, M. A. and Glasberg, R. E. (1982) The nature and consequences of forensic psychiatric decision-making. *Canadian Journal of Psychiatry*, **27**, 463–70.

Miller, M. and Morris, N. (1988) Predictions of dangerousness: An argument for limited use. *Violence and Victims*, **3**, 263–73.

Miller, R. D. (1990) Ethical issues involved in the dual role of treater and evaluator. In *Ethical practice in psychiatry and law* (ed. R. Rosner and R. Weinstock), pp. 129–50. New York: Plenum Press.

Mills, M. J., Sullivan, G. and Eth, S. (1987) Protecting third parties: A decade after Tarasoff. *American Journal of Psychiatry*, **144**, 68–74.

Modestin, J. and Ammann, R. (1996) Mental disorder and criminality: Male schizophrenia. *Schizophrenia Bulletin*, **22**, 69–82.

Monahan, J. (1981) *The prediction of violence behavior: An assessment of clinical techniques.* Beverly Hills, CA: Sage.

Monahan, J. (1992*a*) Mental disorder and violent behavior: Perceptions and evidence. *American Psychologist*, **47**, 511–21.

Monahan, J. (1992*b*) "A terror to their neighbors": Beliefs about mental disorder and violence in historical and cultural perspective. *Bulletin of the American Academy of Psychiatry and the Law*, **20**, 191–5.

Monahan, J. (1993) Limiting therapist exposure to Tarasoff liability: Guidelines for risk containment. *American Psychologist*, **48**, 242–50.

Monahan, J. (1996) Violence prediction: The past twenty and the next twenty years. *Criminal Justice and Behavior*, **23**, 107–20

Monahan, J. (1997) Actuarial support for the clinical assessment of risk. *International Review of Psychiatry*, **9**, 167–9.

Monahan, J. and Steadman, H. J. (1994) Toward a rejuvenation of risk assessment research. In *Violence and mental disorder: Developments in risk assessment* (ed. J. Monahan and H. J. Steadman), pp. 1–17. Chicago: University of Illinois Press.

Monahan, J. and Steadman, H. J.E. (1994) *Violence and mental disorder: Developments in risk assessment.* Chicago: University of Illinois Press.

Mossman, D. (1994) Assessing predictions of violence: Being accurate about accuracy. *Journal of Consulting and Clinical Psychology*, **62**, 783–92.

Mulvey, E. P. (1994) Assessing the evidence of a link between mental illness and violence. *Hospital and Community Psychiatry*, **45**, 663–8.

Mulvey, E. P. and Lidz, C. W. (1984) Clinical considerations in the prediction of dangerousness in mental patients. *Clinical Psychology Review*, **4**(4), 379–401.

Mulvey, E. P. and Lidz, C. W. (1985) Back to basics: A critical analysis of dangerousness research in a new legal environment. *Law and Human Behavior*, **9**, 209–19.

Mulvey, E. P. and Lidz, C. W. (1993) Measuring patient violence in dangerousness research. *Law and Human Behavior*, **17**, 277–88.

Mulvey, E. P. and Lidz, C. W. (1995) Conditional prediction: A model for research on dangerousness to others in a new era. *International Journal of Law and Psychiatry*, **18**, 129–43.

Mulvey, E. and Lidz, C. (1998) Clinical prediction of violence as a conditional judgement. *Social Psychiatry and Psychiatric Epidemiology*, **33**, S107–113.

Mulvey, E., Shaw, E. and Lidz, C. (1996) Why use multiple sources in research on patient violence in the community? *Criminal Behaviour and Mental Health*, **4**, 253–8.

Mulvey, E. P., Geller, J. L. and Roth, L. H. (1987) The promise and peril of involuntary outpatient commitment. *American Psychologist*, **42**, 571–84.

Nicholson, R. A. and Kugler, K. E. (1991) Competent and incompetent criminal defendants: A quantitative review of comparative research. *Psychological Bulletin*, **109**, 355–70.

Nisbett, R. E. and Wilson, T. D. (1977) Telling more than we can know: Verbal reports on mental processes. *Psychological Review*, **84**(3), 231–29.

Otto, R. K. (1992) Prediction of dangerous behavior: A review and analysis of "second-generation" research. *Forensic Reports*, **5**, 103–33.

Otto, R. K. (1994) On the ability of mental health professionals to "predict dangerousness": A commentary on interpretations of the "dangerousness" literature. *Law and Psychology Review*, **18**(43), 68.

Parry, J. W. (1994) Involuntary civil commitment in the 90s: A constitutional perspective. *Mental and Physical Disability Law Reporter*, **18**, 320–36.

Pennington, N. and Hastie, R. (1992) Explaining the evidence: Tests of the Story Model for juror decision making. *Journal of Personality and Social Psychology*, **62**, 189–206.

Petrila, J. (1995) Who will pay for involuntary civil commitment under capitated managed care? An emerging dilemma. *Psychiatric Services*, **46**, 1045–48.

Pflafflin, F. (1979) The contempt of psychiatric experts for sexual convicts: Evaluation of 936 files from sexual offence cases at courts in the state of Hamburg, Germany. *International Journal of Law and Psychiatry*, **2**, 485–97.

Pfohl, S. (1978) *Predicting dangerousness.* Lexington, MA: Lexington Books/Health.

Poythress, N. G. (1990) Avoiding negligent release: Contemporary clinical and risk management strategies. *American Journal of Psychiatry*, **147**(8), 994–7.

Prins, H. (1988) Dangerous clients: Further observations on the limitation of mayhem. *British Journal of Social Work*, **18**, 593–609.

Quinsey, V. L., Harris, G. T., Rice, M. E. *et al.* (1998) *Violent offenders: Appraising and managing risk.* Washington, DC: American Psychological Association.

Regier, D. A., Narrow, W. E., Rae, D. S. *et al.* (1993) The de facto US mental and addictive disorders service system: Epidemiologic Catchment Area prospective 1-year prevalence rates of disorders and services. *Archives of General Psychiatry*, **50**, 85–94.

Rice, M. and Harris, G. (1995) Violent recidivism: Assessing predictive validity. *Journal of Consulting and Clinical Psychology*, **63**, 737–748.

Rice, M. E. and Harris, G. T. (1997) The treatment of mentally disordered offenders. *Psychology, Public Policy and Law*, **3**, 126–83.

Rosch, E. (1977) Human categorization. In *Studies in cross-cultural psychology* (ed. N. Warren), pp. 3–49. London: Academic.

Salekin, R. T., Rogers, R. and Sewell, K. W. (1995) A review and meta-analysis of the Psychopathy Checklist and Psychopathy Checklist—revised: Predictive validity of dangerousness. *Clinical Psychology: Science and Practice*, **3**, 203–15.

Sawyer, J. (1966) Measurement *and* prediction: Clinical *and* statistical. *Psychological Bulletin*, **66**, 178–200.

Schneider, D. J. (1991) Social cognition. *Annual Review of Psychology*, **42**, 527–61.

Segal, S. P., Watson, M. A., Goldfinger, S. M. *et al.* (1988) Civil commitment in the psychiatric emergency room: I. The assessment of dangerousness by emergency room clinicians. *Archives of General Psychiatry*, **45**, 748–52.

Serin, R. C. and Amos, N. L. (1995) The role of psychopathy in the assessment of dangerousness. *International Journal of Law and Psychiatry*, **18**, 231–8.

Shelton versus Tucker (1960) 364 U.S. 479.

Silver, E., Mulvey, E. P. and Monahan, J. (1999) Assessing violence risk among discharged psychiatric patients: Toward an ecological approach. *Law and Human Behavior*, **23**(2), 237–255.

Skeem, J. L., Golding, S. L., Berge, G. *et al.* (1998) Logic and reliability of evaluations of competence to stand trial. *Law and Human Behavior*, **22**, 519–47.

Skeem, J., Mulvey, E. and Lidz, C. (1999) Building clinicians' decisional models into tests of predictive validity: The accuracy of conditional predictions of violence (submitted for publication).

Slobogin, C. (1994) Involuntary community treatment of people who are violent and mentally ill: A legal analysis. *Hospital and Community Psychiatry*, **45**, 685–9.

Slovic, P. and Monahan, J. (1995) Probability, danger and coercion: A study of risk perception and decision making in mental health law. *Law and Human Behavior*, **19**, 49–65.

Slovic, P., Monahan, J. and MacGregor, D. (in press) Violence risk assessment and risk communication: The effects of using actual cases, providing instruction and employing probability versus frequency formats. *Law and Human Behavior*.

Smith, V. L. (1991) Prototypes in the courtroom: Lay representations of legal concepts. *Journal of Personality and Social Psychology*, **61**, 857–72.

Smith, V. L. (1993) When prior knowledge and law collide: Helping jurors use the law. *Law and Human Behavior*, **17**, 507–36.

Steadman, H. J. and Cocozza, J. J. (1974) *Careers of the criminally insane: Excessive social control of deviance*. Lexington, MA: DC Health.

Steadman, H. J., Mulvey, E. P., Monahan, J. *et al.* (1998) Violence by people discharged from acute psychiatric inpatient facilities and by others in the same neighborhoods. *Archives of General Psychiatry*, **55**, 393–401.

Stouffer, S. (1941) Notes on the case-study and the unique case. *Sociometry*, **4**, 349–57.

Strand, S., Belfrage, H., Fransson, G. *et al.* (1999) Clinical and risk management factors in risk prediction of mentally disordered offenders—more important than historical data? *Legal and Criminological Psychology*, **4**, 67–76.

Swanson, J. W. (1993) Alcohol abuse, mental disorder and violent behavior: An epidemiologic inquiry. *Alcohol Health and Research World*, **17**, 123–32.

Swartz, M. S., Swanson, J. W., Hiday, V. A. *et al.* (1998) Violence and severe mental illness: The effects of substance abuse and nonadherence to medication. *American Journal of Psychiatry*, **155**, 226–31.

Tarasoff versus Regents of the University of California (1976) 551 P 2d. 334.

Tardiff, K. (1996) Concise guide to assessment and management of violent patients (2nd edn). Washington, DC: American Psychiatric Press.

Taylor, P. J. (1997) Mental disorder and risk of violence. *International Review of Psychiatry*, **9,** 157–61.

Taylor, P. J., Garety, P., Buchanan, A. *et al.* (1994) Delusions and violence. In *Violence and mental disorder: developments in risk assessment* (ed. J. Monahan and H. J. Steadman), pp. 161–82. Chicago: University of Illinois Press.

Teplin, L. (1984) Criminalizing mental disorder: The comparative arrest rate of the mentally ill. *American Psychologist*, **39,** 794–803.

Thornberry, T. and Jacoby, J. (1979) *The criminally insane: A community followup of mentally ill offenders.* Chicago: University of Chicago Press.

Truscott, D., Evans, J. and Mansell, S. (1995) Outpatient psychotherapy with dangerous clients: A model for clinical decision making. *Professional Psychology: Research and Practice*, **26,** 484–90.

Turk, D. C.E. and Salovey, P. E. (1988) *Reasoning, inference and judgement in clinical psychology.* New York: Free Press.

Wallin, P. (1941) The prediction of individual behavior from case studies. In *The prediction of personal adjustment* (ed. P. Horst). New York: Social Science Research Council.

Way, E. (1997) Connectionism and conceptual structure. *American Behavioral Scientist*, **40,** 729–53.

Webster, C. D. (1997) A guide for conducting risk assessments. In *Impulsivity: theory, assessment and treatment* (ed. C. D. Webster and M. A. Jackson), pp. 251–77). New York: Guilford Press.

Webster, C. D. and Polvi, N. (1995) Challenging assessments of dangerousness and risk. In *Coping with psychiatric and psychological testimony* (ed. J. Ziskin), pp. 221–240). Marina del Rey, CA: Law and Psychology Press.

Webster, C. D., Harris, G. T., Rice, M. E., Cormier, C. and Quinsey, V. L. (1994) *The violence prediction scheme: assessing dangerousness in high risk men.* Toronto, Canada: University of Toronto Centre of Criminology.

Webster, C. D., Eaves, D., Douglas, K. S. and Wintrup, A. (1995) *The HCR-20 Scheme: the assessment of dangerousness and risk.* Simon Fraser University and Forensic Psychiatric Services Commission of British Columbia.

Webster, C. D., Douglas, K. S., Eaves, D. and Hart, S. D. (1997) Assessing risk of violence to others. In *Impulsivity: Theory, assessment and treatment* (ed. C. D. Webster and M. A. Jackson), pp. 251–77). New York: Guilford Press.

Werner, P. D., Rose, T. L. and Yesavage, J. A. (1983) Reliability, accuracy and decision-making strategy in clinical predictions of imminent dangerousness. *Journal of Consulting and Clinical Psychology*, **51,** 815–25.

Wessely, S., Buchanan, A., Reed, A. *et al.* (1993) Acting on delusions: I. Prevalence. *British Journal of Psychiatry*, **163,** 69–76.

Yesavage, J. A., Werner, P. D., Becker, J. M. *et al.* (1982) The context of involuntary commitment on the basis of danger to others: A study of the use of the California 14-day certificate. *Journal of Nervous and Mental Disease*, **170,** 622–7.

Chapter 7

Drug treatment, compliance and risk

Michael J. Travis

Introduction

Schizophrenia, and related disorders, are linked to an increased risk of committing violent criminal offences. As the core symptoms of these illnesses can be relieved by appropriate treatment in the majority of cases it is tempting to suggest that they represent a major preventable cause of violent offending behaviour.

Diagnostically, mentally disordered offenders present a relatively heterogenous group depending on the population studied, for instance in special hospitals in the UK in the first half of 1993, 47% of patients suffered from schizophrenia (mostly paranoid subtype) and a further 6% suffered from either schizoaffective or delusional disorder. Thirty per cent of this total cohort had a primary personality disorder (authors' figures) and less than 4% suffered with a neurotic disorder (Taylor et al. 1998).

There is a growing consensus in the literature that there is an association between psychotic disorders and offending behaviour (Taylor and Gunn 1984; Swanson et al. 1990; Hodgins 1992; Coid 1996). Offending behaviour in this group is often preceded by the onset of psychotic symptoms (Taylor and Hodgins 1994) and the risk of violence is significantly increased by comorbid substance misuse and dependence (Swanson et al. 1990; Taylor et al. 1998), a finding which compliments recent work on the increased risk of relapse in 'dual diagnosis' patients (Swofford et al. 1996).

In this chapter we briefly review the literature on the relationship between psychosis, particularly schizophrenia, and offending behaviour focusing on violence. We will further consider factors which increase the risk of offending such as active symptoms and comorbid substance misuse. The primary role of medication in the acute treatment of schizophrenia and, more particularly, the maintenance phase of treatment will be reviewed. It is clear that compliance with treatment is sometimes essential to the prevention of relapse, therefore the notion of compliance and specific issues with relation to mentally disordered offenders will be discussed.

The last 10 years has seen a resurgence in optimism in the treatment of schizophrenia, mainly due to the advent of these drugs. The pharmacology, impact and potential utility of these drugs to address some of the problems posed by the mentally disordered offender will be addressed. The chapter will focus on the use of anti-psychotic medication, particularly the newer anti-psychotics, in the treatment of schizophrenia and related psychotic disorders with particular emphasis on the specific issues raised in the care of mentally disordered offenders with schizophrenia. Interventions designed to decrease the risk of relapse and therefore the risk of offending behaviour will be reviewed.

Psychosis and risk of violence

For some time there has been a debate on the relationship between mental disorder and offending behaviour, particularly violent behaviour. The public, legal systems and most mental health professionals would acknowledge a clear link between risk of harm and active psychotic symptoms whereas most social science researchers and criminologists would seem to deny a causal link. Nevertheless there is now a substantial literature indicating a statistical association between psychiatric illness, particularly psychotic illnesses, and violent behaviour.

In studies of prison inmates it is estimated that a diagnosis of schizophrenia increases the risk of committing a homicide by about three- to eight-fold (reviewed in Eronen *et al.* 1998). Similar increases in risk are not seen for non-psychotic disorders. In studies of hospital in-patients carried out in a variety of countries, patients with schizophrenia or related disorders were three to seven times more likely to have committed violent offences than matched non-psychiatric cohorts (Lindqvist and Allbeck 1990; Tiihonen *et al.* 1997; Hodgins *et al.* 1996), or indeed matched hospital populations (Wessely *et al.* 1994).

In community studies, which avoid some of the selection bias derived from studying populations in contact with services, rates of violence are consistently higher in patients with serious mental illness. In the epidemiological catchment area (ECA) study, Swanson *et al.* (1990) found that the presence of schizophrenia or major affective disorder was associated with a nearly four-fold increase in the chances of violence in one year, with most of this increased risk being attributable to those with a diagnosis of schizophrenia. Similar studies have been carried out in the Washington Heights area of New York (Link *et al.* 1992), where psychiatric patients as a whole had 2–3 times the rates of violent behaviour; and in Israel (Stueve and Link 1997), where it was noted that patients diagnosed with psychosis of any type were over three times more likely to engage in violent behaviour than either the non-psychotic psychiatric disorder or general populations.

It is salutary to note that in the studies whose results are quoted above, substance misuse had an additive effect in increasing the risk of violence. This will be considered further below.

Psychotic symptoms and risk of violence

In attempting to understand how effective intervention may limit violent offending by people with psychosis it is necessary to consider the evidence linking psychotic symptoms with offending behaviour. A number of studies have highlighted that a particular form of delusional thinking may predict violence. 'Threat control-over-ride' symptoms (Link and Stueve 1994) involve an over-riding of one's internal cognitive controls or the perceived threat of harm from others. When a patient experiences passivity phenomena or perceives others' actions as being a threat, violence may be seen as an understandable response. Link and Stueve (1994) found a significant association between these symptoms and violent behaviour and found no such relationship between violence and other psychotic symptoms. Swanson et al. (1996), using the ECA data, noted that this cluster of symptoms predicted a two-fold increase in the likelihood of violent behaviour in comparison with the risk consequent upon other psychotic symptoms, and a five-fold risk in comparison with those with no psychiatric history. These findings are indirectly supported by other studies which found that paranoid ideation and hostility predicted violence (McNiel and Binder 1994; Mulvey and Lidz 1998) and that violence was more common in the acute phase of schizophrenia (Steadman et al. 1998; Modestin and Ammann 1996).

These findings are at odds with a study by Estroff et al. (1994), focusing on psychiatric in-patients. Estroff and colleagues found that psychotic symptoms and 'threat/control-override' symptoms in particular predicted a lower rate of violence and that social withdrawal and small social networks were associated with violence. In a reanalysis and reappraisal of this data Swanson et al. (1997) have argued that 'perceived threat' per se did predict violence. They argued also that there was a curvilinear relationship between psychotic symptoms and violence and that as patients become more unwell they are less likely to be able to plan and execute violent acts.

This latter finding suggests that patients with psychosis my be at more risk of violent offending during the process of a psychotic relapse, perhaps quite early in relapse, rather than when they have fully relapsed. Thus factors which influence outcome and relapse in schizophrenia should be explored.

Comorbid substance misuse, psychosis and risk

The relationship between substance misuse and schizophrenia is complex. Many drugs of abuse, such as ketamine, amphetamine and lysergic acid diethylamide (LSD) are psychotomimetic and care must be taken to avoid the misdiagnosis of a drug-induced psychosis as schizophrenia. Psychoactive substance misuse both precedes and follows the onset of psychotic symptoms. Substantiation that sub-groups of patients receive transient symptom reduction from some abused drugs further complicates this picture, and it may well be that some patients are 'self medicating' with drugs of abuse (Dixon et al. 1991).

It is estimated that 20–47% of the population with schizophrenia may qualify as 'dual-diagnosis' patients (Barbee *et al.* 1989; Regier *et al.* 1990). Such patients have a higher use of services and worse outcome than patients who are not abusers (Lehman *et al.* 1993). Swofford *et al.* (1996) reported that during an anti-psychotic dose reduction study substance abusers were twice as likely to be hospitalized and had four times as many relapses as the non-user group during the two-year follow-up period. It is interesting to note that patients with schizophrenia seem to suffer significant harm at lower levels of substance use (Drake and Wallach 1993). In a recent study of substance misuse in schizophrenic patients in Camberwell, of the 'dual–diagnosis' patients 20.5% had alcohol problems only, 4.7% had drug problems only and 11.1% had drug and alcohol problems. In this sample men were 2–3 times more likely to abuse substance than women and there was no difference between white and black patients. All of the 'dual-diagnosis' patients had increased lengths of admission to hospital (Menezes *et al.* 1996).

Thus in the general population of patients with schizophrenia comorbid substance misuse predicts a worse outcome in terms of relapse and admissions and we have already seen that psychotic symptoms appear to drive much of the violence seen in psychotic disorders. It is not surprising to note, therefore, that there is a marked additive effect for psychosis and substance misuse in terms of predicting violence and offending behaviour. In a recent community survey in the UK, 'dual-diagnosis' patients were over four times more likely than patients with psychosis alone to commit any criminal offence, three times more likely to be reported as being aggressive and eight times more likely to feel hostile (Scott *et al.* 1998). Swanson *et al.* (1997) note an increase in risk from over three-fold to almost 10-fold for mentally disordered patients with comorbid alcohol abuse. Similarly in a study of patients who had committed homicide, Eronen *et al.* (1996) reported a risk of homicide for patients with schizophrenia of seven times the average. For patients with comorbid alcoholism this risk increased to 17 times. It is interesting to note that in the Swanson study the risk with alcohol alone was about seven times the average and in the Eronin study the risk was about ten times the average. Thus the increased risk of comorbidity is additive rather than synergistic.

These data are reinforced by a recent prospective trial of 'involuntary out-patient commitment' for patients with serious mental illness. Swartz *et al.* (1998) report that in their sample of 331 patients, the majority suffering from schizophrenia, substance misuse alone increased the risk of violence two-fold with an additive effect for non-compliance with anti-psychotic medication. Thus even in 'dual-diagnosis' patients adequate treatment may reduce the risk of violence.

Maintenance drug treatment in schizophrenia

Given the evidence quoted above, it is logical to suggest that with effective amelioration of psychotic symptoms and prevention of relapse the risk of offending will be reduced. There is good evidence to suggest that conventional anti-psychotics are effective for both of these aims

Pharmacotherapy for acute schizophrenia

The fortuitous discovery of chlorpromazine in the early 1950s heralded an era of effective pharmacological treatment for schizophrenia. Since the initial 1952 report of reduction in agitation, aggression and delusional states in schizophrenic patients there has been a wealth of placebo-controlled trials establishing the efficacy of neuroleptic anti-psychotic medication for acute schizophrenia. The best known large-scale clinical trial which gives a good idea of the effect size to be expected was carried out by The National Institute of Mental Health in the USA (1964). This study involved four treatment groups (chlorpromazine, thioridazine, fluphenazine and placebo) with 90 randomly allocated subjects in each. The subjects were treated for six weeks and rated on 14 different symptoms in addition to global clinical improvement. In this study 75% of subjects in the chlorpromazine-, thioridazine-, and fluphenazine-treated groups showed significant improvement, 5% failed to be helped and 2% worsened. In the placebo group only 25% of patients showed significant improvement and over 50% were unchanged or worse. A reanalysis of these results indicated improvements occurred in the active drug-treated groups across all 14 symptom areas, including positive and negative symptoms (Goldberg *et al.* 1965), although there was no difference between the active drugs.

Davis and Andriukaitis (1986) performed a meta-analysis using the trials involving chlorpromazine and investigated the relationship between dose and clinical effect. They noted that a threshold of 400 mg of chlorpromazine is required. This was based on the fact that in 31 trials using a dose of 400 mg of chlorpromazine per day or greater only 1 had failed to show that chlorpromazine was more effective than the reference treatment; whereas in the 31 trials using a dose less than 400 mg of chlorpromazine, 19 had failed to show a significant effect.

Pharmacotherapy as maintenance treatment in schizophrenia

Although it is widely accepted that anti-psychotic medication is the mainstay of treatment in acute schizophrenia its role in long-term maintenance has been more contentious. Nevertheless the importance of maintenance drug therapy in the treatment of chronic schizophrenia has been evident since the early 1960s.

Initial studies indicated that between half and two-thirds of patients with schizophrenia who were stable on medication relapsed following cessation of maintenance pharmacological therapy compared with between 5 and 30% of the patients maintained on medication (Caffey *et al.* 1964; Hogarty *et al.* 1974; Davis 1975) Two recent reviews have collated the information from trials in which neuroleptics were withdrawn from populations of patients with schizophrenia who had responded to medication (Gilbert *et al.* 1995; Viguera *et al.* 1997).

In a review of 66 studies from 1958 through to 1993 Gilbert and colleagues noted that the relapse rate in the medication withdrawal groups was 53.2% (follow-up 6.3–9.7 months) compared with 15.6% (follow-up 7.9 months) in the maintenance groups. There was also a positive relationship between risk of relapse and length of follow-up. Viguera and colleagues used data on 22 patient cohorts and investigated the relationship between gradual (last depot injection or tailing off over 3 weeks or more) and abrupt medication discontinuation. They noted a cumulative relapse rate of about 46% at six months and 56.2% at 24 month follow-up in patients whose medication was stopped abruptly. They calculated that in patients whose medication was stopped gradually the relapse rate at six months was halved. They also described that 50% of in-patients had relapsed by 5 months after cessation of medication whilst in their out-patient group relapse rates remained less than 50% at 4 year follow-up.

Further evidence of the beneficial effect of medication in preventing relapse is provided by the series of studies looking at expressed emotion (EE) within the families of patients with schizophrenia. In these studies the rate of relapse in patients whose medication was discontinued and who were living in a higher EE environment was in the region of 42–92%, whilst for those receiving medication the rates were in the region of 15–53% (Leff and Vaughn 1981)

Thus, although occasional individual patients may remain well without medication, findings from medication discontinuation studies have conclusively shown that as a group patients with schizophrenia fare better if they receive anti-psychotic medication. However, prolonged use of anti-psychotic medication, particularly the older typical anti-psychotics , carries a high risk of adverse effects, particularly tardive dyskinesia. In order to attempt to minimize the risk of these events much recent work has focused on the use of low dose medication regimes and intermittent dosing strategies.

Low-dose anti-psychotics

The rationale underlying the use of low dose regimes is that significantly lower doses of medication are required for the maintenance, as opposed to the acute, treatment of schizophrenia. This assumes that for the patients all major treatment goals have been met by the time of dose reduction. The two major aims are to ensure that the stability of symptomatic improvement is at least maintained and to minimize the risk of neurological side effects and secondary negative symptoms caused by higher doses of, particularly, typical anti-psychotics.

A number of trials have investigated the use of standard doses of depot neuroleptics (between 250 and 500 mg chlorpromazine equivalents) in comparison with continuous 'low dose' regimes, usually at least 50% less (reviewed in Schooler 1993; Barbui et al. 1996). On the whole these studies have indicated that the patients treated with the lower doses of neuroleptics have a higher rate of exacerbations of their psychotic symptoms and higher rates of relapse. Using the results of six selected studies Barbui et al. (1996) quote a relative risk of relapse of 45–65% in the low dose group at 12 months follow-up with the relapse rate highest in the lowest dose group (50mg chlor-promazine equivalents per day). Most of the studies did, however, report a lower incidence of extrapyramidal side effects and fewer symptoms of anxiety or negative symptoms (Schooler 1993). There a number of limitations to these studies, not least that the doses used in the standard groups are in the low to moderate dose range. Also, no systematic evaluation has been carried out of the patient characteristics likely to predict good response to lower dose therapy.

Intermittent or targeted medication

This treatment strategy is based on the assumption that patients can be maintained on low doses of anti-psychotics given intermittently. The most researched strategy is known as 'targeted treatment'. This strategy is based on the assumption that patients only require anti-psychotic medication whilst symptomatic. The rationale is that if the total 'medication load' for the patient can be reduced then rates of tardive dyskinesia will be lower and social functioning may be improved. Targeted treatment relies on a close collaboration between patients and carers and the identification of a signature 'prodrome' that warns of incipient relapse. During this prodrome medication can be given to the patient and a full relapse avoided.

Table 7.1 (adapted from Schooler 1993) shows the results from four trials of targeted treatment. In the Herz et al. (1991) and Carpenter et al. (1990) studies all patients were seen on a weekly basis either in the form of supportive group therapy and family education or on one-to-one. If prodromal signs were noted a known medication was substituted for placebo or started until the patient was restabilized. In both studies the targeted groups received less total medication but had more frequent prodromal signs and relapses, however rehospitalization and psychopathology did not differ between the two groups at two year follow-up. In the Jolley et al. (1990) study patients were seen every four weeks and the families received a one-hour teaching session. At one year the results mirrored those outlined above and side effects were less in the targeted group. However, at two years the targeted groups, whilst still receiving less medication, had a higher rate of relapse and hospitalization. Gaebel et al. (1993) have reported on a cohort of 365 patients using a similar design to the studies mentioned above, with the inclusion of a group of patients who only received medication when 'in crisis' rather than at the identification of prodromal symptoms. This 'crisis' group did significantly less well than the early intervention group with three times as many relapsing in the first six months. The two-year analysis of the continuous medication and targeted groups indicates that there were significantly more relapses in the early intervention targeted groups in comparison with those receiving continuous medication and more frequent hospitalizations (37% versus 24%). Having said this, employment rates over the course of the study in the two groups were similar at about 50%. In confirmation of these results, Schooler et al. (1997) reported data from a large collaborative study comparing continuous with targeted treatment. They found that few patients in

Table 7.1 Maintenance targeted or intermittent treatment studies (adapted from Schooler 1993)

	Herz et al. (1991)	Carpenter et al. (1990)	Jolley et al. (1990)	Gaebel et al. (1993)
Study characteristics[1]				
Number of Patients	101	116	54	365
Patient Population	Out-patients	Recently discharged	Out-patients	Recently Hospitalized
Stabilization	3 months	8 weeks	6 months	3 months post-discharge
Psychosocial support	Weekly support groups	Individual case managers	Monthly visits	Special out-patients clinics
Control features	Random/double-blind	Random/non-blind	Random / double-blind	Random/non-blind
Dosage				
Continued	290[2]	1.7[3]	1,616[4]	208[5]
Targeted early	150	1.0	298	91
Targeted crisis				118
Study results				
12 month relapse %				
Continued	10	33	9	15
Targeted early	29	55	22	35
24 month relapse %				
Continued	17	39	14	23
Targeted early	36	62	54	49

[1] Treatment was 24 months in all studies.
[2] mg/day expressed in chlorpromazine (CPZ) equivalents.
[3] 1 = low, e.g. <300 mg CPZ; 2 = moderate, e.g. 301–600 mg/day.
[4] Mean total dose expressed in haloperidol (HPL) equivalents.
[5] Cumulative dosage over 2 years in (1000 g) CPZ equivalents.

the targeted group did not relapse and therefore as a group they were also rehospitalized more frequently. Again, they received a slightly lower dose of medication over the course of the study.

Thus, in summary, it appears that patients receiving intermittent targeted therapy, whilst receiving less medication than those on continuous therapy, have a higher rate of relapse and also a higher rate of rehospitalization in most studies. At two years, however, there is little difference in social functioning or psychopathology between the two groups, indicating that the lower total dose of medication in the targeted groups is having little effect in improving patients' quality of life. These consistent findings of targeted treatment failing to be effective have led most of the authors to recommend that continued low dose maintenance medication is the best option for the majority of patients (Schooler *et al.* 1997; Davis *et al.* 1994). On the basis of the available evidence, targeted treatment may be considered for individual patients who refuse to take medication but are willing to maintain contact with clinical services provided that their risk to self or others when experiencing a relapse is low.

Compliance and risk

As we have seen, violent offending is linked with psychotic symptoms and acute relapse of illness in addition to substance misuse. It can therefore be suggested that the prevention of relapse in the mentally disordered patient with schizophrenia should lead to lower rates of offending, and perhaps reduced substance misuse if indeed some patients use illicit substances as a form of 'self medication' for the symptoms of schizophrenia. That substance misuse is also associated with medication non-compliance (Kashner *et al.* 1991, Owen *et al.* 1996) both supports and yet confounds this hypothesis. The relationship is by no means simple and there are sparse data available to separate these factors.

As can be seen from the evidence above, complete non-compliance with medication treatment will cause between 50 and 92% of patients with schizophrenia to relapse within 6–24 months. Partial compliance has been less well studied. However it may be inferred from the evidence on low dose treatment strategies (mimicking partial compliance with depot medication) and intermittent treatment (mimicking patients who only take their medication at times of increased symptoms) that even partial non-compliance leads to a significant risk of relapse which is unacceptable in this high risk group.

This assumption is borne out by data from the reanalysis of community derived data carried out by Swanson *et al.* (1997). They noted that in their subjects with schizophrenia the probability of violent acts towards others was reduced from about 70% to less than 50% for subjects who had received mental health treatment in the past 6 months. Previously, other authors, whilst attempting to control for confounding variables, had noted significant relationships between medication non-compliance in patients with serious mental illness and violent acts in the community (Smith 1989) as well as hostility and violence in outpatients (Bartels *et al.* 1991).

Factors in medication compliance

As has been discussed, compliance with treatment is undoubtably crucial in this group of patients and poor compliance is one of the most frequent reasons for readmission to hospital for patients with schizophrenia. Despite this, the literature on factors associated with compliance remains relatively sparse. Non-compliance may be related to a number of variables including the nature of illness, the degree of insight, and, most commonly, the frequency and acceptability of side effects (Lindstrom 1994; Fenton *et al.* 1997).

Rates of non-compliance are high; even in clinical trial populations as many as 30% become non-compliant within one year (Kane 1985). A quarter to a third of patients who discontinue treatment cite medication side effects as the major reason for their non-compliance (reviewed in Fenton *et al.* 1997). The most important side effect from the available literature is akathisia (Buchanan 1992).

In order to aid medication compliance a number of psychosocial interventions have been suggested. Purely psychoeducational or didactic approaches have limited effectiveness. Medication compliance therapy (or medication adherence) is based on a combination of cognitive behaviour therapy (CBT) techniques and motivational interviewing, commonly used in the addictions (Rollnick *et al.* 1993). Compliance therapy has been evaluated by a randomized controlled trial (RCT) and has been found to lead to significant improvements in attitudes to medication, insight and compliance (Kemp *et al.*. 1996). These advantages were maintained over an 18-month period, and global social functioning and time of survival in the community prior to readmission were increased (Kemp *et al.* 1998). The brevity of the therapy (four to six sessions with possible additional booster sessions), combined with its clinical effectiveness, make it relatively cost-effective (Healey *et al.* 1998).

Approaches such as these, however, do require considerable motivation from the individual patient and thus it may be more effective to pursue a reduction in non-compliance rates by vigorous strategies to reduce side effects and enhance patient acceptability, such as reducing medication to the lowest possible dose or switching patients onto the newer anti-psychotics. Switching medications may aid compliance directly, by improving efficacy and decreasing side effects, but may also act indirectly by enhancing cognition and improving negative symptoms such as amotivation.

Impact of the newer anti-psychotics

As we have seen there is overwhelming evidence that anti-psychotic medication is the most effective strategy in preventing the relapse of schizophrenia. However, there is still considerable scope for improvement. Treatment with the older conventional anti-psychotics leads to a number of crippling and stigmatizing side effects and may be ineffective for up to 25% of patients.

A wealth of research has been directed at the optimization of the use of the older anti-psychotics and yet there is no clear consensus on the best dose/frequency/duration strategy to provide a comfortable balance between the risk of unwanted side effects and the aim of protection against relapse. These factors, taken together, make treatment non-compliance, substance misuse, relapse and thereby offending behaviour much more likely. There is increasing evidence that the newer, so called 'atypical', anti-psychotics offer benefits over older drugs.

The re-introduction of clozapine in 1990 and the advent of several new anti-psychotics over the last four years has renewed interest and optimism in the treatment of schizophrenia. These new anti-psychotics have, for want of a better term, been classified as 'atypical anti-psychotics', a phrase which has a variety of definitions, tells us little about the pharmacology of the drug, and does not aid the clinician with prescribing. A possible classification is outlined in Table 7.2. The new 'atypical anti-psychotics' may be better called 'third generation anti-psychotics'. The rationale for this is that the first generation anti-psychotics were developed from the known pharmacology and structure of chlorpromazine and share high D_2 occupancy as their primary mode of action. Second generation anti-psychotics include drugs such as sulpiride, thioridazine and remoxipride. Using current definitions these may be classified as 'atypical anti-psychotics'. They still appear to exert their effects via D_2 receptor antagonism, however, and do not seem to confer the benefits of the third generation drugs. The third generation of anti-psychotics have been developed using clozapine, rather than chlorpromazine, as a prototype. Although they have a variable pharmacology they may exert their effects via other receptors, such as the $5\text{-}HT_{2A}$ receptor, in addition to the D_2 receptor. The third generation drugs may be sub-divided further, on the basis of their relative affinities for a range of receptors, into 'broad spectrum third generation', such as clozapine, olanzapine and quetiapine, and 'serotonin–dopamine antagonist (SDA) third generation', such as risperidone, sertindole and ziprasidone (see Fig. 7.1 derived from Schotte *et al.* 1996). As can be seen in the figure the term SDA does not infer that these drugs are selective for serotonin and dopamine receptors but rather that they have a very high affinity for dopamine D_2 and serotonin $5\text{-}HT_{2A}$ receptors—it is via action at those receptors that they exert their primary effect.

The use of the novel third generation anti-psychotics, risperidone, sertindole, olanzapine and quetiapine, for prophylactic treatment has not yet been the subject of the

Table 7.2 Classification of anti-psychotics

First generation anti-psychotics (formerly known as typical anti-psychotics)
Based on the structure and pharmacology of chlorpromazine
i.e. chlorpromazine, haloperidol, zuclopenthixol, stelazine, etc.

Second generation anti-psychotics
Next stage in drug development, may be 'atypical' by some definitions
i.e. sulpiride, remoxipride, thioridazine

Third generation anti-psychotics (formerly the 'atypical' anti-psychotics)
Based on the structure and/or pharmacology of clozapine, i.e

Broad spectrum
 clozapine
 olanzapine
 quetiapine

Serotonin/dopamine antagonist
 risperidone
 sertindole
 ziprasidone

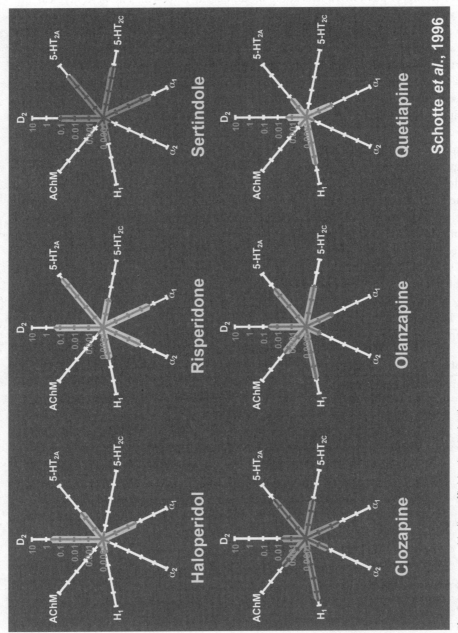

Fig. 7.1 Receptor binding affinities in $1/K_i$ (nM)

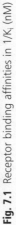

type of RCTs described above for the older anti-psychotics. However several long-term treatment comparisons have been carried out.

There are a number of reasons to make the assumption that third generation anti-psychotics should be at least equal to older anti-psychotics in prophylaxis. Firstly, all of the older anti-psychotics investigated in RCTs have been shown to be equally effective maintenance treatments. Secondly, it can be argued that as the third generation are at least as efficacious as first generation anti-psychotics in acute treatment, it would follow that they will also be adequate long-term treatments. Importantly, all of the newer anti-psychotics show a reduced propensity to cause extrapyramidal side effects at clinical doses, one of the major causes of non-compliance. This and other preliminary data suggest that the third generation anti-psychotics will be better for long term therapy (see Weiden *et al.* 1996). Although we still do not know precisely how clozapine exerts its effect, all of the third generation anti-psychotics share a high 5-HT$_{2A}$/striatal D$_2$ receptor blockade ratio as part of their pharmacodynamic profile. It has been suggested that this is why these drugs exhibit a lower incidence of neurological side effects and secondary negative symptoms at optimum doses (Kapur and Remington 1996). It may be hypothesized that if adverse effects and negative symptoms are indeed minimized with the third generation anti-psychotics then compliance and rehospitalization rates will be lower than with first generation anti-psychotic maintenance treatment (see Weiden *et al.* 1996). It is useful to review the pharmacology and early clinical data on each of the newer anti-psychotics and then focus on specific areas where they may have advantages: compliance, side effects, negative symptoms, cognition and affective symptoms in schizophrenia.

Clozapine

Clozapine, the prototypical third generation anti-psychotic, has been used since the 1960s for treatment of schizophrenia but after reports of several deaths from neutropenia its use has become restricted. According to the UK data sheet, clozapine can only be used for patients unresponsive to two other anti-psychotics given at an adequate dose for an adequate duration, or those with tardive dyskinesias (TD) or severe extrapyramidal symptoms, and only with blood monitoring (Clozaril Patient Monitoring Service 2001). Each patient has to be registered and the drug is only dispensed after a normal white cell count. In the UK a blood count is performed every week for 18 weeks, then every two weeks for the next year and thereafter monthly. In the USA blood monitoring is weekly throughout treatment. Clozapine is contraindicated in those with previous neutropenia.

Important aspects of clozapine's pharmacology include its low affinity for the D$_2$ receptor, in comparison with older anti-psychotics. Clozapine has higher affinity at the D$_1$ and D$_4$ receptors than at the D$_2$ receptor. Clozapine also binds to the extrastriatal D$_2$-like receptor, the D$_3$ receptor. It is thought that the low incidence of extrapyramidal side effects is due to the low activity at the D$_2$ receptor. Clozapine also has antagonistic activity at the $5HT_{1A}$, $5HT_{2A}$, $5HT_{2C}$ and $5HT_3$ receptors. It is postulated that it is the balance between the blockade of these receptors that underlies clozapine's clinical efficacy in improving positive and negative symptomatology. Clozapine also is an antagonist at the alpha1 receptor, less so at the alpha2 receptor, resulting in sedation and hypotension. Clozapine's antagonism of the histamine H_1 receptor adds to the sedative effects and may be responsible for weight gain. Other side effects include hypersalivation, tachycardia, sedation and hypotension. More rarely clozapine can produce seizures (approximately 1%) and blood dyscrasias. The risk of neutropenia is 1–2%. In most cases this is reversible. The majority of cases (83%) occur within the first 20 weeks of treatment. Risk of agranulocytosis decreases to 0.07% after the first year of treatment. Agranulocytosis probably results from toxic and immunologic factors (reviewed in Travis 1997). It is this latter potentially fatal side effect that has led to the limits on clozapine's use and the requirement for blood monitoring. Interestingly clozapine does not increase serum prolactin.

Clozapine has been investigated in few RCTs of maintenance therapy. This is due to the restrictions imposed on its use. In one of the few studies published Essock *et al.* (1996) followed up a sample of 227 patients randomized to either clozapine or treatment as usual. They reported that those treated with clozapine had significantly greater reductions in side effects, disruptiveness, hospitalization and readmission after discharge. Furthermore, clozapine's clinical efficacy in relapse prevention is well established, naturalistically, at 1–2 years of treatment and there have been reports of good maintenance efficacy for up to 17 years of treatment (for a review see Travis 1997).

Risperidone

Risperidone was the first of the serotonin–dopamine atypical anti-psychotics. This drug has high affinity for the $5 HT_{2A}$ receptor, with a similar affinity at the D_2 receptor to most typical anti-psychotics. It is an antagonist at both receptors. In the acute phase of treatment, risperidone appears more effective than haloperidol in terms of improvement in positive and especially negative symptom scores; interestingly in this analysis of the data from two trials of 513 patients, risperidone was also superior to haloperidol at reducing hostility/excitement and anxiety/depression (Marder *et al.* 1997).

The optimal dose of risperidone appears to be between 4 and 6 mg per day. At doses higher than 8–12 mg per day risperidone can cause the extrapyramidal side effects (EPS) of tremor, rigidity and restlessness with a similar frequency to 'classical' anti-psychotics. Risperidone can increase serum prolactin which may lead to sexual dysfunction.

Risperidone has been assessed for long-term efficacy and safety in a number of long-term open label studies. The earlier data of Mertens (1991), Bressa *et al.* (1991) and Lindstrom *et al.* (1995) suggested that long-term therapy with risperidone was associated with meaningful reduction in psychopathology, amelioration of EPS and improved social functioning from baseline measures or against placebo.

However trials such as these tell us little about any additional benefits of the newer medications over standard treatments. For this, trials need to be conducted comparing the newer agents with active comparators. For the purpose of this chapter 'comparator' will be used to refer to any medication with proven anti-psychotic efficacy with which the performance of one of the newer medications has been compared.

The first active comparator controlled study compared risperidone (mean 9mg per day) with haloperidol (mean 8.9 mg per day) over a twelve-month period. There were 91 subjects in the risperidone-treated group and 99 in the haloperidol group. There were similar reductions in symptom ratings in both groups with a trend in favour of risperidone. Relapse rates were similar at between 14–16%, as were EPSs (Lopez-Ibor 1996). However it must be remembered that the dose of risperidone in this trial was higher than that now recommended.

More recently, a meta-analysis of 11 of the risperidone/conventional anti-psychotic comparator RCTs has been performed (Song 1997). The author reports that significantly more patients on risperidone showed clinical improvement than with comparator (57% versus 52%) and that patients on risperidone used significantly less medication for EPS (29.1% versus 33.9%).

Sertindole

As well as high affinity for the 5-HT$_{2A}$ receptor, sertindole is thought to specifically target D$_2$-like receptors in the limbic region and this has been demonstrated in rats. Sertindole is also a potent alpha1 adrenoreceptor antagonist.

Sertindole leads to the prolongation of the QT$_{C2}$ interval on electrocardiogram (ECG). This interval represents cardiac ventricular repolarization and prolongation has been associated with potentially fatal ventricular tachyarrhythmias, in particular torsades-de-pointes. Thus patients need an ECG prior to starting sertindole and regular ECGs thereafter. Caution with concomitant use of local and general anaesthetics is recommended. Early clinical studies have indicated similar EPS rates to placebo at clinical doses. Sertindole has been reported not to increase plasma prolactin levels with long-term usage.

Sertindole has been demonstrated to be effective in the maintenance treatment of schizophrenia. Daniel et al. (1998) reported on a twelve-month double blind trial of sertindole 24 mg per day versus haloperidol 10mg per day in 282 stable out-patients with schizophrenia. Although the sertindole and haloperidol groups were similar in terms of total positive and negative syndrome scale (PANSS) scores, there was a trend for enhanced efficacy for sertindole on negative symptoms that did not reach statistical significance. The sertindole group was also less frequently hospitalized (10/140 versus 16/142 for haloperidol) and had a lower use of anti-cholinergic medication (15% versus 35%).

Due to safety concerns the manufacturers suspended the use of sertindole in December 1998.

Olanzapine

A broad-spectrum atypical anti-psychotic, olanzapine has a side effect profile similar to clozapine but with a higher incidence of EPS at doses above 15–20mg per day. Olanzapine also demonstrates antagonistic effects at a wide range of receptors but has a higher affinity for D_2 and 5 HT_{2A} receptors than clozapine and a lower affinity at the D_1 receptor sub-type. In acute phase studies olanzapine is definitely efficacious for positive and secondary negative symptoms and is superior to haloperidol on overall improvement according to the Brief Psychiatric Rating Scale (BPRS) and every other secondary measure (Tollefson *et al.* 1997). Olanzapine may also be effective for the primary negative symptoms of schizophrenia.

Standard dose olanzapine (5–15mg per day) is effective maintenance treatment for schizophrenia in comparison with placebo and olanzapine (1 mg per day) (Dellva *et al.* 1997). This was demonstrated in a 46 week extension of acute phase studies. There were 93 patients overall in the standard dose group, 14 patients in the olanzapine-treated group and 13 patients in the placebo-treated group, respectively. The estimated one-year risk of relapse with olanzapine was 19.6–28.6% for standard dose olanzapine in comparison with a 45.5% risk with very low dose olanzapine and a 69.9% risk of relapse with placebo.

Initial data, from a meta-analysis of three studies using haloperidol-treated patients as a test group, indicates that 80.3% of patients receiving olanzapine maintain their response at one year in comparison with 72% for haloperidol-treated patients (Tran *et al.* 1998).

Quetiapine

Another broad-spectrum atypical, quetiapine has a similar receptor-binding profile to clozapine. In comparison with clozapine it has relatively lower affinity for all receptors with virtually no affinity for muscarinic receptors. Quetiapine is effective in acute phase studies for the treatment of positive and secondary negative symptoms. In a RCT involving a group of 106 patients quetiapine treatment was significantly better than placebo over six weeks across all treatment domains (Borison *et al.* 1996). Response rates to quetiapine in comparison with chlorpromazine were similar across all symptom domains (mean dose 407mg quetiapine versus 384 mg for chlorpromazine). Using the criterion of greater than a 50% reduction in BPRS scores, 65% of quetiapine-treated patients were responders in comparison with 52% in the chlorpromazine group (Peuskens and Link 1997). Arvanitis and Miller (1997) have reported a dose ranging study comparing 12 mg of haloperidol with doses of quetiapine from 75 mg to 750 mg per day involving a total of 361 patients. At six weeks the response rates were significantly better in the haloperidol group and groups treated with a dose of 150 mg per day of quetiapine or higher. Response rates between these haloperidol- and quetiapine-treated groups were similar. In all of these studies the rates of EPS with quetiapine are similar to those seen in placebo-treated groups and significantly lower than in conventional anti-psychotic comparator groups. Most common side effects are somnolence and dry mouth. Quetiapine demonstrates a lower potential to cause weight gain than clozapine and olanzapine and does not increase serum prolactin.

In the open label extensions of the acute trials 265 responders to quetiapine were considered suitable for one year of treatment. Of these, 33% were still on quetiapine at 12 months with a sustained level of symptomatic improvement (Rak *et al.* 2000). This is similar to continuation rates in similar trials with olanzapine and sertindole.

Ziprasidone

Not yet released in the UK, ziprasidone has a high $5HT_{2A}/D_2$ blockade ratio and a similarly high affinity for the $5HT_{2A}$ receptor as other SDAs. It is an agonist at the $5HT_{1A}$ receptor. Ziprasidone also has potent affinity for D_3 and moderate affinity for D_4 receptors. It exhibits weak serotonin and noradrenergic reuptake inhibition.

Ziprasidone appears to have relatively low levels of side effects. These may include somnolence, headache and mild weight gain but results of full clinical studies remain to be published.

An initial clinical trial of ziprasidone versus haloperidol, 15 mg per day over 4 weeks, suggested that ziprasidone, 160 mg per day, was as effective as haloperidol at reducing positive symptom scores but produced fewer side effects (Goff *et al.* 1998). In two placebo-controlled trials involving 139 and 301 patients over four and six weeks respectively (Keck *et al.* 1998; Daniel *et al.* 1999) the pooled data indicated that 80–160 mg ziprasidone was consistently significantly more effective than placebo and lower doses of ziprasidone. Improvements in positive and negative symptoms were similar in magnitude to those seen in patients treated with risperidone, olanzapine or quetiapine. Interestingly, 160 mg of ziprasidone was associated with a greater than 30% decrease in depressive symptoms in the subgroup of patients with significant depression at the outset of the trials.

Ziprasidone has also been used in a one-year, placebo-controlled trial in order to assess its utility for relapse prevention. A total of 294 patients were studied and randomized to placebo treatment or ziprasidone at 40–160 mg per day. Of the 117 patients who were maintained on ziprasidone at 6 months, only 6% had experienced an exacerbation of their symptoms by one year compared with 35% of the 23 patients remaining on placebo; this compares favourably with the available data on the older anti-psychotics (Arato *et al.* 1999).

Adverse events

The issue of side effects or adverse events is closely linked to tolerability and acceptability and therefore to both compliance and relapse prevention. Often the most debilitating and obvious side effects of conventional anti-psychotics are motor. As described above, all of the newer anti-psychotics demonstrate a lower propensity to cause EPS at clinically effective doses. In addition to the classical psuedo-parkinsonian side effects of tremor, bradykinesia and rigidity, these drugs may provide benefits for patients who suffer from akathisia and tardive dyskinesia.

Akathisia develops in 18–75% of patients treated with typical anti-psychotics. Although an early study with clozapine failed to show a significant difference between clozapine and other drugs (Cohen *et al.* 1991) this was probably due to an inadequate washout time for previous therapy. Later studies have indicated that over a twelve week period there is a striking reduction in akathisia (Safferman *et al.* 1992; Cheng-appa *et al.* 1994) with rates of less than 10%. Indeed, clozapine leads to a reduction in akathisia (18–75% down to 10%) (Chengappa *et al.* 1994). Moller *et al.* (1997) have reported that risperidone at 4–8mg/day produces a significantly lower incidence than haloperidol. Olanzapine treatment groups have improved akathisia ratings from baseline (Beasley *et al.* 1997) and quetiapine shows similar akathisia rates to placebo and leads to improvements in akathisia ratings in switch-over studies (Small *et al.* 1997; Arvanitis *et al.* 1997).

It is in the area of TD that clozapine appears to have its most marked effect. On conventional treatments TD develops in between 5 and 60% of patients with an increased risk of 3–5% per year of treatment (Malhotra *et al.* 1993; Fleischhacker and Whitworth 1994; Jeste *et al.* 1995). Clozapine treatment has a very low risk of causing TD. Case reports of TD with clozapine treatment are rare (De Leon *et al.* 1991) and may reflect the natural occurrence of TD. Cases of TD have been reported in controlled studies. Gerlach and Peacock (1994) reported nine from 100, and Kane *et al.* (1994) two from 28 patients treated for over a year. However it is possible that these patients had questionable TD at the outset (Wagstaff and Bryson 1995; Cunningham-Owens 1996). There is far more evidence supporting a decrease in TD for patients commenced on clozapine. Liebermann *et al.* (1991) report a 50% reduction of symptoms over 28 months of treatment in 43% of patients and Gerlach and Peacock (1994) a resolution of TD in 54% of patients after five years of clozapine treatment. Furthermore, Tamminga *et al.* (1994) reported a significant difference in reduction of TD scores in a clozapine group versus a haloperidol-treated group and that this difference began after about four months of treatment. There have also been case reports of switching to clozapine being effective in reducing tardive dystonia (Shapleske *et al.* 1996).

Given that an increased risk of tardive dyskinesia is associated with more profound EPS at treatment commencement there are *a priori* reasons for assuming lower rates of TD with all the newer medications. In risperidone-treated groups at <8 mg/day there are EPS benefits which increase over time with a rate of TD at approximately 0.3% per year (Lindstrom *et al.* 1995). Additional evidence comes from the large-scale controlled studies with olanzapine, which has a 0.52% one year risk of TD versus 7.45% for haloperidol (13.5 mg versus 13.9 mg) (Beasley *et al.* 1999). These findings tie in with early studies on quetiapine versus haloperidol and ziprasidone versus placebo which both show placebo rates of TD (Arvanitis and Miller 1997; Arato *et al.* 1999).

Table 7.3 Relative side-effects of the newer antipsychotics

	Typicals	Clozapine	Risperidone	Olanzapine	Quetiapine	Ziprasidone
Anti-cholinergic	±	+++	±	+	±	±
Orthostatic hypotension	± to +++	+++	+	±	+	±
Prolactin elevation	++ to +++	0	++	±	±	±
QT prolongation	± to +	+	± to +	± to +	± to +	± to +
Sedation	+ to +++	+++	+	++	++	+
Seizures	±	++ to +++	±	±	±	±
Weight gain	± to ++	+++	+ to ++	+++	+ to ++	±

From Jibson and Tandon 1998.

The rate of other side effects may vary between each of the newer drugs, although fully adequate comparison studies remain to be published. A comparison based on the available literature is shown in Table 7.3 (from Jibson and Tandon 1998).

Compliance

Supporting these findings and the notion that compliance may be enhanced in patients receiving the newer anti-psychotics, patients on clozapine have low non-compliance rates of approximately 7% (Lindstrom et al. 1994). It can be hypothesized that reasons for this reduced rate include a combination of the reduced EPS seen with clozapine and the frequent contact required for blood monitoring (Carpenter 1996a). However, the commitment to blood monitoring has been suggested by some authors to lead to a 30–50% drop-out rate from clozapine therapy (Hirsch and Puri 1993) and this suggests a balance between the two factors. It can be argued that clozapine's low EPS profile may make patients more committed to the necessary blood tests. Since all of the newer anti-psychotics share with clozapine a lower likelihood of causing EPS, it seems reasonable to assume that compliance with the newer drugs will be higher. Data on drop-out rates from clinical trials of the newer anti-psychotics support this assumption. In a meta analysis of risperidone RCTs (Song 1997), risperidone-treated groups were significantly less likely to drop out than groups treated with conventional antipsychotics (29.1% versus 33.9%). In one trial comparing risperidone with haloperidol, 52% of risperidone-treated patients dropped out of treatment versus 63% for haloperidol, and risperidone-treated patients stayed on treatment for longer before dropping out (Lopez-Ibor et al. 1996). Tollefson et al. (1997) report that in the acute phase of treatment 53% of patients treated with haloperidol (mean daily dose 11.8 mg) dropped out of treatment and only 33% of patients treated with olanzapine (mean daily dose 13.2 mg). In a comparison of chlorpromazine and quetiapine, patients receiving quetiapine were half as likely to drop out of treatment because of an adverse event (Peuskens and Link 1997). In comparison with haloperidol, patients treated with quetiapine were four times less likely to drop out of treatment because of adverse events (Arvanitis and Miller 1997). Although total drop-out rates did not differ in these two studies, a pilot treatment satisfaction study of patients treated with quetiapine reported a very high rate of satisfaction with, and acceptability of, quetiapine with over 90% of the study group preferring quetiapine over their previous medication treatment (Hellewell *et al.* 1999).

Negative symptoms

It is postulated that clozapine has an almost unique action against the negative symptoms of schizophrenia, out of proportion to its effect on positive symptoms (Meltzer 1990, 1991), but the evidence for this is by no means clear. Tandon *et al.* (1993) found that the improvement in negative symptoms covaried with the improvement in positive symptoms, and Hagger *et al.* (1993) found no improvement in negative symptoms. A more recent finding is that in comparison with haloperidol clozapine has a significant effect on negative symptoms in patients with non-deficit schizophrenia but not in those with deficit schizophrenia, i.e. those with enduring negative symptoms (Breier *et al.* 1994; Conley *et al.* 1994). It has therefore been suggested that clozapine's seemingly beneficial effect on negative symptoms may simply be a reflection of its reduced tendency to cause extrapyramidal side effects (Kane *et al.* 1994). The weight of current evidence suggests that clozapine has an excellent effect on the secondary but not primary negative symptoms (Carpenter 1996*b*). All of the newer anti-psychotics appear to have an effect on secondary negative symptoms. All of the available trials have indicated a modest but significant advantage for all of the newer medications over conventional anti-psychotics in negative symptom improvement (Song 1997; Tollefson *et al.* 1997; Small *et al.* 1997; Tandon *et al.* 1997). The data from trials of risperidone and olanzapine have been assessed using a path-analytical approach, which attempts to control for changes in negative symptoms which are simply related to a reduction in adverse effects. At 6 mg risperidone has a direct effect on PANSS negative symptoms in chronic schizophrenia (Moller et *al.* 1997). Olanzapine has been reported to have an effect on core primary negative symptoms at doses of 15 mg to 25 mg per day (Tollefson and Sanger 1997). It could be suggested that as the data for quetiapine in relation to negative symptoms are similar to the olanzapine and risperidone data then a similar analysis would yield similar results for quetiapine-treated groups. However path-analytical methods cannot prove cause and effect and further work will need to performed in this area with careful delineation of primary and secondary negative symptoms.

Cognition

The older anti-psychotics have limited impact on the neurocognitive deficits which are a core feature of schizophrenia, are apparent at the onset of illness and may deteriorate during the first few years of illness, although inconsistent long-term improvements have been noted (Meltzer *et al.* 1996; Bilder 1997). There has been increasing interest in the role that the newer anti-psychotics may have in ameliorating these problems which are linked to poor outcome and future unemployment. Clozapine may lead to improvements in attention, memory and executive function over six to twelve months (Lee *et al.* 1994). Risperidone appears to improve frontal function and spatial working memory when compared with haloperidol (Gallhofer *et al.* 1996, Green *et al.* 1997). Olanzapine improves a variety of measures of function including psychomotor speed, verbal fluency and memory (McGurk and Meltzer 1998). It has recently been reported that quetiapine improves attentional performance to the level of that seen in a matched control group over two months of treatment (Sax *et al.* 1998). A preliminary study comparing quetiapine ($n = 24$) and haloperidol ($n = 15$) in a randomized double blind trial demonstrated that patients treated with quetiapine showed significant improvements in overall cognitive performance, verbal fluency and verbal contextual memory (Velligan *et al.* 1999).

It is still not clear how relevant the modest improvements reported in these studies are to long-term outcome. However, it is likely that the benefits will become increasing apparent as longer term studies are performed.

Affective symptoms and use in other disorders

Patients with schizophrenia are significantly more likely than the general population to suffer from other psychiatric disorders such as depression and conventional anti-psychotics are used to treat psychotic disorders other than schizophrenia. It is useful, therefore to look at the possible benefits of the newer medications in limiting co-morbid disorders and the possibility of using them outside of schizophrenia.

Clozapine has efficacy in a number of other disorders where traditionally typical anti-psychotics have been used. Clozapine has been reported to be effective in patients with treatment resistant schizoaffective or manic illnesses (Zarate *et al.* 1995 and reviewed in Kimmel *et al.* 1994). In one study clozapine reduced baseline mania ratings by greater than 50% in 72% of a group of patients suffering from either mania or schizoaffective disorder and 32% had a significant improvement in BPRS scores. The latter finding was more frequent in the bipolars and the non-rapid cycling patients (Calabrese *et al.* 1996). In depressive disorders clozapine has a more equivocal response. Although seemingly effective against depressive symptoms occurring co-morbidly with schizophrenia (Meltzer and Okayli 1995), there has been little work showing a particular use for clozapine in the treatment refractory depression (Banov *et al.* 1994; Rothschild 1996).

Conventional anti-psychotics may both improve and contribute towards depressive symptoms. Clozapine reduces both depressive features and suicidality (Meltzer and Okali 1995). Risperidone produces significantly greater reduction in anxiety/depression sub-scales in comparison with haloperidol (Marder *et al.* 1997). Olanzapine has significant anti-depressant effects in comparison with haloperidol (Tollefson *et al.* 1998).

The finding that clozapine, in patients resistant to previous classical anti-psychotic treatment, reduces the incidence of suicidality (suicidal ideation, planning, attempts and suicide completion) from that seen at baseline is of particular interest in the UK because of recent government targets. Meltzer and Okali (1995) reported a reduction of suicidality in 40% of their patients and the number of patients with no reported suicidality increased from 54 to 88%. Further evidence for decreased suicidality is that the rates of suicide amongst the 50 000 plus patients in the USA who have received clozapine is one-tenth of that seen in the general schizophrenic population (0.09% versus 0.8%) (Meltzer and Okali 1995; Cohen *et al.* 1990).

Pharmacoeconomics

The high cost of clozapine and other atypical anti-psychotics, when compared with classical anti-psychotics, has sparked an increasing interest in analysing the cost of drug treatment as a function of the cost of total care, i.e. number of hospitalizations, residential care, number of out-patient attendances and intensity of community input. The area of clozapine pharmacoeconomics has been extensively reviewed by Fitton and Benfield (1993). In summary, schizophrenia was estimated to directly and indirectly cost the UK, in 1987, £1600 million pounds of which the annual direct cost is estimated to be £1669 per patient. In the USA it is estimated that the annual direct cost of treatment-resistant schizophrenia is $11 300–22 600 million.

Analyses of the cost effectiveness of clozapine treatment in the USA indicated that on the whole clozapine was more expensive during the initiation of treatment but that over and after the first year there were substantial savings, savings more marked in insured or self-funding patients than in those paid for with public funds. These savings were mainly due to a reduced number of days in hospital for the clozapine-treated groups (Reid *et al.* 1994). A similar analysis in the UK indicated that clozapine treatment was either slightly cheaper or cost the same as conventional treatment with an estimated saving to the NHS of £91 per patient per year (Davies and Drummond 1993).

The largest part of the savings with clozapine appears to be in reducing the amount of time that patients with schizophrenia spend in hospital. It is therefore interesting to note that during one year's treatment with risperidone the number of days that the patients spent in an in-patient bed (bed-days) reduced to 13 from 54 bed-days on the treatment the patients had been receiving in the year prior to starting risperidone (Addington *et al.* 1993). Olanzapine has been reported to offer similar cost savings (Tollefson 1997). A more recent study comparing the costs of risperidone and haloperidol treatment in Australia has indicated that risperidone cost two-thirds as much as haloperidol per expected favourable outcome and five-sixths as much as haloperidol over two years (Davies *et al.* 1998).

Conclusion

The mentally disordered offender presents treatment difficulties to most clinicians. Balancing the needs and rights of the patients with issues such as relapse prevention and the safety of the community at large can often be difficult. In the UK there is not yet legislation which can force a patient to comply with medication when outside of a hospital setting. Therefore the issue of compliance with medication becomes one of creating a 'concordance' with the individual patient such that they will willingly receive treatment.

The work with older first generation conventional anti-psychotics has demonstrated that they have clear benefits in preventing psychotic relapse and thus by inference violent offending. However, the frequent lack of efficacy and the side effects of these medications, in some people, may promote non-compliance with treatment and the use of substances of abuse as self medication.

The issue of compliance in the mentally disordered offender is particularly pertinent. The need to ensure compliance with treatment and thus prevent relapse and possible offending is a crucial part of any individual risk assessment. This may lead clinicians to favour long acting injectable medications over oral medication for this group. There is considerable evidence from controlled and naturalistic out-patient based studies that depot injection medication reduces relapse rates by a half to one-third with a consequent significant reduction in hospital bed occupancy (reviewed in Davis *et al.* 1994). The primary reason for this is thought to be covert non-compliance in the groups continued on oral mediation. This is borne out by studies comparing oral and depot medications where compliance with oral medications is assured. In these studies there is no difference between the two routes of administration in the prevention of relapse. It can therefore be argued that the primary benefits of depot medications is that they simply allow the clinician to know what medication the patient has received and when. The patient may still refuse the injection and under current UK legislation cannot be forced unless legally detained. This may change in the future if community compulsory treatment orders are legislated in the UK. These orders would allow patients to be forced to receive anti-psychotic medication even if not detained in hospital. However, it is likely that the practical limitations of this approach would mean that few patients would be subject to such orders (Burns *et al.* 1993; Burns 1999). Given this, it seems likely that most patients receiving depot will not be compulsorily treated and therefore may refuse depot injection medication at any time.

It can be suggested that the intra-muscular route of administration alone may make patients less willing to continue with medication in the long term, but this along with the fact that the only currently available long acting injectable anti-psychotics are conventional anti-psychotics, with all the attendant side effects, makes it intuitive that patient acceptability of these medications will be lower than that of an oral medication with fewer side effects. Additionally, a patient may prefer oral medication with occasional plasma drug level monitoring, as is now carried out routinely with clozapine treated patients in some centres, to a weekly or fortnightly injection. This step would still allow clinicians dealing with mentally disordered offenders to be sure that their patients are receiving adequate treatment but be more acceptable to the patient.

It can also be argued that because our knowledge of the psychopharmacology of schizophrenia has moved on considerably over the last 10 years and because we now have anti-psychotic medications with far fewer debilitating side effects, clinicians should be able to discuss the effects and side effects of the medication they are prescribing with greater confidence and knowledge and enter into more of a dialogue with their patients over the pros and cons.

Although the evidence that the newer anti-psychotics are more effective in the maintenance treatment and prevention of relapse in schizophrenia is preliminary, it is becoming increasingly clear that the rational use of these medications offers mild to moderate advantages over older anti-psychotic medication in a number of different spheres of schizophrenia treatment and considerable advantages in terms of minimizing extrapyramidal side effects. Cumulatively the benefits may be substantial. The data presented here indicate that the newer anti-psychotics offer enhanced efficacy for positive and negative symptoms, reduced short- and long-term side-effects, are more acceptable to patients suffering from schizophrenia and offer improvements in mood and cognition in comparison with older anti-psychotics. These effects may be additive or synergistic, combining to allow patients to enter more into the mainstream of rehabilitation, psychological therapies and employment, which could lead to a 'snow-ball' effect of greatly reduced risk of offending behaviour and consequent enhanced improvement in quality of life for mentally disordered offenders.

References

Addington, D. E., Jones, B., Bloom, D. *et al.* (1993) Reduction of hospital days in chronic schizophrenic patients treated with risperidone: a retrospective study. *Clinical Therapeutics*, 15(5), 917–26.

Angermeyer, M. C., Cooper, B. and Link, B. G. (1998) Mental disorder and violence: results of epidemiological studies in the era of de-institutionalization. *Social Psychiatry and Psychiatric Epidemiology*, 33(1), S1–6.

Arato, M., O'Connor, R., Meltzer, H. *et al.* (1999) The Ziprasidone extended use in Schizophrenia (ZEUS) Study: A propective, double blind, placebo controlled, 1 year clinical trial. Data on file, Pfizer Pharmaceutical Group.

Arboleda-Florez, J., Holley, H. and Crisanti, A. (1998) Understanding causal paths between mental illness and violence. *Social Psychiatry and Psychiatric Epidemiology*, 33 (Suppl. 1), S38–46.

Arvanitis, L. A. and Miller, B. G. (1997) Multiple fixed doses of "Seroquel" (quetiapine) in patients with acute exacerbation of schizophrenia: a comparison with haloperidol and placebo. The Seroquel Trial 13 Study Group. *Biological Psychiatry*, 42(4), 233–46.

Banov, M. D., Zarate, C. A. J., Tohen, M. *et al.* (1994) Clozapine therapy in refractory affective disorders: polarity predicts response in long term follow up. *Journal of Clinical Psychiatry*, 55(7), 295–300.

Barbee, J. G., Clark, P. D., Crapanzano, M. S. *et al.* (1989) Alcohol and substance abuse among schizophrenic patients presenting to an emergency psychiatric service. *Journal of Nervous and Mental Disease*, 177(7), 400–7.

Barbui, C., Saraceno, B., Liberati, A. *et al.* (1996) Low-dose neuroleptic therapy and relapse in scchizophrenia: metaanalysis of randomised controlled trials. *European Psychiatry*, 11, 306–13.

Bartels, S. J., Drake, R. E., Wallach, M. A. *et al.* (1991) Characteristic hostility in schizophrenic outpatients. *Schizophrenia Bulletin*, 17(1), 163–71.

Beasley, C. M., Jr, Tollefson, G. D. and Tran, P. V. (1997) Efficacy of olanzapine: an overview of pivotal clinical trials. *Journal of Clinical Psychiatry*, 10, 7–12.

Beasley, C. M., Jr, Dellva, M. A., Tamura, R. N. *et al.* (1999) Randomised double-blind comparison of the incidence of tardive dyskinesia in patients with schizophrenia during long-term treatment with olanzapine or haloperidol. *British Journal of Psychiatry*, 174, 23–30.

Bilder, R. M. (1997) Neurocognitive impairment in schizophrenia and how it affects treatment options. *Canadian Journal of Psychiatry—Revue Canadienne de Psychiatrie*, 42(3), 255–64.

Borison, R. L., Arvanitis, L. A. and Miller, B. G. (1996) ICI 204,636, an atypical antipsychotic: efficacy and safety in a multicenter, placebo-controlled trial in patients with schizophrenia. U.S. SEROQUEL Study Group. *Journal of Clinical Psychopharmacology*, 16(2), 158–69.

Breier, A., Buchanan, R. W., Waltrip, R. W. I. *et al.* (1994) The effects of clozapine on plasmanorepinephrine: relationship to clinical efficacy. *Neuropsychopharmacology*, 10, 1–7.

Bressa, G. M., Bersani, G., Meco, G. *et al.* (1991) One years follow-up study with risperidone in chronic schizophrenia. *New Trends in Experimental and Clinical Psychiatry*, 7(4), 169–77.

Buchanan, A. (1992) A two-year prospective study of treatment compliance in patients with schizophrenia. *Psychological Medicine*, 22(3), 787–97.

Burns, T. (1999) Invited Commentary: Community treatment orders. *Psychiatric Bulletin*, 23, 647–8.

Burns, T., Goddard, K. and Bale, R. (1993) Mental Health Professionals favour community supervision orders. *British Medical Journal*, 307, 803.

Caffey, E. M., Diamond, L. S., Frank, T. V. *et al.* (1964) Discontinuation or reduction of chemotherapy in chronic schizophrenics. *Journal of Chronic Diseases*, 17, 347–58.

Calabrese, J. R., Kimmel, S. E., Woyshville, M. J. *et al.* (1996) Clozapine for treatment-refractory mania. *American Journal of Psychiatry*, 156(6), 759–64.

Carpenter, W. T. Jr (1996*a*) Maintainence Therapy of Persons with schizophrenia. *Journal of Clinical Psychiatry*, 57 (Suppl. 9), 10–18.

Carpenter, W. T. Jr. (1996*b*) The treatment of negative symptoms: pharmacological and methodological issues. *British Journal of Psychiatry* Suppl. 29, 17–22.

Carpenter, W. T., Jr, Hanlon, T. E., Heinrichs, D. W. *et al.* (1990) Continuous versus targeted medication in schizophrenic outpatients: outcome results (published erratum appears in *American Journal of Psychiatry* 148(6), 819). *American Journal of Psychiatry*, 147(9), 1138–48.

Chengappa, K. N., Shelton, M. D., Baker, R. W. *et al.* (1994) The prevalence of akathisia in patients receiving stable doses of clozapine. *Journal of Clinical Psychiatry*, 55(4), 142–5.

Cohen, L. J., Test, M. A. and Brown, R. L. (1990) Suicide and schizophrenia: data from a prospective community treatment study. *American Journal of Psychiatry*, 147(5), 602–7.

Cohen, B. M., Keck, P. E., Satlin, A. *et al.* (1991) Prevalence and severity of akathisia in patients on clozapine. *Biological Psychiatry*, 15(29), 1215–19.

Coid, J. W. (1996) Dangerous patients with mental illness: increased risks warrant new policies, adequate resources, and appropriate legislation. *British Medical Journal*, 312(7036), 965–6.

Conley, R., Gounaris, C. and Tamminga, C. (1994) Clozapine response varies in deficit versus non-deficit schizophrenic subjects. *Biological Psychiatry*, **35**, 746–47.

Cunningham and Owens, D. G. (1996) Adverse effects of antipsychotic agents. Do newer agents offer advantages? *Drugs*, **51**(6), 895–930.

Daniel, D. G., Wozniak, P., Mack, R. J. *et al.* (1998) Long-term efficacy and safety comparison of sertindole and haloperidol in the treatment of schizophrenia. The Sertindole Study Group. *Psychopharmacology Bulletin*, **34**(1), 61–9.

Daniel, D. G., Zimbroff, D. L., Potkin, S. G. *et al.* (1999) Ziprasidone 80 mg/day and 160 mg/day in the acute exacerbation of schizophrenia and schizoaffective disorder: a 6-week placebo-controlled trial. Ziprasidone Study Group. *Neuropsychopharmacology*, **20**(5), 491–505.

Davies, A., Adena, M. A., Keks, N. A. *et al.* (1998) Risperidone versus haloperidol: I. Meta-analysis of efficacy and safety. *Clinical Therapeutics*, **20**(1), 58–71.

Davies, L. M. and Drummond, M. F. (1993) Assessment of costs and benefits for treatment resistant schizophrenia in the U.K. *British Journal of Psychiatry*, **162**, 38–42.

Davis, J. M. (1975) Overview:maintenance therapy in psychiatry—I. Schizophrenia. *American Journal of Psychiatry*, **132**, 1237–45.

Davis, J. M. and Andriukaitis, S. (1986) The natural course of schizophrenia and effective maintainence treatment. *Journal of Clincal Psychopharmacology*, **6** (Suppl.), 2–10.

Davis, J. M., Matalon, L., Watanabe, M. D. *et al.* (1994) Depot antipsychotic drugs—place in therapy. *Drugs*, **47**(5), 741–73.

de Leon, J., Moral, L. and Camunas, C. (1991) Clozapine and jaw dyskinesia: a case report. *Journal of Clinical Psychiatry*, **52**(12), 494–5.

Dellva, M. A., Tran, P., Tollefson, G. D. *et al.* (1997) Standard olanzapine versus placebo and ineffective-dose olanzapine in the maintenance treatment of schizophrenia. *Psychiatric Services*, **48**(12), 1571–7.

Dixon, L., Haas, G., Weiden, P. J. *et al.* (1991) Drug abuse in schizophrenic patients: clinical correlates and reasons for use. *American Journal of Psychiatry*, **148**(2), 224–30.

Drake, R. E. and Wallach, M. A. (1993) Moderate drinking among people with severe mental illness. *Hospital and Community Psychiatry*, **44**(8), 780–2.

Eronen, M., Tiihonen, J. and Hakola, P. (1996) Schizophrenia and homicidal behavior. *Schizophrenia Bulletin*, **22**(1), 83–9.

Eronen, M., Angermeyer, M. C. and Schulze, B. (1998) The psychiatric epidemiology of violent behaviour (review, 60 references). *Social Psychiatry and Psychiatric Epidemiology*, **33** (Suppl. 1), S13–23.

Essock, S. M., Hargreaves, W. A., Covell, N. H. *et al.* (1996) Clozapine's effectiveness for patients in state hospitals: results from a randomized trial. *Psychopharmacology Bulletin*, **32**(4), 683–97.

Estroff, S. E., Zimmer, C., Lachicotte, W. S. *et al.* (1994) The influence of social networks and social support on violence by persons with serious mental illness. *Hospital and Community Psychiatry*, **45**, 669–79.

Estroff, S. E., Swanson, J. W., Lachicotte, W. S. *et al.* (1998) Risk reconsidered: targets of violence in the social networks of people with serious psychiatric disorders. *Social Psychiatry and Psychiatric Epidemiology*, **33** (Suppl. 1), S95–101.

Fenton, W. S., Blyler, C. R. and Heinssen, R. K. (1997) determinants of medication compliance in schizophrenia: empirical and clinical findings. *Schizophrenia Bulletin*, **23**(4), 637–51.

Fitton, A. and Benfield, P. (1993) Clozapine: An appraisal of its pharmacoeconomic benefits in the treatment of schizophrenia. *PharmacoEconomics*, **4**(2), 131–156.

Fleischhacker, W. W. and Whitworth, A. B. (1994) Adverse effects of antipsychotic drugs. *Current Opinions in Psychiatry*, 7, 71–5.

Gaebel, W., Frick, U., Kopcke, W. *et al.* (1993) Early neuroleptic intervention in schizophrenia: are prodromal symptoms valid predictors of relapse? *British Journal of Psychiatry* (Suppl. 21), 8–12.

Gallhofer, B., Bauer, U., Lis, S. *et al.* (1996) Cognitive dysfunction in schizophrenia:comparison of treatment with atypical antipsychotic agents and conventional neuroleptic drugs. *European Neuropsychopharmacology*, 6 (Suppl. 2), S13–20.

Gerlach, J. and Peacock, L. (1994) Motor and Mental side effects of clozapine. *Journal of Clinical Psychiatry*, 55(9) (Suppl. B), 107–9.

Gilbert, P. L., Harris, J., McAdams, L. A. *et al.* (1995) Neuroleptic withdrawal in schizophrenic patients. *Archives of General Psychiatry*, 52, 173–88.

Goff, D. C., Posever, T., Herz, L. *et al.* (1998) An exploratory haloperidol-controlled dose-finding study of ziprasidone in hospitalized patients with schizophrenia or schizoaffective disorder. *Journal of Clinical Psychopharmacology*, 18(4), 296–304.

Goldberg, S. C., Klerman, G. L. and Cole, J. O. (1965) Changes in schizophrenic psychopathology and ward behaviour as a function of phenthiazine treatment. *British Journal of Psychiatry*, 111, 120–33.

Green, M. F., Marshall, B. D., Jr., Wirshing, W. C. *et al.* (1997) Does risperidone improve verbal working memory in treatment-resistant schizophrenia? *American Journal of Psychiatry*, 154(6), 799–804.

Hagger, C., Buckley, P., Kenny, J. T. *et al.* (1993) Improvement in cognitive functions and psychiatric symptoms in treatment refractory schizophrenic patients receiving clozapine. *Biological Psychiatry*, 34, 702–12.

Healey, A., Knapp, M., Astin, J. *et al.* (1998) Cost-effectiveness evaluation of compliance therapy for people with psychosis. *British Journal of Psychiatry*, 172, 420–4.

Hellewell, J. S. E., Langham, S., Hurst, B. *et al.* (1999) Treatment with seroquel:patient satisfaction and acceptability. *The International Journal of Neuropsychpharmacology*, 2 (Suppl. 1), S112-S113.

Herz, M. I., Glazer, W. M., Mostert, M. A. *et al.* (1991) Intermittent vs maintenance medication in schizophrenia. Two-year results. *Archives of General Psychiatry*, 48(4), 333–9.

Hiday, V. A., Swartz, M. S., Swanson, J. W. *et al.* (1998) Male-female differences in the setting and construction of violence among people with severe mental illness. *Social Psychiatry and Psychiatric Epidemiology*, 33 (Suppl. 1), S68–74.

Hirsch, S. R. and Puri, B. K. (1993) Clozapine: progress in treating refractory schizophrenia. *British Medical Journal*, 306, 1427–8.

Hodgins, S. (1992) Mental Disorder, intellectual deficiency and crime. *Archives of General Psychiatry*, 49, 476–83.

Hodgins, S., Mednick, S. A., Brennan, P. A. *et al.* (1996) Mental disorder and crime. Evidence from a Danish birth cohort. *Archives of General Psychiatry*, 53, 489–96.

Hodgins, S. (1998) Epidemiological investigations of the associations between major mental disorders and crime: methodological limitations and validity of the conclusions. *Social Psychiatry and Psychiatric Epidemiology*, 33 (Suppl. 1), S29–37.

Hogarty, G. E., Goldberg, S. C., Schooler, N. R. *et al.* (1974) Drug and sociotherapy in the aftercare of schizophrenic patients. II: two year relapse rates. *Archives of General Psychiatry*, 31, 603–8.

Jeste, D. V., Caliguri, M. P., Paulsen, J. S. *et al.* (1995) Risk of tardive dyskinesia in older patients: a prospective longitudinal study of 266 outpatients. *Archives of General Psychiatry*, 52(9), 756–65.

Jibson, M. D. and Tandon, R. (1998) New atypical antipsychotic medications. *Journal of Psychiatric Research*, 32(3–4), 215–28.

Jolley, A. G., Hirsch, S. R., Morrison, E. *et al.* (1990) Trial of brief intermittent neuroleptic prophylaxis for selected schizophrenic outpatients: clinical and social outcome at two years. *British Medical Journal*, 301(6756), 837–42.

Kane, J. M. (1985) Compliance issues in outpatient treatment. *Journal of Clinical Psychopharmacology*, 5, 22S–27S.

Kane, J. M., Safferman, A. Z., Pollack, S. *et al.* (1994) Clozapine, negative symptoms, and extrapyramidal side effects. *Journal of Clinical Psychiatry*, 55(9) (Suppl. B), 74–7.

Kapur, S. and Remington, G. (1996) Serotonin-dopamine interaction and its relevance to schizophrenia. *American Journal of Psychiatry*, 153, 466–76.

Kashner, T. M., Rader, L. E., Rodell, D. E. *et al.* (1991) Family characteristics, substance abuse, and hospitalization patterns of patients with schizophrenia. *Hospital and Community Psychiatry*, 42(2), 195–6.

Keck, P., Jr, Buffenstein, A., Ferguson, J. *et al.* (1998) Ziprasidone 40 and 120 mg/day in the acute exacerbation of schizophrenia and schizoaffective disorder: a 4-week placebo-controlled trial. *Psychopharmacology*, 140(2), 173–84.

Kemp, R., Hayward, P., Applewhaite, G. *et al.* (1996) Compliance therapy in psychotic patients: randomised controlled trial. *British Medical Journal*, 312 (7027), 345–9.

Kemp, R., Kirov, G., Everitt, B. *et al.* (1998) Randomised controlled trial of compliance therapy. 18-month follow-up. *British Journal of Psychiatry*, 172, 413–9.

Kimmel, S. E., Calabrese, J. R., Woyshville, M. J. *et al.* (1994) Clozapine in treatment-refractory mood disorders. *Journal of Clinical Psychiatry*, 55 (Suppl. B), 91–3.

Kullgren, G., Tengstrom, A. and Grann, M. (1998) Suicide among personality-disordered offenders: a follow-up study of 1943 male criminal offenders. *Social Psychiatry and Psychiatric Epidemiology*, 33 (Suppl. 1), S102–6.

Lee, M. A., Thompson, P. A. and Meltzer, H. Y. (1994) Effects of clozapine on cognitive function in schizophrenia. *Journal of Clinical Psychiatry*, 55 (Suppl. B), 82–7.

Leff, J. and Vaughn, C. (1981) The role of maintenance therapy and relatives' expressed emotion in relapse of schizophrenia: a two-year follow-up. *British Journal of Psychiatry*, 139, 102–4.

Lehman, A. F., Myers, C. P., Thompson, J. W. *et al.* (1993) Implications of mental and substance use disorders. A comparison of single and dual diagnosis patients. *Journal of Nervous and Mental Disease*, 181(6), 365–70.

Liebermann, J. A., Saltz, B. L., Johns, C. A. *et al.* (1991) The effects of clozapine on tardive dyskinesia. *British Journal of Psychiatry*, 158, 503–10.

Lindqvist, P. and Allebeck, P. (1990) Schizophrenia and crime. A longitudinal follow-up of 644 schizophrenics in Stockholm. *British Journal of Psychiatry*, 157, 345–50.

Lindstrom, L. H. (1994) Long term clinical and social outcome studies in schizophrenia in relation to the cognitive and emotional side effects of antipsychotic drugs. *Acta Psychiatrica Scandinavia*, 380 (Suppl.), 74–6.

Lindstrom, E., Eriksson, B., Hellgren, A. *et al.* (1995) Efficacy and safety of risperidone in the long-term treatment of patients with schizophrenia. *Clinical Therapeutics*, 17(3), 402–12.

Link, B. G. and Stueve, C. A. (1994) Psychotic symptoms and the violent/illegal behaviour of mental patients compared to community controls. In *Violence and Mental disorder: Developments in Risk Assessment* (ed. J. Monahan and H. Steadman), pp. 137–160. Chicago: University of Chicago Press.

Link, B. G., Stueve, A. and Cullan, F. T. (1992) The violent and illegal behavior of mehtal patients reconsidered. *American Sociological Review*, 57, 275–92.

Link, B. G., Stueve, A. and Phelan, J. (1998) Psychotic symptoms and violent behaviors: probing the components of "threat/control-override" symptoms. *Social Psychiatry and Psychiatric Epidemiology*, 33 (Suppl. 1), S55–60.

Lopez-Ibor, J. J., Ayuso, J. L., Gutierrez, M. *et al.* (1996) Risperidone in the treatment of chronic schizophrenia: multicenter study comparative to haloperidol. *Actas Luso-Espanolas de Neurologia, Psiquiatria y Ciencias Afines*, 24(4), 165–72.

Malhotra, A. K., Litman, R. E. and Pickar, D. (1993) Adverse effects of antipsychotics drugs. *Drug Safety*, 9, 429–36.

Marder, S. R., Davis, J. M. and Chouinard, G. (1997) The effects of risperidone on the five dimensions of schizophrenia derived by factor analysis: combined results of the North American trials. *Journal of Clinical Psychiatry*, 58(12), 538–46.

McGurk, S. R. and Meltzer, H. Y. (1998) The effects of atypical antipsychotic drugs on cognitive functioning in schizophrenia. *Schizophrenia Research*, 29, 160.

McNeil, D. E. and Binder, R. L. (1994) The relationship between acute psychiatric symptoms, diagnosis, and short term risk of violence. *Hospital and Community Psychiatry*, 45(2), 133–7.

Meats, P. (1997) Quetiapine (Seroquel); An effective and well-tolerated atypical antipsychotic. *International Journal of Psychiatry in Clinical Practice*, 1, 231–9.

Meltzer, H. Y. (1990) Pharmacologic treatment of negative symptoms. In *Negative Schizophrenic Symptoms: Pathophysiology and Clinical Implications* (ed. J. F. Greden and R. Tandon), pp. 215–231. Washington, DC: American Psychiatric Press.

Meltzer, H. Y. (1991) The effect of clozapine and other atypical drugs on negative symptoms. In *Negative Versus Positive Schizophrenia* (ed. A. Marneros, N. C. Andreasen and M. T. Tsuang), pp. 365–376. Berlin, Germany: Springer.

Meltzer, H. Y. and Okayli, G. (1995) Reduction of suicidllity during clozapine treatment of neuroleptic-resistant schizophrenia: impact on risk benefit assessment. *American Journal of Psychiatry*, 152, 183–90.

Meltzer, H. Y., Thompson, P. A., Lee, M. A. *et al.* (1996) Neuropsychologic deficits in schizophrenia: relation to social function and effect of antipsychotic drug treatment. *Neuropsychopharmacology*, 14(3) (Suppl.), 27S-33S.

Menezes, P. R., Johnson, S., Thornicroft, G. *et al.* (1996) Drug and alcohol problems among individuals with severe mental illness in south London. *British Journal of Psychiatry*, 168, 612–19.

Mertens, C. (1991) Long term treatment of schizophrenic patients with risperidone. *Biological Psychiatry*, 29, 413S–414S.

Modestin, J. and Ammann, R. (1996) Mental disorder and criminality: male schizophrenia. *Schizophrenia Bulletin*, 22, 69–82.

Moller, H. J., Bauml, J., Ferrero, F. *et al.* (1997) Risperidone in the treatment of schizophrenia: results of a study of patients from Germany, Austria, and Switzerland. *European Archives of Psychiatry and Clinical Neuroscience*, 247(6), 291–6.

Mulvey, E. P. and Lidz, C. W. (1998) Clinical prediction of violence as a conditional judgment. *Social Psychiatry and Psychiatric Epidemiology*, 33 (Suppl. 1), S107–13.

National Institutes of Mental Health Psychophrmacology Service Centre Study Group (1964) Phenothiazine treatment in schizophrenia. *Archives of General Psychiatry*, 10, 246–226.

Owen, R. R., Fischer, E. P., Booth, B. M. *et al.* (1996) Medication noncompliance and substance abuse among patients with schizophrenia. *Psychiatric Services*, 47(8), 853–8.

Peuskens, J. and Link, C. G. (1997) A comparison of quetiapine and chlorpromazine in the treatment of schizophrenia. *Acta Psychiatrica Scandinavica*, 96(4), 265–73.

Phelan, J. C. and Link, B. G. (1998) The growing belief that people with mental illnesses are violent: the role of the dangerousness criterion for civil commitment. *Social Psychiatry and Psychiatric Epidemiology*, 33 (Suppl. 1), S7–12.

Regier, D. A., Farmer, M. E., Rae, D. S. *et al.* (1990) Comorbidity of mental disorders with alcohol and other drug abuse. Results from the Epidemiologic Catchment Area (ECA) Study. *Journal of the American Medical Association*, 264(19), 2511–8.

Reid, W. H., Mason, M. and Toprac, M. (1994) Savings in hospital bed-days related to treatment with clozapine. *Hospital and Community Psychiatry*, 45(3), 261–4.

Rollnick, S., Kinnersley, P. and Stott, N. (1993) Methods of helping patients with behaviour change. *British Medical Journal*, 307(6897), 188–90.

Rothschild, A. J. (1996) Management of psychotic, treatment resistant depression. *Psychiatric Clinics of North America*, 19(2), 237–52.

Safferman, A. Z., Lieberman, J. A. and Pollack, S. (1992) Clozapine and akathisia. *Biological Psychiatry*, 31, 733–4.

Sax, K. W., Strakowski, S. M. and Keck, P. E., Jr (1998) Attentional improvement following quetiapine fumarate treatment in schizophrenia. *Schizophrenia Research*, 33(3), 151–5.

Schooler, N. A. (1993) Reducing dosage in maintainence treatment of schizophrenia. *British Journal of Psychiatry*, 163 (Suppl. 22), 58–65.

Schooler, N. R., Keith, S. J., Severe, J. B. *et al.* (1997) Relapse and rehospitalization during maintenance treatment of schizophrenia. The effects of dose reduction and family treatment. *Archives of General Psychiatry*, 54(5), 453–63.

Scott, H., Johnson, S., Menezes, P. *et al.* (1998) Substance misuse and risk of aggression and offending among the severely mentally ill. *British Journal of Psychiatry*, 172, 345–50.

Shapleske, J., Mickay, A. P. and Mckenna, P. J. (1996) Successful treatment of tardive dystonia with clozapine and clonazepam. *British Journal of Psychiatry*, 168(4), 516–18.

Small, J. G., Hirsch, S. R., Arvanitis, L. A. *et al.* (1997) Quetiapine in patients with schizophrenia. A high- and low-dose double-blind comparison with placebo. Seroquel Study Group. *Archives of General Psychiatry*, 54(6), 549–57.

Smith, L. D. (1989) Medication refusal and the rehospitalized mentally ill inmate. *Hospital and Community Psychiatry*, 40(5), 491–6.

Song, F. (1997) Risperidone in the treatment of schizophrenia: a meta-analysis of randomized controlled trials. *Journal of Psychopharmacology*, 11(1), 65–71.

Steadman, H. J., Mulvey, E. P., Monahan, J. *et al.* (1998) Violence by people discharged from acute psychiatric inpatient facilities and by other in the same neighborhoods. *Archives of General Psychiatry*, 55, 1–9.

Stueve, A. and Link, B. G. (1997) Violence and Psychiatric Disoredrs: results from an epidemiological study of young adults in Israel. *Psychiatry Quarterly*, 68, 327–42.

Stueve, A. and Link, B. G. (1998) Gender differences in the relationship between mental illness and violence: evidence from a community-based epidemiological study in Israel. *Social Psychiatry and Psychiatric Epidemiology*, 33 (Suppl. 1), S61–7.

Swanson, J. W., Borum, R., Swartz, M. S. *et al.* (1996) Psychotic symptoms and disorders and the risk of violent behaviour. *Criminal Behaviour and Mental Health*, 6, 317–38.

Swanson, J., Estroff, S., Swartz, M. *et al.* (1997) Violence and severe mental disorder in clinical and community populations: The effects of psychotic symptoms, comorbidity and lack of treatment. *Psychiatry*, 60, 1–22.

Swanson, J., Swartz, M., Estroff, S. *et al.* (1998) Psychiatric impairment, social contact, and violent behavior: evidence from a study of outpatient-committed persons with severe mental disorder. *Social Psychiatry and Psychiatric Epidemiology*, 33 (Suppl. 1), S86–94.

Swartz, M. S., Swanson, J. W., Hiday, V. A. *et al.* (1998) Taking the wrong drugs: the role of substance abuse and medication noncompliance in violence among severely mentally ill individuals. *Social Psychiatry and Psychiatric Epidemiology*, 33 (Suppl. 1), S75–80.

Swason, J. W., Holzer, C. F., Ganju, V. K. *et al.* (1990) Violence and psychiatric disorder in the community: evidence from the Epidemiologic Catchment Area Surveys. *Hospital and Community Psychiatry*, 41, 761–70.

Swofford, C. D., Kasckow, J. W., Scheller-Gilkey, G. *et al.* (1996) Substance use: a powerful predictor of relapse in schizophrenia. *Schizophrenia Research*, 20(1–2), 145–51.

Tamminga, C. A., Thaker, G. K., Moran, M. *et al.* (1994) Clozapine in tardive dyskinesia: Observations for human and animal model studies. *Journal of Clinical Psychiatry*, 55(9) (Suppl. B), 102–6.

Tandon, R., Ribeiro, S. C., DeQuardo, J. R. *et al.* (1993) Covariance of positive and negative symptoms during neuroleptic treatment in schizophrenia: a replication. *Biological Psychiatry*, 34(7), 495–7.

Tandon, R., Harrigan, E. and Zorn, S. H. (1997) Ziprasidone: A novel antipsychotic with unique pharmacology and therapeutic potential. *Journal of Serotonin Research*, 4, 159–77.

Taylor, P. J. (1998) When symptoms of psychosis drive serious violence. *Social Psychiatry and Psychiatric Epidemiology*, 33 (Suppl. 1), S47–54.

Taylor, P. J. and Gunn, J. C. (1984) Violence and psychosis. *British Medical Journal*, 288, 194–9.

Taylor, P. J. and Hodgins, S. (1994) Violence and psychosis: critical timings. *Criminal Behaviour and Mental Health*, 4, 267–89.

Taylor, P. J., Leese, M., Williams, D. *et al.* (1998) Mental disorder and violence. A special (high security) hospital study. *British Journal of Psychiatry*, 172, 218–26.

Tehrani, J. A., Brennan, P. A., Hodgins, S. *et al.* (1998) Mental illness and criminal violence. *Social Psychiatry and Psychiatric Epidemiology*, 33 (Suppl. 1), S81–5.

Tiihonen, J., Isohanni, M., Rasanen, P. *et al.* (1997) Specific major mental disorders and criminality: a 26-year prospective study of the 1966 northern Finland birth cohort. *American Journal of Psychiatry*, 154, 840–45.

Tollefson, G. D. and Sanger, T. M. (1997) Negative symptoms: a path analytic approach to a double-blind, placebo- and haloperidol-controlled clinical trial with olanzapine. *American Journal of Psychiatry*, 154(4), 466–74.

Tollefson, G. D., Beasley, C. M., Jr, Tran, P. V. *et al.* (1997) Olanzapine versus haloperidol in the treatment of schizophrenia and schizoaffective and schizophreniform disorders: results of an international collaborative trial. *American Journal of Psychiatry*, 154(4), 457–65.

Tollefson, G. D., Sanger, T. M., Lu, Y. *et al.* (1998) Depressive signs and symptoms in schizophrenia: a prospective blinded trial of olanzapine and haloperidol (published erratum appears in *Archives of General Psychiatry* 55(11), 1052). *Archives of General Psychiatry*, 55(3), 250–8.

Tran, P. V., Dellva, M. A., Tollefson, G. D. *et al.* (1998) Oral olanzapine versus oral haloperidol in the maintenance treatment of schizophrenia and related psychoses. *British Journal of Psychiatry*, 172, 499–505.

Travis, M. J. (1997) Clozapine. A review. *Journal of Serotonin Research*, 4(2), 125–44.

Velligan, D. I., Newcomer, J., Pultz, J. *et al.* (1999) Changes in cognitive functioning with quetiapine fumarate versus haloperidol. Abstract presented at the American Psychiatric Association's annual meeting May 15–20 1999.

Viguera, A. C., Baldessarini, R. J., Hegarty, J. D. *et al.* (1997) Clinical risk following abrupt and gradual withdrawal of maintenance neuroleptic treatment. *Archives of General Psychiatry*, **54**, 49–55.

Wagstaff, A. J. and Bryson, H. M. (1995) Clozapine: A review of its pharmacological properties and therapeutic use in patients with schizophrenia who are unresponsive to or intolerent of classical antipsychotic agents. *CNS Drugs*, **4**(5), 370–400.

Weiden, P., Aquila, R. and Standard, J. (1996) Atypical antipsychotic drugs and long-term outcome in schizophrenia. *Journal of Clinical Psychiatry*, **57** (Suppl. 11), 53–60.

Wessely, S. (1998) The Camberwell study of crime and schizophrenia. *Social Psychiatry and Psychiatric Epidemiology*, **33** (Suppl. 1), S24–8.

Wessely, S. C., Castle, D., Douglas, A. J. *et al.* (1994) The criminal careers of incident cases of schizophrenia. *Psychological Medicine*, **24**(2), 483–502.

Zarate, C. A. J., Tohen, M., Banov, M. D. *et al.* (1995) Is clozapine a mood stabilizer? *Journal of Clinical Psychiatry*, **56**(3), 108–12.

Chapter 8

Out-patient psychotherapy and mentally disordered offenders

Kingsley Norton and Jonathan Vince

Introduction

The aim of out-patient psychotherapy with mentally disordered offenders is to improve their mental health or prevent its deterioration. This is to enable them to exercise maximally their potential for rational judgement. Optimally, this helps them to refrain from criminal behaviour which is under their conscious control. How, and how far, these aims are achieved is influenced by many factors. Some are related to the patients themselves, some to the professionals involved and others to the interactions between them or between other individuals with whom patients or staff come into regular contact.

At one end of the spectrum, mentally disordered offenders comprise those who have never been admitted to a psychiatric hospital nor to prison. At the other end are those who have been in either or both institutions and who are out-patients as part of a lengthy period of psychiatric treatment and rehabilitation. The size and nature of the psychotherapeutic task thus varies considerably, as does the degree of coercion involved in their receiving treatment. In the UK, for example, some mentally disordered offender out-patients will be subject to recall to hospital or prison depending upon their observed or reported attitudes and behaviour and the legal framework which applies to them. Some relevant information regarding such attitudes and behaviour may be available to the psychotherapist. How the latter evaluates and responds to such information may thus affect offender patients in profound ways, including through the loss of their liberty.

Staff range from individual psychotherapists to cotherapists working with groups of offenders or with offenders' families in the context of a multi-agency treatment package. Some staff have no formal statutory obligations or responsibilities beyond those which are stated in or implied by the tenets of their profession and their job description. Others have a range of statutory duties which are dictated by the legal framework within which the therapy is taking place.

As a consequence of the interaction of the various clinical and criminal justice factors, the potential range and combination of out-patient treatments is vast and the complexity of the therapeutic contact is variable. In this chapter, therefore, general treatment principles of out-patient psychotherapy are emphasized but necessarily at the expense of a detailed exposition of any particular treatment modality. The legal framework within which the therapy occurs is also considered but only in general terms and insofar as it may complicate the clinical task. Finally, there is a need to be selective about the patient population whose treatment issues are discussed. The focus chosen is those offenders who suffer from severe personality disorder, since they form the major diagnostic grouping of mentally disordered offenders receiving out-patient psychotherapy within the forensic health care system of the UK.

Severe personality disorder

Severe personality disorder (SPD) is an elusive concept (Kernberg 1984; Norton and Hinshelwood 1996). It has been defined as the fulfilling of the criteria for membership of PD diagnostic sub-categories from more than one of the so-called 'clusters' of the DSM personality disorder category (Tyrer and Johnson 1996). It may be present in 2–4% of the adult population (Tyrer 1988). Although imprecise, SPD is a notion which makes sense to most practising clinicians (Holmes 1999). SPD is relevant to mentally disordered offenders because such patients often present with disturbed behaviour or other manifestations of interpersonal conflict. Initially, therefore, they may not complain directly about themselves, their behaviour, thoughts or feelings. It falls to society, because of the patient's law-breaking or perceived dangerousness, to lodge the 'complaint'. However, although it may appear that SPD patients do not wish to communicate their difficulties verbally, many of them lack a capacity so to do (Norton and McGauley 1998). The lack of motivation for treatment perceived by the therapist thus may be more apparent than real (Norton 1997), since early adverse experiences have not only disallowed these patients acquisition of effective communication skills but also impaired their belief in others' willingness to listen and respond sympathetically. Various psychological theories of abnormal personality development attempt to account for SPD in adulthood and inform appropriate therapy.

Within psychoanalysis, some suggest that it is a failure of 'mirroring' (Winnicott 1965) or an insufficiently responsive interpersonal environment (Kohut 1971) which underlies the disorder—a 'deficit' model. In adulthood, there is a resulting psychological distortion, with extreme and contradictory views of the self and others prevailing. Alternatively, SPD is construed as the result of an inadequate metabolism of aggression during the formative years (Kernberg 1984). Within this 'conflictual' model, the developing child's excessive aggressive impulses remain insufficiently metabolized by care givers (for example, being met by retaliatory, rather than empathic, responses), giving rise to intrapsychic conflict which evokes a range of primitive defence mechanisms. The latter eventually become installed as part of the future SPD patient's adult personality. Such defences distort the perception of self and others and, as a consequence, a range of interpersonal and psychosocial problems ensue, including criminal behaviour.

Attachment theorists suggest that disruption, frank abuse or neglect during childhood lead to the formation of 'insecure attachments' (Bowlby 1973). In adulthood, these are reflected in excessively clinging interpersonal relationships or else an intense fear of closeness (accompanied by a contemporaneous longing for it), leading to the SPD patient's alienating or rejecting interpersonal behaviour (Holmes 1999). Sometimes there is an oscillation between the two styles of relating to others within the same relationship. Regardless of style, there may be an associated wide range of crimes committed, against the person or property.

It has been hypothesiszed that SPD patients have an inadequately developed 'theory of mind' (Fonagy 1991). As a result they have an impoverished sense of others and a consequent tendency to 'use' other people, rather than to relate more maturely and respectfully to them. The patient's body is, at times, also perceived and treated as 'other'. Consequently, it is misused in a number of perverse ways, for example via deliberate self-harm or certain sado-masochistic practices. Some of the SPD patient's psychosocial difficulties and criminal behaviour can be understood as originating from such a basis.

Cognitive therapists conceive of cognitive distortions or 'schemas' underpinning the maladaptive attitudes and criminal behaviour of SPD patients (Beck *et al.* 1990; Young 1990). The offender patient's different self-schemas may themselves be incompatible and the consequent instability of self and its associated feelings of emptiness may lead SPD patients to oscillate between two or more 'self-states' (Ryle and Marlowe 1995), for example, a compulsively caring and, alternatively, cruel and withholding self (Norton 1995). Such patients are confusing both to themselves and also to others with whom they relate.

Managing anxiety: the interpersonal context

As described above, the clinical encounter between the SPD patient and psychotherapist can itself be complicated and confusing, on account of the patient's unstable and extreme perceptions of self and others. Such confusion also derives from the absence of a presented complaint, since SPD patients tend to present 'of' themselves, rather than 'from within' (Brooke 1994). This means that their problem is often enacted interpersonally and not articulated. Thus a patient with problems of anger control may not ask for help with this but merely present a belligerent attitude which alienates the therapist. The latter is thus burdened with the task of elucidating the patient's symptom as well as responding to it. Feeling frustrated, therapists may unwittingly behave so as to disallow personal disclosure or escalate their patient's aggression. Patients may then perceive treatment as more part of their problem than its solution (Lockwood 1992) and the therapist may become anxious or frustrated through a sense of professional failure.

A crucial clinical task therefore is to identify when and how the clinical transaction deviates from the straightforward path of appropriate presentation, expectations and responses and to manage any attendant anxiety in the therapist, the patient or both (Norton and McGauley 1998). So important is the management of anxiety that the aim of treatment could be reformulated as being to *improve the SPD patient's capacity to contain anxiety and hence to inhibit its discharge through anti-social or criminal behaviour.* In forensic psychiatric practice, it is often difficult for staff to provide an interpersonal environment which accurately identifies and sufficiently contains anxiety, thereby facilitating personality maturation.

The more anxious are therapists themselves, the less well can they identify and manage the anxiety within the system of the patient–therapist interaction. Managing therapist anxiety depends partly upon locating its source. Therapists' anxiety can derive from: (1) uncertainty about the patient's mental state, especially in respect of psychosis or dangerousness; (2) concerns about their own physical safety in relation to the patient; (3) wider considerations of safety in relation to the patient's family or others inhabiting their social environment; (4) fear of criticism of their own professional judgement and competence (from peers, supervisors, inquiries, the media or the criminal justice system), especially in relation to the assessment of risk. The psychotherapist may need to attend to all of the above sources in order to understand and manage his or her anxiety level.

To manage the anxiety successfully, the therapist requires accurate and up-to-date information about the offender patient and also his or her interpersonal and social environment. Potentially, learning about what is actually happening with the patient between therapy sessions, as well as during them, makes the therapist's task more straightforward and less anxiety-provoking. Of equal importance, however, is therapists' awareness of their own (especially interpersonal) context and any aspects which may threaten its integrity and effectiveness in containing anxiety, including contradictory demands from the dual responsibility to both clinical and criminal justice 'systems' (Davies 1995).

In dealing with SPD patients, the psychotherapist needs to be vigilant, continually looking for interpersonal evidence of inconsistencies of treatment delivery and of 'splitting' between professionals in the multi-disciplinary team or between members of any different professional agencies involved with the same out-patient (Gabbard 1998). This may be revealed in acrimonious argument and hostile disagreements or, alternatively, by a lack of communication and an absence of conflict resolution. Good communication, through frequent and regular contact between these professionals, is required if as complete as possible a psychosocial picture of the offender patient is to emerge and the relevant areas of conflict or dissent among professionals identified and resolved or minimized (Davies 1995).

How relevant information concerning the patient's mental state and behaviour between sessions is collected will vary according to the complexity of the case (i.e. the size of risk posed by the patient and number of involved professionals or other 'informants'). In principle, however, the matter is so important that it needs to be considered with *all* offender patients. Therefore, in the treatment of SPD offenders, therapists should always ask themselves if there is an adequate network of communication established in relation to the clinical task, taking into account its complexity (as defined above). Ideally, the communication network is effectively in place before therapy begins. Deciding upon the precise nature and form of the network should thus be considered as part of the patient's assessment of suitability for psychotherapy.

Engaging the patient: the therapeutic alliance

SPD is usually conceived as the result of damaging or other adverse experiences in the patient's formative years, together with any genetic endowment which might predispose to anti-social or aggressive behaviour. Consequently the patient has difficulties with forming a basically trusting attitude to others (Erikson 1959) and this translates into difficulties in forming a therapeutic alliance with the psychotherapist. Establishing a therapeutic alliance may not occur at all or may take a considerable period of time, perhaps a year or even more. This period and process should be considered as one of the most important aspects of therapy.

There needs to be a reasonably robust therapeutic alliance before direct and effective communication, to and from the patient, can be established (Frank 1991). Even then it should not be assumed that any alliance will continue without further attention being paid to it. To secure an authentic, as opposed to an 'illusory', therapeutic alliance may not be possible (Meloy 1988). Even when it is, there may need to be an extensive educating of the offender patient to achieve it. This will need to include imparting information about what is expected of him or her by the therapeutic process and, likewise, what he or she is entitled to expect from others involved in the treatment. It may be useful to draw up a therapeutic contract with the SPD patient which specifies these aspects (see Fig. 8.1), even before difficulties have been encountered, tempers lost and anxiety levels raised (Miller 1990). Many treatment contracts fail to help because they are instituted at a time when trust has been lost or when anxiety levels are excessively high.

How relevant information about the proposed treatment and the importance of a therapeutic alliance is conveyed will vary according to the intellectual, psychological and social circumstances of the patient, as well as the complexity of the overall clinical task. In addition to verbal discussion, written material can be used to provide the patient with details about the therapeutic technique to be deployed and also about the nature of the personality disorder from which he or she suffers (Linehan 1992). In particular, how the latter can impact negatively on therapy through the patient's ambivalence, mistrust and low or fluctuating self-esteem can be explained (Norton 1996). When such unhelpful attitudes are prominent, an extended period of assessment may

An effective contract

- is mutually agreed by all parties
- makes clear specific responsibilities (including both what is allowed and what will not be tolerated)
- has the minimum of structure
- provides alternative strategies for managing intolerable feelings
- provides positive reinforcement for beneficial change
- should be strictly enforced, allowing for reasonable negotiated modification
- aims to foster a therapeutic alliance
- requires updating with clinical change
- may fail because of
  - being unduly restrictive
  - becoming a substitute for therapy
  - being used as a means of defence or punishment.

After Miller 1989, 1990.

Fig. 8.1 Treatment contracts.

be required in order to facilitate the processing and assimilation of the information provided and the developing of a therapeutic alliance, with or without a treatment contract (Norton and McGauley 1998).

> Mr X was on probation following release from prison where he had served three years of a six year sentence for rape. A condition of his licence was that he attended for a course of psychotherapy. He was initially reluctant to allow his psychotherapist access to his current partner and his probation officer. The therapist had wished to be able to obtain information from both of these sources on a regular basis. Mr X believed he was entitled to the same treatment and confidentiality as anybody else. Most of the first year of 'therapy' was spent in discussion about the importance of the setting up of a network of communication which was considered by the therapist to be sufficiently open.

An element of coercion, implied by the legislative framework in which the psychotherapy is taking place (as with Mr X), can mean that the topic of coercion is used by the patient to avoid disclosing relevant, and potentially painful, personal issues. Concern or anger about the involuntary nature of attendance or loss of confidentiality may thus surface to impair emotional engagement and mar the establishing of a therapeutic alliance. There may need to be long and careful uncovering of the patient's ambivalence, mistrust, and low or fluctuating self-esteem to reach an acknowledgement that endless talking about coercion may be ultimately a self-defeating strategy.

Conversely, the element of coercion to receive psychotherapy can sometimes be facilitative, assisting an ambivalent patient to pursue a course of engagement without having to fully own motivation, at least initially. This can be useful in patients with a particularly poor capacity to trust, who may long for a close relationship but fear being hurt through an abuse of trust were intimacy to be established. That there is an element of coercion usually means there is, in effect, a third party (usually, the Probation Service or the Home Office). Potentially, this situation can be exploited to benefit the therapeutic alliance. Thus, the therapist can creatively use the third party as an external agent in relation to whose stern authority the patient's collaboration is enlisted. They become reluctant allies who, in effect, combine forces in order to defeat a common 'enemy'. Such triangulation can also protect a vulnerable therapeutic alliance in the early stages. However, extreme care must be taken to avoid actually colluding with the patient against a third party, which would imply that the therapist condoned the criminal behaviour. The aim is not to contribute to the creation of an 'illusory' alliance (Meloy 1988) but to convey to the patient a genuine concern that the latter is being supported to act in their own best interests, avoiding further criminal behaviour and hence punishment and restrictions on the patient's freedom.

Establishing effective communication: external networks

The therapeutic alliance may be inadequate to sustain psychotherapy (Horwitz 1974). Recognizing this, however, requires the detection of the signs of a failing alliance. Such signs may be obvious; for example, the patient does not attend, leaves sessions early or displays disruptive or unco-operative behaviour during the session itself. However, the relevant signs may not necessarily be obvious or detectable during therapy sessions (see 'countertransference' below), but only in between, hence the relevance of a network of communication external to the therapy. Establishing such communication requires negotiation with (and, depending upon the legal framework, the agreement of) the patient. If the usual professional code of confidentiality is to be broken, the potential negative implications of this for the therapeutic alliance need to be thoroughly discussed at the outset. Ideally the patient will have been educated about such aspects as part of the development of the therapeutic alliance.

Evidence of a failing alliance may surface initially via adverse aspects in the relationships with others who are external to the therapy itself, including other staff (e.g. staff from the hostel where the patient lives). Every effort should be made by the out-patient psychotherapist to monitor the integrity of the network, regularly 'sampling' the views of all relevant professional personnel. This can reveal disagreements or other discordant attitudes among participating staff in respect of the choice or delivery of treatment.

Delivering out-patient psychotherapy

Almost all mentally disordered offenders suffering from SPD who are seen in forensic psychiatry will at some time receive *supportive psychotherapy*. Its aim is to improve the offender's psychosocial adaptation or prevent deterioration. Supportive psychotherapy usually requires regular individual sessions (sometimes weekly) and needs to focus on expected obstacles (including any foreseeable temptations to commit crime) which will confront the patient in the following weeks. The aim is to support or develop the patient's adaptive coping strategies and defences, through a discussion of the likely forthcoming events, and to inhibit the habitual ways in which the patient might be self-defeating, self-destructive or otherwise engaged in anti-social or criminal behaviour in relation to those future events. Delivering supportive psychotherapy is not necessarily straightforward. It requires skills which can be obtained through appropriate training (Rockland 1989; Hartland 1991). Few mental health workers receive the requisite training. Successful supportive psychotherapy can cement a therapeutic alliance and pave the way for the subsequent deployment of one of a range of specific psychotherapeutic interventions (see below). It is often required for a period of years—patients need to be aware of this timescale from the start.

Some SPD patients are skilled at diverting their therapists' attention from a previously agreed clinical task, even when this involves achieving no change. Thus, patients may 'seduce' their therapists to delve into their pasts, as might be appropriate were achieving personality change one of the aims, when this is explicitly not the agreement. If such a situation passes unnoticed, a failure to change may worsen the patient's self-esteem or encourage disappointment in the therapist and hence weaken the therapeutic alliance. Shifting focus away from support needs to be resisted or else discussed and agreed as part of an explicit review of progress.

Psychoanalytic psychotherapy is only for selected SPD patients and is intensive, i.e. usually two or more sessions per week, and long-term—lasting for years (Kernberg 1984). Considerable motivation, adequate psychosocial support and some psychological-mindedness are required. These requirements rule out this treatment for many SPD offenders. The aim is more ambitious than with supportive psychotherapy, since it includes at least some reorganization of the patient's personality. Depending upon the psychoanalytic model, change is construed as occurring via the resolution of intrapsychic structural conflicts or through corrective emotional experiences which rectify the fundamental deficit (see above).

Identifying and understanding the transference–countertransference relationship between SPD patient and therapist is usually a central task. However, there remains controversy over the use and value of transference interpretations early in therapy and over how the negative transference is managed. There is increasing agreement, however, that transference interpretations need to be modified with those SPD patients who have been significantly abused during their earlier lives (Gunderson and Sabo 1993). With such patients, therefore, it can be important to recognize, and to state to them, the earlier survival value of defensive and self-defeating behaviour and interpersonal styles (even though these may have involved criminal behaviour) prior to interpreting their current maladaptive or even destructive potential within the clinical interaction.

Family therapy is mainly used to sustain individual out-patient therapy of whatever kind. It is seldom considered to be a sufficient therapy on its own (Gunderson and

Sabo 1993). It tends to be used only for those intact families marked by overinvolvement or in which there is a history of significant abuse and neglect. As an adjunct to other psychological treatments, it tends to be deployed on an 'as required' basis, i.e. not at times when the individual therapy is progressing. One advantage of family therapy, where this involves another therapist(s), is the possibility for conjoint sessions with family, family therapist(s) and individual therapist. In providing a greater professional presence there is the potential for greater wisdom and diversity of views. However, with an increased number of therapists comes the potential for 'splitting' of the staff, the destructive effects of which can go unnoticed or unresolved (see below).

Group therapy may be beneficial for some SPD patients, particularly those showing prominent demandingness, egocentricity, social isolation or withdrawal and socially deviant behaviour (Horwitz 1987). It therefore has a potential place in the treatment of mentally disordered offenders, many of whom will show all of the above features. It offers advantages over individual therapy since the group setting permits the therapist to observe the patient interpersonally—interacting with others. It may be that maladaptive behaviour can be more easily and safely confronted within the group setting. Certainly issues concerning dependency and manipulation are easier for the therapist to identify within the group and there may be greater success in helping the patient to view such aspects as maladaptive and requiring change than is the case with individual approaches. The group setting provides each individual patient with a chance to view others interacting, witnessing their adaptive and not just their maladaptive coping strategies and styles. Peer support during a session can be available through the other members of the group when this is required. However, controversy remains over whether there should be more than one SPD patient per out-patient group and whether concurrent individual out-patient psychotherapy is superior to group therapy alone (Gunderson and Sabo 1993). Therapists who have little experience of treating SPD patients or who know little of group dynamics might do well to avoid group approaches with SPD patients altogether. If they do attempt therapy in a group setting, they should ensure that sufficient support and supervision is available (see below).

Behaviour therapy is seldom advocated. However, it can address the SPD patient's impulsivity, self-destructiveness and the maladaptive expression of their aggression. As an adjunct to other psychological therapies, it can provide an understanding of positive and negative reinforcers of the patient's behaviour, including those which may be operating via any other concurrent out-patient treatment approaches. It can also inform skills training, for example, social skills, assertiveness and anger management.

Dialectical behavioural therapy has been developed specifically to deal with self-destructiveness in women with borderline personality disorder (Linehan 1992). It is delivered in weekly individual sessions but with an ongoing twice weekly group. It is a highly structured programme with clear goal- and task-setting. It includes a didactic package with teaching about general problem-solving skills, emotional regulation strategies, interpersonal skills and distress tolerance. It is one of the few out-patient psychotherapy treatments for PD to have evidence for efficacy based upon a random-ized controlled study.

Cognitive therapy embraces a range of therapies, all of which aim to identify and rectify the patient's major cognitive schemas or self-states (Young 1990; Ryle and Marlowe 1995). Various cognitive strategies are deployed (including daily thought records and the eliciting of personal constructs) in order to identify how schemas are reiterated and reinforced in everyday life. The collaborative nature of the clinical enter-prise with SPD patients is emphasized. Increasingly, however, notice is taken of the impact of events in the patient's history. Also, transference and countertransference issues are considered as important aspects to which the therapist should attend. Such an approach represents a narrowing of the gap between cognitive therapy and psycho-dynamic psychotherapy (Young 1990).

The role of medication

Pharmacotherapy can be deployed alongside psychotherapy. However, the prescribing of drugs to patients with SPD needs to be undertaken with care, particularly to those who have a history of parasuicide or drug addiction (Norton 1996). It is wiser to dispense small amounts of medication frequently than large amounts spaced widely apart. The latter increases the likelihood of the conjunction of an increase in risk of suicide and the ready availability of a means to carry it out. The use of medicines which are particularly dangerous in overdose or which require significant compliance from the patient (for example monoamine oxidase inhibitors or lithium carbonate) should be avoided if safer alternatives are available. Prescribing single drugs rather than 'cocktails' lessens the risk of serious adverse side effects. As with psychotherapy, it is important to engage patients in a therapeutic alliance and to encourage their active collaboration in treatment.

The SPD patient can sometimes be involved with the prescribing therapist as if in a methodical, scientific 'experiment' with the medication. Relevant pharmacological information can be shared with the patient concerning likely or possible side effects. It can be helpful to acknowledge, in advance, that negative side effects could outweigh potential benefits. This kind of approach, which contrasts with that which simply re-inforces the doctor's authority (through the latter's attempts to maximize the 'placebo' response) can render the therapeutic alliance more robust. It may also lower the patient's anxiety and overall level of distress. Consequently, the amount and duration of medication which is required can sometimes be lessened. For some patients, medication is said to have a beneficial symbolic significance, in being a concrete reminder of the therapeutic relationship—perhaps part of the placebo phenomenon (Singer 1987).

Evaluating the transference–countertransference relationship

Understanding the inter-related concepts of transference and countertransference and recognizing their manifestation within the clinical encounter with SPD offender patients is crucial to the out-patient therapeutic endeavour, regardless of the type of psychotherapy deployed, i.e. including supportive psychotherapy and also the non-analytic psychological therapies. Since obvious signs of a lack of emotional containment or a threat to the therapeutic alliance may not surface other than in the patient's gross and obvious behaviour during a session, fluctuations or unusual features detected in the countertransference of therapists may be the only relevant evidence which is available early and/or directly to them.

> Initially Dr A had not paid attention to the fact that he locked the consulting room door after a particular patient left his weekly session. Although receiving regular weekly supervision from a consultant psychotherapist, he had not mentioned this fact. Even when Dr A had become concerned by the size of risk of his patient's violence he had not volunteered this information, yet the locking of the door occurred only in relation to this particular patient.
>
> The matter was brought to light almost by chance when the patient had left a session early and the supervisor had asked for specific details of what had actually happened in the consulting room. This revelation prompted an in-depth discussion of the effects of this patient on Dr A and in particular how unconscious of his own high anxiety level Dr A was, especially while the patient was in the room with him.

As in the above case, the therapist's identification and understanding of an important countertransference reaction can occur outside of the actual clinical encounter, for example during supervision. Given that the countertransference has its roots in the unconscious mind, therapists need to remain alert to the varied and subtle ways in which it may become manifest, including through unwitting alterations in their own attitudes and behaviour, as with Dr A. Most therapists develop relatively fixed routines of working, some of which can be disturbed by the interaction with a particular SPD patient. It is therefore important that any such disturbance is not dismissed or ignored but viewed in the light of its potential relevance to the overall transference–countertransference situation with a given patient.

When more than one therapist (or other professionals) are involved in the treatment of an individual patient there is the possibility, if not likelihood, that distinctly different clinical views of the 'shared' patient will emerge. This development can be invaluable in allowing all to modify their own formulations, leading overall to a more complex and accurate appraisal. Hence, erroneous or partial views can be corrected through discussion and argument. For such positive outcomes to occur, however, not only is effective communication required but a readiness to entertain the other's viewpoint—not necessarily easy to achieve in practice (see Davies 1995).

The failure of one or other of the parties involved in the joint treatment of an SPD patient to modify their views, however, does not necessarily have any sinister clinical significance. Two (or more) staff members may 'agree to differ'; they carry on, nevertheless, with an acceptably high regard and respect for their professional colleagues and are open-minded enough to accept the other's viewpoint at another time and with another patient. However , the above situation does not always obtain. Sometimes disagreements are so hostile or intense that they leave a residue which has an adverse effect on future dealings. Alternatively, there may appear to be an apparent cessation of hostilities but these continue in private, sometimes reported to others but not to the target of the hostility. In each of these two scenarios there is a great potential for the delivery of the SPD patient's treatment to be compromised. Hence, such disagreements and their aftermath should be within the scope of the out-patient psychotherapist's field of regular scrutiny.

> Mr B. was a physically imposing and large man referred to the forensic service by a community mental health team because of his feeling tormented by violent and sadistic nightmares and intrusive images of sadistic violence. He was unable to sleep for fear of nightmares. The initial management had included a psychological assessment and pharmacotherapy. Unfortunately, neither had been helpful to Mr B.
>
> A female clinical psychologist carried out the initial assessment on behalf of the forensic team. This was prolonged over a period of several sessions. During this time Mr B was observed to be agitated. He repeatedly left his seat in the consulting room to pace around, as if unable to contain himself. He conveyed an air of menace. Because she feared Mr B to be potentially violent, the psychologist invited a psychiatrist colleague (male) to join her to involve him in an assessment of risk and to consider a change to Mr B's existing medication. The psychologist and psychiatrist thus arranged to interview Mr B jointly as part of an extended assessment phase.
>
> What the two cotherapists discovered, in their regular discussions of the subsequent sessions, was that one or other of them would have felt anxious and threatened by Mr B's behaviour during the session, while the other felt quite disconnected and unconcerned, believing that the assessment was progressing unremarkably. They were interested to note that they could each take up either position in terms of 'countertransference'. They realized that neither of their views of Mr B on its own could represent the full state of affairs and that Mr B could not simultaneously be at high risk of violence and at low risk. They were each therefore vigilant about how they felt during and after sessions and wary about the fact that Mr B evoked such different reactions from them. This latter fact in itself was considered to be of concern, potentially representing aspects of Mr B's unintegrated personality.

What this vignette demonstrates is how good working relationships between two professionals can mitigate a partial or extreme formulation of a potentially violent patient and, in theory at least, lead to an appropriately cautious appraisal which derives from the integration of apparently conflicting items of information. In the case of Mr B the cotherapists decided to interview Mr B's partner and GP to corroborate and clarify some of the worrying aspects of his recent history, the nature of his premorbid personality and also his mood state and behaviour between sessions. Minimizing or exaggerating the extent of Mr B's difficulties (on the basis of one or other extreme and partial view of the cotherapists) could have increased the risk of his actually being violent. It was the cotherapists' mutual respect, open communication and willingness to note and value countertransference which prevented extreme perceptions being sustained and enabled risk to be assessed accurately and managed appropriately. The combination of this approach, cognitive therapy and low doses of neuroleptic medication optimized the outcome.

Such an optimal state of affairs will not always occur. There may be many reasons for this. The differing views of professionals may fuel existing personality clashes between them. Failing to value countertransference evidence may lead to such aspects remaining undetected or undisclosed. Working relationships dominated by mistrust or suspicion remove the possibility of airing such responses. The absence of a shared treatment philosophy which values such a response may mean that the 'personal' views of professionals are either not admissible as relevant information or are relegated in importance, hence they cannot influence formulations of the patient's difficulties nor its management. In some instances this is because the team is dysfunctional, with poor communication and a lack of co-ordination of its members' therapeutic endeavours. At other times, it may reflect the interaction between those involved in treatment and a particular SPD patient (Main 1957). In the latter case the situation is referred to as 'splitting' (see Gabbard 1988).

Splitting represents an interesting but complex phenomenon occurring interperson-ally among involved professionals but exquisitely reflecting aspects of an individual (in this context SPD) patient whose care is shared among them. It is as if dominating aspects of the patient's internal world of thoughts, attitudes and feelings become acti-vated in the wider interpersonal environment (Stanton and Schwartz 1954; Main 1957; Kernberg 1998). Such a phenomenon has been observed for at least the past fifty years and yet its discovery within the work situation can still mystify those caught up in the process. This not least is because such 'splits' often occupy or exploit existing lines of cleavage or 'cracks' which exist in and between all groups of professionals and thus it may be difficult to distinguish it from an ordinary or habitual intra- or inter-disciplinary disagreement. Initially at least, the splitting may be undisclosed on account of a reluctance to express strong negative feelings and views about a colleague's profes-sional performance. In as much as its origins are unconscious, it may be felt to be too irrational to disclose to colleagues who might be critical on account of the lack of an adquate rationale to account for it.

How the process of splitting is conceived is a matter of view and conjecture (Gab-bard 1998). Why some members involved in treatment of a particular SPD patient and yet not others become embroiled in the process is not always clear. It is posited that characteristics of individual staff, as well as of the particular SPD patient, play a part and it is likely that any staff might become involved in the splitting and that none is totally immune. Indeed, it has been suggested that staff involved in the treatment of offender patients should expect to fulfil roles which are unconsciously assigned to them by the patient (Davies 1995). Consequently, an important, though not neces-sarily simple, clinical task is the identification of the relevant (often reciprocal) roles played.

The patient's presentation of different self-states results in staff perceiving different, potentially conflictual or complementary, aspects of that patient (Ryle and Marlow 1995). Erroneously, they may be convinced that they have seen the 'whole' picture. Discovering that others do not share their own passionately held view is thus difficult to countenance. If, following discussion, such differences of opinion and perception can be acknowledged then a clear and more complete picture of the patient can emerge, as with Mr B. The latter scenario does not reflect staff being 'split'. Splitting develops from a more profound and prolonged identification (via projective identification) with the patient and reflects the therapist's inability to lose face and to be free of views which they feel impelled to hold. The strength of the grip of such views on the therapist is maintained because of its personal, as opposed to professional, relevance. It is this which results in the view being so tenaciously held in spite of others' contrary opinions.

In the case of Mr B, his early life had been unstable and marked by abuse and neglect. His mother suffered from schizophrenia and was frequently psychotic and hospitalized. Mr B and his siblings were thus left to the untender care of a physically abusive stepfather. Mr B was highly ambivalent about his mother and initially refused to discuss his stepfather at all during the assessment period. Simplistically, his unintegrated internal world, occupied alternately by a sadistic and aggressive self-state or a cut-off and 'absent' self-state, could be seen as lying at the root of the cotherapists' differing, but complementary, views. Their good working relationship allowed them to avoid their interpersonal splitting becoming entrenched with each of them locked into reciprocal positions.

Distinguishing improvement from deterioration

Regression during psychotherapy is an expectable, potentially positive, phenomenon (Freud 1936) which in terms of overt behaviour may be difficult to distinguish from deterioration. This can pose a dilemma for forensic psychotherapists which represents an understandable cause of concern and source of anxiety to them, as well as to wider society. Many patients habitually behave so as to alienate and distance the therapist because of an intense, albeit ambivalent and inadequately acknowledged, fear of intimacy, especially during the assessment phase. Such defensiveness may involve physical threat, intimidation or criminal 'acting out', even though the effect of this could be self-defeating to the patient, e.g. if it were to result in the therapist terminating treatment or reporting significant concerns to others in the criminal justice system. This maladaptive behaviour can also occur during established therapy, particularly when previously avoided emotional conflict is encountered as a result of the therapy. Taken at face value, such behaviour may be indistinguishable from similar behaviour occurring prior to or early in therapy. Optimally, the therapist can distinguish the one from the other.

Trying to appraise accurately the psychological status of patients during out-patient psychotherapy and the risk they pose (to themselves or others) is of crucial importance and may be literally vital. The complexity of this situation, however, presents the therapist with an essential but difficult question: 'Is the patient doing badly or well-enough?' To answer this question, the therapist's countertransference may sometimes provide important clues and represent the most sensitive indicator. However, it is difficult for therapists to be sufficiently confident in such a 'soft' sign, which is so subjective.

Ms Y was serving a long probation order with a condition to attend for treatment following a prison sentence for grievous bodily harm towards a boyfriend during the break-up of their relationship. At the instigation of her probation officer, she had embarked upon psychoanalytic psychotherapy with a male therapist. During the course of this treatment, which was extremely stormy, with frequent temper outbursts during the sessions, she had understood more of the antecedents to her violent attacks on men. Part of this appeared to stem from her relationship with her father, who had been a distant and cool figure during her childhood, only ever showing emotion under extreme provocation from Ms Y. In the therapy, the latter experienced her therapist's silence as being withholding and provocative and she frequently reacted with an angry tirade about how useless he was to her.

In the first year or so of the therapy the therapist felt emotionally battered by the encounters with this patient. He felt Ms Y did not at all value his efforts to understand her. At times he believed that he might be physically attacked but he never was and he did not view her as a particular threat to anybody outside of therapy, her father being by now dead. Towards the end of the second year of therapy Ms Y reported that she had again been violent, this time to a man with whom she had attempted to flirt at a party. He had not risen to her sexually provocative bait, preferring the male company he was keeping.

On hearing of this recent violence, the therapist was initially concerned that Ms Y was deteriorating and viewed her behaviour as evidence that therapy was in fact unhelpful. He thus entertained the idea of contacting Ms Y's probation service urgently to alert them to the recent violence. On further reflection, however, he realized that Ms Y was recounting the violent episode, about which she could have remained silent, without her usual belligerence. He then recalled that he had not felt emotionally abused during the recent weeks, even though Ms Y still displayed her anger for some part of each session. Sensing this to be a benign shift in the transference–countertransference relationship, he ventured to make a comment to Ms Y about the upset she might be feeling behind her obvious anger. She began to weep, sustaining this during a period of her therapist's silence (which itself in the past might have evoked an angry outburst).

Following this session, angry outbursts disappeared from the sessions and Ms Y was regularly in tears about a range of issues past and present. Her therapist felt that he had been right to keep an open mind about the violence, not maintaining his initial conclusion that this necessarily represented a deterioration. He was helped through examining his countertransference reaction, realizing that the patient had developed beneficially in the months leading up to the violent behaviour at the party. It was this which allowed him to avoid mistaking a surface behavioural manifestation of violence for the whole complex picture. (In fact, it transpired that Ms Y's violence had merely been a slap in the face, which she had chosen to exaggerate, fearing that without exaggeration her therapist would not have been interested.) Gradually, in the third year of psychoanalytic psychotherapy, Ms Y was freer to accept that she could not control the emotions of others to the extent that she wanted to. She felt less angry and was not violent. Eventually, even the emotional provocation posed by the ending of the therapy did not evoke an aggressive response.

This example demonstrates the potential utility of an examination of the therapist's countertransference reaction as part of a transference–countertransference relationship, to help decide whether the overall trend is towards personality integration or not. It would have been relatively easy for Ms Y's therapist, given the regularity of his patient's angry outbursts, simply to construe her violent behaviour as deterioration and a lack of any psychological maturation. He might even have terminated therapy, as if the violence had been simply what it appeared to be. If he had not been aware of the dynamics in the relationship with Ms Y, his interventions, and hence the outcome of therapy, would therefore have been quite different. A face valid construing of the violent behaviour may itself have led to more violence because of a weakened therapeutic alliance caused by his failure to recognize the progress Ms Y had made and the lack of accurate empathy which this implied. Empathic failure, based on the therapist's past experience of this patient, would have inflamed her and increased the likelihood of further violent behaviour. To utilize the countertransference reaction therapeutically, however, requires not only a grounding in the relevant theory but also supervised practice in its application. To this end, a personal experience of psychoanalytic psychotherapy is useful.

Therapists should maintain a low threshold for asking for consultation or supervision, especially where the risk of violence is known to be high and/or when countertransference reactions are problematic—whether negative or positive (Gunderson and Sabo 1993). As part of a strategy for identifying and managing risk, therapists also need to bear in mind the patient's psychosocial environment and also their own professional environment, including the security of the consulting room used, *at the time* it is used. The former can be assessed by involving family members or friends to provide support or information and sometimes both. The latter (i.e. other professionals) may need to be alerted to any change in the perceived level of dangerousness or be involved in providing supervision, further treatment or custodial care.

Assuming there has been relevant prior communication, both the patient and others can be involved in trying to make the distinction between regression and deterioration in collaboration and within a climate of enquiry rather than interrogation. This means that the patient's propensity to be aggressively defensive can be minimized. Nevertheless, many patients will not have an investment in collaborating with their therapist in pursuing this clarificatory task. The former may have reoffended and be unwilling to divulge relevant information for fear of a custodial disposal. Others external to the therapy may therefore need to be contacted and asked for relevant information regarding anti-social or criminal behaviour and attitudes as part of a previously agreed procedure or contract (see above). Where there is regression, as opposed to deterioration, the patient may be able to divulge information, especially when the possibility of reoffending as part of regression has been discussed during the assessment phase. Although the therapist's countertransference may be the most reliable indicator with which to distinguish regression from deterioration, this subjective marker should not be taken in isolation and considered sufficient (i.e. separately from other evidence deriving from others inhabiting the patient's external world), especially in forensic patients with a history of serious violence or parasuicidal activity.

It can be important for therapists to convene a case conference of all relevant parties in order to establish more completely the patient's actual state of affairs. In this way different elements from the patient's internal and external worlds can be brought together with the aim of arriving at a more objective view.

Terminating therapy

How therapy ends will depend upon many variables, in particular whether the patient has changed for the better or not. If treatment success is the reason for considering termination, the usual therapeutic considerations will apply, in terms of issues likely to be reawakened and needing to be addressed in relation to the ending. Thus past losses or privations may be rekindled and resurface during this phase. A range of guises may be assumed which can be manifest variously, within sessions, between them and in terms of the transference–countertransference relationship. Sufficient time needs to be set aside to process adequately relevant aspects, especially when the therapeutic relationship has been a long one. Since the patient's initial presentation involved anti-social or other law-breaking behaviour there is a risk of its returning or threatening to return during the terminal phase, as if to undo the beneficial effect of the psychotherapeutic work. It may therefore be that there is an unspoken or even unconscious invitation to collude with the patient's view that little or nothing has been achieved (as with Ms Y).

Even though such 'normal' terminations with SPD patients can be difficult to deal with, terminations due to failure make it likely that the ending will be much more problematic. Failure, however defined, will inevitably be accompanied by negative feelings for both therapist and patient. Dealing with such feelings serves to increase the amount of anxiety within the therapist–patient system and this increases the likelihood of destructive 'acting out' by the patient. Assessing the size of the risk of a dangerous enactment is thus important. However, it may be difficult to undertake objectively on account of the high levels of anxiety. Again, information from others external to the clinical situation may need to be sought to reduce uncertainty, hence to lower anxiety, in order to assess accurately the risk (see above).

Termination due to a change in external circumstances, including that initiated by the therapist, can provoke the resurfacing of issues concerning past traumatic losses. Depending upon its stage within therapy, and the degree of notice of it, there may be a risk of serious enactment, as when there is obvious therapeutic failure. The shorter the notice of the ending or period of therapy to process the relevant leaving issues, the more the termination is likely to be damaging to the patient or others. Other professionals may need to be involved to provide a continuation of therapy, to aid with termination via providing support, for instance by the initiating of supportive psychotherapy to prevent deterioration. Sometimes professionals external to the clinical situation, because of their statutory responsibilities, will need to know that the particular SPD patient is no longer receiving treatment. They may need to act in accordance with the dictates of the legal framework, for example, to recall the patient into custody or to some other 'secure' destination.

Relationship of out-patient to in-patient psychotherapy

Failure of out-patient psychotherapy may be one indicator of referral to in-patient (or day hospital) psychotherapy (Norton and Hinshelwood 1996). However, it may not be so much that treatment itself has failed but that the risks associated with its continuing are considered too high. In such a circumstance referral to a unit specializing in the psychological treatment of SPD patients might be properly entertained. Specialist psychotherapy units, at least in the UK, are few in number. Partly on account of the scarcity of such resources therefore, and partly upon clinical grounds, they are selective, choosing those SPD patients most likely to benefit. Criteria suggesting good outcome include some educational success, relationship stability, employment record (Whiteley 1970) or the patient's memory of a confiding relationship during childhood (Healy and Kennedy 1993).

Having SPD patients as day patients or in-patients confers certain advantages over the out-patient setting. Both individual and group treatments can be more safely deployed because of the ready availability of support and supervision. Consolidating a therapeutic alliance between patient and staff may be more achievable. In some specialist SPD units, there is no individual psychotherapy and all therapy is delivered via a range of group meetings (Norton 1992; Wilberg et al. 1998; Campling 1999). In other units there is a range of individual and group treatments (Muir 1986).

Another advantage over out-patient psychotherapy for SPD offender patients is the potential for monitoring the patient between the formal psychotherapy sessions and also for setting up a network of communication (about patients' attitudes and behaviour) during this social time (Norton 1997). What insight is gained from the psychotherapy can be put into practice during the social time (Mahony 1979). Such 'experimentation' can yield more material for discussion and verbal feedback in the formal psychotherapy programme and lead to further exploration, insight and experimentation (Whiteley 1986).

This process of interacting, exploring and experimenting is emotionally arduous and the SPD patient's peer group is required to support as well as to challenge and confront maladaptive attitudes and behaviour (see Fig. 8.2). A highly structured treatment programme, which provides alternatives to 'acting out', as well as a sophisticated

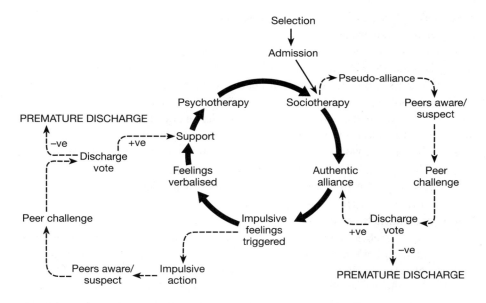

Fig. 8.2 In-patient sociotherapeutic and psychotherapeutic processes.

system of responding to emergencies occasioned by violence or untoward emotional events, is required in order to assess and manage risk to ensure that this complex treatment environment remains sufficiently containing and safe (Norton 1997).

Deploying a single, albeit complex treatment intervention (which blends psychotherapy with sociotherapy, i.e. the exploitation of the non-treatment and unstructured 'social' time for therapeutic gain) means that staff can become more expert at it than they could be if they were dealing simultaneously with different approaches to an heterogeneous patient population within a single setting. The greater degree of consistency which this affords in terms of treatment delivery allows patients to feel that they are in a predictable environment which is also sensitive and responsive to their needs.

Predictability and responsiveness encourages the development of trust and enhances the patient's self-esteem (Norris 1983). This leads to a greater containment of anxiety than is usually possible in the out-patient setting. Less ambivalent attitudes towards treatment in general, and professionals in particular, slowly follow. This is especially so when the staff delegate aspects of their usual power and authority to their patients as part of the treatment programme. The latter are thus enabled to take charge of some treatment as well as some day-to-day matters pertaining to the running of the unit, for example shopping for food, preparing and cooking it. Such a treatment regime is aptly termed the 'therapeutic community' (Main 1946; Jones 1952). Within such an environment, through an enhancement of the therapeutic alliance, deeper exploration of relevant issues (for example concerning sexual abuse and violence), as perpetrators and/or victims, can ensue.

Working in prolonged contact with SPD in-patients, especially within a residential setting, is demanding. As in the out-patient setting, issues concerning countertransference, its understanding and potential benefit to therapy, are of central importance (Gabbard 1986). The task is for staff to sustain such reactions, in order to understand their significance for the patient rather than to dismiss or otherwise relegate them in importance (Rosenbluth 1991). Since the reactions are usually, but by no means always, negative (Yeomans 1993), this may be hard to do. In the specialist in-patient situation support and supervision is provided which encourages the ventilation of countertransference reactions with the idea of harnessing the insights derived to the therapeutic needs of the patient. How this is enacted varies from unit to unit (Gabbard 1988; Norton and Hinshelwood 1996).

One of the beneficial consequences of sustaining countertransference reactions is that the intensely held opposing or complementary views of different members of the staff involved (multi-disciplinary or multi-agency) can be observed. This is the first step. It allows further evaluation of these views so that their potential significance for the patient, to whom such views apply, can be ascertained. The second step is for staff to understand their shared patient more completely via this interpersonal, and frequently polarizing, enactment. This second step is difficult to achieve and may not occur, even within the specialist setting. The staff may identify 'splitting' but not attempt or succeed at the next step. When this is so, they fail to convert that which is so intellectually constraining into something creative and in the interests of both the patient and staff.

The out-patient psychotherapist may need to know about the specialist psychotherapy environment since it often differs markedly from that of a traditional psychiatric hospital (Norton 1992). It is important for the out-patient therapist to understand something of the specialist regime, its method and rationale, to ensure that some consistency prevails. This enables the transition from day or in-patient to be as smooth as possible. Following successful therapy, the SPD patient may be able to use rather than misuse the out-patient psychotherapeutic service; indeed, such appropriate usage may itself be a marker of successful specialist treatment.

Patients may leave prematurely from the specialist setting. In such a situation a careful risk assessment should form part of any decision to offer out-patient psychotherapy. The focus of the out-patient work can be re-referral to the same specialist service so that the difficulties encountered, which led to the premature termination, can be tackled thereby making a second specialist admission more likely to succeed. Indeed, preparing offender patients for admission or readmission to a specialist SPD treatment unit may itself be an appropriate, albeit limited, goal of out-patient psychotherapy.

Conclusions

The level of risk posed by many mentally disordered offender out-patients is related, in part, to the amount of anxiety to which they are exposed during and outside therapy. This is because elevated anxiety levels impair their adaptive interpersonal and social functioning, through taxing their usual coping strategies and increasing their overall defensiveness, including that expressed as violent behaviour. Such high anxiety may derive from: sources internal to them; the interpersonal situation (including that of the out-patient psychotherapy); and aspects in their wider external world. Therefore, to an extent, the out-patient management of SPD patients is an exercise in identifying and managing anxiety (both within the system of the therapist–patient interaction and within the wider 'supra-system') so as to maximize the patients' healthy psychological state, while minimizing their risk to others.

Identifying and managing anxiety (emotional containment) is a standard part of a psychodynamic approach to patient care. The wider societal need for containment of mentally disordered offenders, therefore, is not necessarily at odds with that of the psychotherapeutic transaction nor, in some instances, with the personal wishes of the individual patient. Patients may be aware of feelings of being out of control and uncontainable, on account of an incapacity to curb their impulsive urges. Often, however, they will be ambivalent about asking for help and mistrustful of professionals.

Before the anxiety can be managed it must be identified. It may not always be obviously present during the clinical interaction, being manifest elsewhere in time and place, including in the wider interpersonal environment of patient and therapist. Therefore, it may reveal itself indirectly through the behaviour of others who, unwittingly, may undermine treatment. In order to locate the anxiety, the psychotherapist needs to monitor continually both the clinical transaction with the patient and also the other interpersonal transactions which impinge upon it.

Monitoring relationships external to the clinical transaction requires communication with relevant individuals from the patient's and therapist's respective professional and social networks. These 'others' not only represent sources of information about the patient's mental state, attitudes towards therapy and any anti-social attitudes or behaviour, but may also enact aspects of the patient's inner world. Their co-operation and support is often needed therefore to preserve therapy, through facilitating the patient to gain a better understanding of its aims and methods, to obtain a more complete understanding of the patient's internal world, and to maximize the safety of all involved.

The therapist's examination of his or her countertransference, a standard part of psychodynamic psychotherapy, may also be an important ingredient of other therapies deployed within the out-patient setting. Certain episodes of overt behavioural disturbance may be better understood through an examination of the overall trend, over time, in the countertransference reactions to a particular SPD patient. They can contribute to an accurate answer to the question of whether there is a clinically useful regression or whether there is deterioration. However, it must be emphasized that evidence from the countertransference represents but one of a number of relevant sources of information. Information from as many sources as possible, including from the wider interpersonal environments of the patient and therapist, needs to be collected and sifted in order to complement such subjective evidence.

The establishing of an authentic therapeutic alliance may enable an appropriate referral to a specialist day or in-patient unit which deals with SPD patients. Such units have some advantages over the out-patient setting; for example, they can deploy individual, group and family treatments with a degree of safety that is not achievable outside. Their staff can become expert at the specialism and derive support and education particularly in the area of identifying and creatively using countertransference information. Successful specialist treatment may lead to SPD patients who can use, rather than abuse, out-patient services.

Acknowledgements

We wish to thank Rob Hale, Maggie Hilton and Martin Wrench for helpful comments on an earlier draft of this chapter and to remind readers that the personal and clinical details of all patients and therapists referred to have been disguised so as to make them, in effect, fictional.

References

Beck, A. T. , Freeman, A. and associates (1990) *Cognitive therapy of personality disorders.* New York: The Guilford Press.

Bowlby, W. R. (1973) *Attachment and loss, Vol. 2, Separation: anxiety and anger.* New York: Basic Books.

Brooke, R. (1994) Assessment for psychotherapy: clinical indicators of self-cohesion and self pathology. *British Journal of Psychotherapy,* **10,** 317–30.

Campling, P (1999) Chaotic Personalities: maintaining the therapeutic alliance. In *Therapeutic communities: past, present and future* (ed. P. Campling and R. Haigh). London: Jessica Kingsley.

Davies, R. (1995) The inter-disciplinary network and the internal world of the offender.

In *Forensic psychotherapy* (ed. C. Cordess and M. Cox). London: Jessica Kingsley.

Erikson, E. H. (1959) Growth and crises of the healthy personality. In *Identity and the life cycle: psychological issues.* New York: International University Press.

Fonagy, P. (1991) Thinking about thinking: some clinical and theoretical considerations in the treatment of a borderline patient. *International Journal of Psychoanalysis,* 7(2), 63–9.

Frank, A. F. (1991) The therapeutic alliances of borderline patients. In *Borderline personality disorder: clinical and empirical perspectives* (ed. J. Clarkin, E. Marziali and H. Munroe-Blum). New York: Guildford.

Freud, A. (1936) *The ego and the mechanisms of defense.* New York: International University Press.

Gabbard, G. O. (1986) The special hopsital patient. *International Review of Psychoanalysis,* **13,** 333–47.

Gabbard, G. O. (1988) A contemporary perspective on psychoanalytically informed hospital treatment. *Hospital Community Psychiatry,* **39,** 1291–5.

Gunderson, J. and Sabo, A. N. (1993) Treatment of borderline personality disorder: a critical review. In *Borderline personality disorder: etiology and treatment* (ed. J. Paris).Washington, DC: American Psychiatric Press.

Hartland, S. (1991) Supportive psychotherapy. In *Textbook of psychotherapy in psychiatric practice* (ed. J. Holmes). London: Churchill Livingstone.

Healey, K. and Kennedy, R. (1993) Which families benefit from in-patient psychotherapuetic work at the Cassel Hospital? *British Journal of Psychotherapy*, 9, 394–404.

Holmes, J. (1999) Psychotherapeutic approaches to the management of severe personalilty disorder in general psychiatric settings. Rila Publications, *CPD Bulletin Psychiatry*, 1(2), 29–68.

Horwitz, L. (1974) *Clinical prediction in psychotherapy.* New York: Jason Aronson.

Horwitz, L. (1987) Indication for group psychotherapy with borderline and narcissistic patients. *Bulletin of the Menninger Clinic*, 52(3), 248–60.

Jones, M. (1952) *Social psychiatry.* London: Tavistock.

Kernberg, O. (1984) *Severe personality disorders: psychotherapeutic strategies.* New Haven, London: Yale University Press.

Kohut, J. (1971) *The analysis of the self.* New York: International Universities Press.

Linehan, M. M. (1992) Cognitive–behavioural treatment for borderline personality disorder: the dialectics of effective treatment. New York: Guilford.

Lockwood, G. (1992) Psychoanalysis and the cognitive therapy of personality disorders. *Journal of Cognitive Psychotherapy*, 6, 25–42.

Mahony, N. (1979) My stay and change at the Henderson Therapeutic Community. In *Therapeutic communities: reflections and progress* (ed. R. D. Hinshelwood and N. Manning). London: Routledge and Kegan Paul.

Main, R. (1957) The ailment. *British Journal of Medical Psychology*, 30, 129–45. Reprinted in Main, T. (1989) *The ailment and other psycho-analytic essays.* London: Free Association Books.

Main, T. F. (1946) The hospital as a therapeutic institution. *Bulletin of the Menninger Clinic*, 19, 66–70.

Meloy, J. R. (1988) *The psychopathic mind: origins, dynamics and treatment.* New Jersey: Jason Aronson, Inc.

Miller, L. J. (1990) The formal treatment contract in the inpatient management of borderline personality disorder. *Hospital and Community Psychiatry*, 41(9), 985–7.

Muir, B. (1986) Is in-patient psychotherapy a valid concept? In The family as in-patient: families and adolescents at the Cassel Hospital (ed. R. Kennedy, A. Heymans and F. Tischler). London: Free Association Books.

Norton, K. R.W. (1996) Management of difficulty personality disorder patients. *Advances in Psychiatric Treatment*, 2, 202–10.

Norton, K. R.W. and Hinshelwood, R. (1996) Severe personality disorder: treatment issues and selection for in-patient psychotherapy. *British Journal of Psychiatry*, 168, 723–31.

Norton, K. R.W. (1997) In the prison of severe personality disorder. *The Journal of Forensic Psychiatry*, 8(2), 285–98.

Norton, K. R.W. and McGauley, G. (1998) *Counselling Difficult Clients.* London: Sage.

Norton, K. R.W. (1995) Personality disordered forensic patients and the therapeutic community. In *Forensic psychotherapy* (ed. C. Cordess. C. and M. Cox). London: Jessica Kingsley.

Norton, K. R.W. (1997) Inpatient psychotherapy: integrating the other 23 hours. *Current Medical Literature—Psychiatry*, 8(2), 31–7.

Norton, K. R.W. (1992) Personality disordered individuals: the Henderson Hospital model of treatment. *Criminal Behaviour and Mental Health*, 2, 80–191.

Norris, M. (1983) Changes in patients during treatment at Henderson Hospital Therapeutic Community during 1977–1981. *British Journal of Medical Psychology*, 56, 135–43.

Rockland, L. H. (1989) *Supportive psychotherapy: a psychodynamic approach*. New York: Basic Books.

Rosenbluth, M. (1991) New uses of countertransference for the in-patient treatment of borderline personality disorder. *Canadian Journal of Psychiatry*, 36, 280–84.

Ryle, A. and Marlow, M. (1995) Cognitive analytic therapy of borderline personality disorder: theory, practice, and the clinical and research uses of the self states sequential diagram. *International Journal of Short-Term Psychotherapy*, 10, 21–34.

Singer, M. (1987) Inpatient hospitalization for borderline patients—process and dynamics of change in long- and short-term treatment. In *The borderline patient* (Ed. J. Grotstein, M. Soloman and J. Lang). New Jersey: Analytic Press.

Stanton, A. H. and Schwartz, M. S. (1954) *The mental hospital*. New York: Basic Books.

Tyrer, P. (1988) London, Wright.

Tyrer, P. and Johnson, T. (1996)*Personality disorder, diagnosis, management and care*. Establishing the severity of personality disorder. *American Journal of Psychiatry*, 153, 1593–7.

Wilbert T., Karterud, S., Urnes, O., Pederson, G. and Friis, S. (1998) Outcomes of poorly functioning patients with personality disorders in a day treatment program. *Psychiatric Services*, 49(11).

Winnicott, D. W. (1965) The theory of the parent–infant relationship. In *The maturational processes and the facilitating environment: studies in the theory of emotional development*. (ed. D. W. Winnicott). London: The Hogarth Press and the Institute of Psychoanalysis.

Whiteley, J. S. (1986) Sociotherapy and psychotherapy in the treatment of personality disorder. Discussion paper. *Journal of the Royal Society of Medicine*, 79, 721–5.

Yeomans, F. (1993) When a therapist over-indulges a demanding borderline patient. *Hospital and Community Psychiatry*, 44, 334–6.

Young, J. (1990) *Cognitive therapy for personality disorders: a scheme-focused approach*. Sarasota, FL: Professional Resources Exchange.

Chapter 9

Involuntary out-patient commitment in the USA: practice and controversy

Marvin S. Swartz and Jeffrey W. Swanson

Introduction

In almost every community in the USA, a population of severely mentally ill (SMI) individuals can be identified who manifest complex problems in multiple areas of life and who come into contact with a variety of public agencies and institutions—including community mental health centres, public hospitals, substance abuse treatment programs, civil and criminal courts, police, jails and prisons, emergency medical facilities, social welfare agencies, and public housing authorities (see the reviews by Geller 1992; Schalock *et al.* 1995; Osher and Drake 1996; Borum *et al.* 1997). The growth of this SMI sub-population, often termed 'revolving door patients', is attributable to increasingly restrictive criteria for involuntary in-patient commitment, limited availability of effective in-patient care, a paucity of effective community-based services and lack of other needed community supports. Many of these patients derive little benefit from low-intensity or office-based treatment programs because they often do not adhere to medication regimens or keep scheduled appointments, may abuse substances, and tend to live in impoverished, dangerous environments with inadequate social support.

The revolving door syndrome is a vicious cycle for patients and families, but also mental health systems, because state and local governments must often continue to fund in-patient programs to the detriment of aggressive, outreach-based treatment. Strategies to enhance treatment adherence in community-based mental health programs, such as court-ordered community treatment or involuntary out-patient commitment (OPC), have gained increasing interest as a means to reduce relapse, reduce hospitalizations and enhance the effectiveness of out-patient care (Swartz *et al.* 1995; Swanson *et al.* 1997).

Violence among individuals with SMI in the community has also become an increasing focus of concern among clinicians, policy makers, and the general public, often as a result of rare, but highly publicized violent acts committed by SMI individuals (Mulvey 1994; Monahan *et al.* 1994; Torrey 1994). Efforts to reduce violence risk by SMI individuals in the community have focused on a variety of interventions, including OPC, designed to improve treatment adherence and thereby reduce violence

(Hiday and Scheid-Cook 1991; Torrey 1994; Swartz *et al.* 1995; Buchanan and David 1994). This chapter discusses the USA experience with OPC, the controversy surrounding coercion in out-patient treatment, and the empirical evidence of the effects of OPC on treatment outcomes.

The statutory background of involuntary out-patient commitment

Involuntary OPC is a legal intervention intended to benefit SMI individuals who need ongoing psychiatric care and support to prevent relapse and hospital readmissions, but who are reluctant to or have difficulty following through with community-based treatment. Virtually all states in the USA permit some form of court-mandated mental health treatment in out-patient care settings. Thirty-eight states and the District of Columbia have explicit OPC statutes, while half a dozen states are currently considering enacting or modifying existing OPC legislation (McCafferty and Dooley 1990; Hiday 1992; Swartz *et al.* 1995; Torrey and Kaplan 1995). OPC has also been enacted or is being considered in several other countries including Israel, Canada and the UK.

OPC should be distinguished from other mechanisms for court-mandated treatment including conditional release or guardianship. Under conditional release, an involuntarily committed patient is released to community care under the ongoing supervision of the hospital. Most patients remain on the hospital census, often for 90 or more days, and may be returned to the hospital if functioning poorly, at risk for relapse or non-adherent with treatment. As a result, this mechanism for mandated treatment is usually restricted to previously hospitalized and involuntarily committed patients. A limited number of naturalistic studies of conditional release indicate that it does appear to be effective in reducing rehospitalization and violent behaviour (O'Keefe *et al.* 1997). Under guardianship the court appoints a guardian for a patient adjudicated to be incompetent. The guardian consents to treatment for the patient who then may be compelled to adhere to treatment, including forced medication and hospitalization. Geller *et al.* (1998) found that mandated treatment under guardianship appeared to reduce rehospitalizations and total hospital days.

OPC currently has at least three variants: a variant of conditional release for involuntarily hospitalized patients, an alternative to involuntary hospitalization for patients who meet in-patient commitment criteria, and an alternative for patients who do not meet criteria for in-patient commitment but are at risk for decompensation without treatment. This latter, lower threshold variant of OPC allows for a preventative form of OPC. In all but a small minority of US states, however, the criteria for commitment to OPC are identical to in-patient commitment criteria, limiting the preventative use of OPC.

Theoretically, OPC permits increased autonomy in a less restrictive community environment, while monitoring compliance and early signs of regression. OPC thus can exercise the two powers or duties of the state embodied in civil commitment:

parens patriae, the duty to care for the gravely disabled and police powers, the duty to prevent harm. Although OPC is sanctioned by most US states, its use and application varies dramatically between and within states (Fernandez and Nygard 1990; Swartz *et al.* 1995), in part due to poor operationalization of commitment criteria, weak enforcement mechanisms, and concerns on the part of providers that the legal directive of responsibility for particular patients could increase legal liability should treatment go awry (Appelbaum 1986). In some states, OPC laws lack explicit enforcement mechanisms for treatment non-adherence and, when required, enforcement often requires burdensome paperwork and staff effort (Torrey and Kaplan 1995). Another pervasive problem is simply the lack of resources for effective treatment. As one critic of OPC has put it succinctly: 'There are simply not enough community services to which people can be involuntarily committed' (Fulop 1995).

Out-patient commitment orders typically require compliance with recommended out-patient treatment, i.e. keeping scheduled appointments with a mental health provider. Some OPC statutes, as in North Carolina, stop short of permitting forced medication of legally competent individuals. In every jurisdiction OPC orders are of limited duration. In North Carolina, a psychiatrist may recommend to the court that an individual be placed on OPC initially not longer than 90 days, after which a hearing must be held to renew the order for up to 180 days. When a person under OPC fails to comply with treatment, the responsible clinician may request that law officers transport the individual to an out-patient facility for persuasion to accept treatment or evaluation for in-patient commitment. Some clinicians are reluctant to petition for OPC because they perceive that its enforcement 'lacks teeth' and it usually does not allow forced medications. However, patients in a North Carolina study believed the law legally required medication adherence and believed non-compliance could result in strong sanctions (Borum *et al.* 1999).

The existing North Carolina OPC statute (NC General Statute, Section 122S) was modified in 1984 to allow less restrictive use of mandated out-patient treatment. Criteria for OPC in North Carolina now include: the presence of serious mental illness, the capacity to survive in the community with available supports, a clinical history indicating a need for treatment to prevent deterioration that would predictably result in dangerousness, and a mental status that limits or negates the individual's ability to make informed decisions to seek or to comply voluntarily with recommended treatment. This latter criterion may suggest the requirement of evidence of a lack of capacity to consent to treatment, but the legislative intent was simply to emphasize evidence of non-compliance in the presence of a serious mental illness (Swartz *et al.* 1997). While similar to other states in encouraging OPC as a less restrictive alternative to hospitalization, North Carolina is unusual in lowering the threshold for OPC to allow its use as a preventive measure to avert relapse and hospitalization (Swartz *et al.* 1995). A recent pilot statute tested in New York City includes similar criteria allowing preventative interventions (Steadman *et al.* 1999).

Understanding how out-patient commitment works

Many policy makers treat OPC as a 'black box', assuming the key issue is its effectiveness regardless of its putative mechanism of action. Swanson *et al.* (1997) proposed an empirically testable conceptual model of OPC in an effort to 'unpack' OPC's potential mechanisms of action. The conceptual model depicted in Fig. 9.1 incorporates several mechanisms by which OPC may improve treatment outcomes for people with SMI. The primary independent variable in this model is the court order to comply with out-patient treatment (OPC), i.e. a formal, legally sanctioned use of coercion applied to the behaviour of mentally ill individuals. However, the model also assumes that other (less formal) coercive influences may act simultaneously (along with the formal coercive force of OPC), to shape the behaviour of patients, care givers, clinicians, case managers and service systems as well.

The model suggests that OPC may exert its primary direct effect on the adherence behaviour of the patient through threat of force to be applied if the individual fails to comply with a regimen of out-patient treatment as mandated by the court. By changing adherence behaviour, however, OPC may produce an indirect effect in any or all of the variables represented in the latter stages of the model. That is, improved compliance should lead to increased mobilization of community mental health

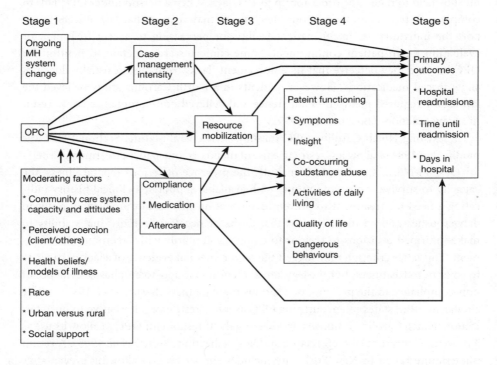

Fig. 9.1 Conceptual model of direct and indirect effects of OPC.

resources and supportive services on the client's behalf (Stage 3), which may then produce improvement in the patient's overall functioning (Stage 4), i.e. decreased psychiatric symptomatology and comorbid substance abuse, improvements in self-care skills, improved quality of life, and reduced dangerousness. These changes in patient functioning should, finally, be evident in decreased hospital readmissions, increased time to readmission and a reduction in total days in the hospital.

Hence, by these pathways, OPC exerts key effects through improved patient compliance with medications and aftercare. However, an equally plausible mechanism—and not a mutually exclusive one—posits that OPC succeeds through the intensification of clinician or case management activity. Here, the model suggests that the court order *stimulates the service system* to engage the patient in treatment through more aggressive follow-up. These intensified efforts may also act as a lever to mobilize resources on the patient's behalf—which may, in turn, lead to improvements in the patient's social function, and eventually to decreased reliance on repeated hospitalization. Also testable is a reciprocal relationship between case management intensity and compliance, whereby the case manager increases or decreases his/her efforts in response to the patient's varying level of compliance.

The conceptual model also proposes a set of moderating factors, which may alter the relationship between OPC and various outcomes. For example, the effects of OPC on rehospitalizations may be greater for severely mentally ill sub-groups known to be especially non-compliant and/or underserved: racial and ethnic minority groups, rural residents, those who do not view themselves as mentally ill or needing treatment, and those with poor social supports. Additional moderating factors include the capacity of relevant community care systems, providers' attitudes towards coercive treatment, and perceptions of coercion on the part of the patient.

In sum, the model shown in Fig. 9.1 suggests three central ideas as a framework for debate about the potential effectiveness of OPC: (1) reduced hospital utilization is a *distal* outcome removed from OPC by several key intervening variables, or *proximal* outcomes, and is also likely to be affected by external systemic factors and secular trends; (2) in OPC, coercion acts with dual prongs—applying the power of law to mandate individuals' compliance with treatment, but also creating an obligation for case managers, clinicians, care givers and the mental health system in general to facilitate treatment; (3) at some level, OPC presupposes that community-based mental health programmes have the wherewithal to enforce commitment orders, provide adequate direct services and mobilize other supportive and therapeutic resources in the community.

Readmission to a mental hospital is perhaps the most commonly studied outcome variable in mental health services research (Kent et al. 1995). While often oversimplified as a proxy measure of illness relapse or treatment failure, the meaning of hospital use for a conceptual model of OPC is more complex. Ideally, the effects of OPC on hospital utilization should be specified using several different measures: time until readmission, average length of stay, total number of admissions, and total number of in-patient days within a given period. As discussed below, in examining the empirical studies of OPC, this conceptual model is being tested in a randomized trial of OPC in North Carolina (Swartz *et al.* 1995). However, before proceeding to empirical evidence, a discussion of the controversy surrounding OPC in the USA will help put the evidence in context.

Controversy about coerced treatment

Despite the potential effectiveness of OPC in reducing involuntary in-patient treatment, many mental health consumers and mental health law advocates oppose any coercion in out-patient treatment, arguing that it broadly infringes on civil liberties and alienates mental health consumers from treatment (Mulvey *et al.* 1987; Schwartz and Costanzo 1987; Stefan 1987; Swartz *et al.* 1997).

Proponents of OPC assert that it works by exerting reasonable pressure on two sets of actors, in two important ways: (1) as a lever on the individual behaviour of persons with mental illness—motivating adherence to treatment under threat of coercion and greater confinement; (2) as a lever on the mental health service system—mobilizing supportive services, outreach and clinical surveillance, thus improving timely access to scarce treatment resources for persons most in need, including hospitalization when necessary. In theory, OPC provides greater autonomy than would otherwise be enjoyed by a segment of the population with SMI at risk for dangerous relapse and rehospitalization. Viewed most optimistically, insofar as OPC effectively reduces hospitalization in this population at risk, it should conserve resources for reinvestment to extend and improve community-based services (Swartz *et al.* 1995; Swanson *et al.* 1997). Nonetheless, as the comments from both sides of the issue illustrate, the intensity of the debate about OPC is considerable:

> [The] medication militia ... have embarked on a deadly Chemical Crusade to forcibly inject many of us—especially homeless and African Americans—with these powerful neurotoxins, sometimes for life ... IOC [Involuntary Out-patient Commitment] is literally fascism ... a profound violation of core values of liberty and freedom (Support Coalition website—www.efn.org/~dendron)

> People recover when they have choice among alternative treatments and services, when they are empowered to make their own decisions and take responsibility for their lives, and when they are offered hope. These conditions are impossible under out-patient commitment (Coalition to Stop Out-patient Commitment website—www.madnation.org)

> Civil libertarians have made it almost impossible to treat psychotic individuals who refuse care. These misguided activists have created a morass of legal obstacles that prevents us from helping many psychotic individuals until they have a finger on a trigger or have attempted suicide ... It's time to reverse course. Mandatory treatment for those too ill to recognize they need help is far more humane than our present mandatory nontreatment. The legal standard for assisted treatment should be the need for medical care, not dangerousness. Society should save people from degradation, not just death. Our law enforcement officials should not be the frontline caregivers for those Americans trapped by psychoses (Torrey and Zdanowicz 1999)

We prevent people suffering from Alzheimer's disease from living on the streets because we understand they have a brain disorder that prevents them from sufficiently caring for themselves. We mandate assisted treatment for individuals with tuberculosis who refuse to take medication because we understand they are potentially dangerous to other people. People suffering from the debilitating effects of neurobiological brain disorders deserve no less. Out-patient commitment programs ... will enable thousands ... once held hostage by their disease to escape their symptoms and enjoy real recovery (Jaffe 1998)

If adequate community care resources were available, it is quite likely that coercive intervention would not be necessary. By offering real support in the community, many of the problems which preventive out-patient commitment is supposed to solve could be remedied through voluntary participation (Tavolaro 1992)

It is important to try to gain a better understanding of the actors in this debate—and the sources of their conflict—if OPC is to be applied in a manner that is measured, warranted, broadly acceptable and ultimately beneficial to key stakeholders. Opponents argue that coerced out-patient treatment infringes on civil liberties, damages the self esteem of persons with mental illness, undermines therapeutic relationships, and ultimately drives people away from needed services and treatment (Mulvey *et al.* 1987; Schwartz and Costanzo 1987; Stefan 1987; Campbell and Schraiber 1989). Proponents of OPC argue that what is regarded as 'coercive' depends largely on the frame of reference: compared to voluntary treatment, OPC is coercive; compared to involuntary hospitalization, OPC diminishes coercion. Moreover, they argue that the loss of autonomy under OPC must be compared to the limited autonomy enjoyed by SMI individuals in many areas of life, the sense of having little say in what happens, the feeling of being too dependent on others, the fear of being vulnerable to harm, or of being abandoned when help is needed. Whether—and under what conditions—various sorts of limits on autonomy are harmful, necessary, beneficial or simply unavoidable, is a discussion at the heart of the OPC controversy.

Clearly, evidence of whether OPC 'works' should be an important consideration in these debates. However, objections on principle to OPC on the part of many patients, legal advocates and clinicians could trump the scientific evidence about its effectiveness or lack thereof. Many stakeholders view involuntary treatment as an unmitigated harm and wrong, while others may perceive it as a benefit. At a December 1997 conference on Involuntary intervention and coerced treatment of people with mental health disorders, organized by the US Substance Abuse and Mental Health Services Administration (SAMHSA) and Center for Mental Health Services (CMHS), key stakeholders voiced sharply contrary interests, suggested dissimilar research priorities and recommended disparate policy goals relevant to concerns about involuntary treatment. The meeting's 'executive summary' states that 'while there was substantial disagreement on whether involuntary treatment should ever be provided, the group agreed that problems and abuses occur in the current system and that change is desirable' (Mancuso 1997).

Patients

A prime exemplar of patient opposition to OPC that is organized and vocal (if perhaps not broadly representative) is the Coalition to Stop Out-patient Commitment in New York State, with endorsements to date from 24 US mental health consumer organizations. Citing respected civil-libertarian legal scholars (e.g. Stefan 1987), the coalition states its case as follows:

> Out-patient commitment means that people who have committed no crime and who do not meet the standards for in-patient commitment can be told where and with whom they may live, how they must spend their days, and what drugs they must take ... Coercion is bad for people's mental health ... It can result in damage to self-esteem and motivation for recovery and the re-triggering of problems associated with past violence and abuse ... Out-patient commitment is not effective ... Out-patient commitment interferes with people's right to choice ... Rather than put scarce resources into a coercive program that hasn't been proven effective, the Coalition favors increasing voluntary access to a range of services that promote recovery and rehabilitation. People with psychiatric diagnoses must be free to choose among respectfully provided services that genuinely meet their needs (excerpts from statement of Coalition to Stop Out-patient Commitment—www.madnation.org)

Family members

The families of persons with severe mental illness bring a different perspective to the OPC debate, insofar as they bear the strain of caring for loved ones with disabling psychiatric conditions exacerbated by lack of treatment. Families represented by the National Alliance for the Mentally Ill (NAMI) have opposed OPC in the past, but in 1995 offered qualified endorsement:

> NAMI recognizes that involuntary out-patient commitment is a serious infringement on the personal autonomy of individuals with severe brain disorders and therefore takes the position that it should be considered only under extreme circumstances when other interventions are not available or appropriate (NAMI 1995)

More recently, however, NAMI former Executive Director Laurie Flynn affirmed OPC in stronger terms, after two Capitol police officers were shot to death in 1998 by a man diagnosed with schizophrenia who reportedly was not receiving treatment at the time. Consumer groups accuse Flynn of using the fear of violence as a flashpoint to focus media and public attention on the most extreme and rare consequences that may follow lack of treatment for psychotic illness, and thereby to justify coercive treatment as benevolent protection—as when Flynn refers to 'what families already know ... the agony of wanting to help loved ones with severe, untreated mental illnesses, while at the same time fearing them' (NAMI press release, May 14, 1998—www.nami.org/pressroom).

Mental health clinicians, service providers and systems

From the point of view of mental health service providers and systems, OPC appears to offer a strategy to reduce hospitalization, manage risk and enhance the effectiveness of treatment technologies and therapies that depend on continuity and sustained adherence. With the advent of managed care in both public and private mental health systems, and with clinicians increasingly held liable for the behaviour of SMI patients inadequately treated, concerns about violence risk collide with pressures to limit high-cost services (Dixon *et al.* 1998; Thienhaus and Piasecki 1998). OPC is of interest in this context potentially for several reasons: (1) OPC may enhance treatment effectiveness in less restrictive and less costly settings by extending community tenure and improving adherence among SMI patients who might otherwise require repeated hospitalization; (2) OPC may prevent violence by improving compliance with medications that mitigate high-risk psychotic symptoms and by increasing access to treatment for co-occurring substance abuse which is often the key ingredient in violent behaviour; (3) OPC may help monitor high-risk cases in the community and identify need for more intense intervention when acute relapse does occur, e.g. providing improved access to crisis services or short-term hospitalization for stabilization as necessary; (4) OPC may help immunize clinicians from perceived liability in rare cases where violent acts are committed by SMI individuals in the community and clinicians may be held to account for not taking steps to ensure adherence with treatment that (presumably) could have prevented such acts.

Nevertheless, there is yet little consensus among clinicians about the value and appropriate role of OPC. Some professionals side with patients in the view that coercive treatment is intrinsically not effective. Their argument is that OPC undermines not only the autonomy of the person with mental illness—autonomy which is important for recovery—but also the basis of trust that is crucial for a therapeutic relationship to assist in that recovery. Some of these clinicians assert that any need for OPC could be obviated by a serious social investment in a continuum of enhanced services including psychiatric treatment, rehabilitation, housing, transportation, adequate income and other supports as needed by persons with SMI. Mullen (1997) articulates this view even while acknowledging the risk of violent behaviour in some SMI individuals:

> The most effective response to the risks of dangerous behaviour in the mentally ill is not to return to policies of greater control and containment but to improve the care, support and treatment delivered to patients in the community. Those at high risk need to be targeted for priority follow-up and intensive support ... (Mullen 1997).

At the other extreme is the position represented most prominently by E. Fuller Torrey and the Stanley Foundation's Treatment Advocacy Center (TAC). Torrey argues explicitly for a return to policies of greater control and containment, i.e. broadening civil commitment criteria on a state-by-state basis and aggressively promoting OPC, including provisions for involuntary administration of medication in out-patient settings. Torrey's position assumes 'lack of insight' is a hallmark of severe mental illness:

Getting good treatment is especially difficult for individuals with brain disorders who lack insight into their illness and need for treatment. In these cases, it is sometimes necessary to legally mandate treatment using such mechanisms as involuntary out-patient commitments, conservatorships, and conditional release (Torrey 1998)

The Public

A recent analysis of data from the 1996 General Social Survey (GSS), from a nationally representative sample ($N = 1444$) of the US population, found that 74% of the public believe that persons with schizophrenia are unable to make treatment decisions and 60% believe persons with schizophrenia are likely to commit violent acts toward others. Nearly 50% of the population say they favour laws to force persons with schizophrenia to visit a clinic or doctor, while 42% favour legally forcing people with this diagnosis to take prescription medication. In cases where persons with schizophrenia pose a danger to others, 95% of the population favours involuntary commitment to a hospital (Pescosolido et al. 1999). Such opinions may or may not be based on scientific evidence. Nevertheless, the general public—taxpayers and voters through elected state representatives—may have a strong say in the fate of OPC: how broadly or narrowly it will be implemented; what forms of coercive treatment will be considered acceptable under what circumstances; what consequences of untreated mental disorder will be tolerated in the name of individual autonomy; and what resources will be available for 'leveraging' services on behalf of SMI individuals in the community. Understanding public opinion about OPC and related issues is thus quite relevant to the task of translating evidence for OPC effectiveness into policy recommendations and guidelines.

Recent events surrounding an experimental OPC program in New York City, discussed in some detail below, illustrate the importance of public perceptions as well as stakeholders' viewpoints as key ingredients in state policy decision-making—and how research findings may be interpreted in different ways to influence opinion and thereby shape policy. In 1994, the New York State legislature passed a bill to establish a three-year pilot programme to test and evaluate OPC combined with enhanced treatment coordination services in Bellevue Hospital (Steadman et al. 1999). The evaluation was designed as a first step toward considering permanent OPC legislation for the state and found no significant statistical differences between control and experimental groups in follow-up hospitalizations, arrests, quality of life, symptoms, homelessness or other outcomes. It would seem the study findings did not make a case that OPC should be adopted in New York on the basis of its likely effectiveness. Nevertheless, the state legislature enacted a statewide OPC statute in response to other considerations: positive appraisal of OPC by clinicians who oversaw the Bellevue program, and timely mass-media coverage of several violent crimes committed by persons with schizophrenia, which focused public attention on OPC as a possible solution to such horrifying events. The heated controversy regarding OPC still begs the questions: is OPC effective in reducing hospitalizations, violent behaviour and improving treatment outcomes? If effective, how does OPC exert its effects? The following sections review naturalistic, quasi-experimental and randomized controlled trials (RCTs) of OPC in the USA.

Naturalistic and quasi-experimental studies of out-patient commitment

Assessing outcomes of OPC poses the problems of separating effects of legal coercion (e.g. the effect of the moral power of court) from other attempts to influence behaviour, the effects of treatment and other factors such as selection effects. Myriads of attempts to influence behaviour are brought to bear on SMI individuals in an effort to improve compliance with treatment. A family member may insist on treatment compliance as a condition of further financial support. Another may offer inducements, such as special amenities, if compliance is achieved. A clinician may threaten in-patient commitment when compliance is poor. These forms of informal coercion may exert powerful effects in concert with or independent of OPC. Selection and treatment factors are also important potential confounds in interpreting empirical evidence regarding OPC. Not all patients eligible for OPC are placed on an order. In naturalistic studies of OPC, patients studied have been selected for OPC for clinical reasons separate from legal criteria.

In an early study based in North Carolina, the first to report effects of OPC, patients were selected for OPC because of characteristics such as family support and employment that were likely to increase patients' likelihood of success in treatment (Hiday and Goodman 1982). Only 12.5% of the patients were involuntarily hospitalized during a 90-day commitment period. However, inextricable confounding of selection effects with the effects of OPC made it impossible to assess the effectiveness of the court order. A second study in North Carolina found that clinicians in a mental health center rated OPC effective in 46% of cases in a six-month follow-up period (Miller and Fiddleman 1984). However, inconsistent enforcement of the order when patients failed to comply makes the findings difficult to evaluate.

Greeman and McClellan (1985) compared the community adjustment of three groups: patients whose involuntary hospitalization was stayed and who were ordered by the court to receive community-based treatment, patients who were released after 72-h emergency admissions and patients involuntarily hospitalized. Few patients in any group did well at one-year follow-up on measures of compliance with medication, appointments kept and absence of disruptive symptoms. However, a higher proportion of patients in court-ordered community treatment (24%) did well compared to patients held for 72 h (14%) and those involuntarily admitted to the hospital (4%). As in the study above, Greeman and McClellan's results are confounded by selection bias (Greeman and McClellan 1985).

The positive effects of OPC are more clearly seen in a study by Zanni and deVeau (1986) who compared patient's hospital experiences one year before and after receiving an OPC order. This pretest–posttest study design avoided selection bias. Patients who received both in-patient and out-patient treatment from the same team and hospital ($N = 42$) had significantly fewer hospitalizations per patient (0.95 versus 1.81) and shorter hospital stays (38 versus 55 days) during the year after OPC compared to the year prior.

Van Putten *et al.* (1988) evaluated OPC by comparing outcomes for three groups of patients identified at various time periods before and after implementation of new legislation authorizing OPC in Arizona in 1983. Group 1 comprised patients involuntarily hospitalized in a county hospital in the six months before the legislation's enactment. Group 2 was made up of patients who were involuntarily hospitalized and eligible for OPC in the first six months after changes in the law. Group 3 consisted of patients who were involuntarily hospitalized and eligible for OPC in the second six months after changes in the law. Positive outcomes in the study included shorter hospital stays for groups 2 and 3 following initial OPC and a lack of incidents of violent acts or being victimized while the patients were under the court order. In addition, a higher proportion of patients in groups 2 and 3 voluntarily used community mental health services after their court orders, compared with patients in group 1. After the new legislation was enacted both patients who were and were not on OPC had significant increases in voluntary community aftercare. Therefore, it is likely that improved services for both groups partly account for the outcomes.

Hiday and Scheid-Cook (1987) reported on a new, lower-threshold OPC statute in North Carolina that allows preventative commitment. No differences in living situation, rates of rehospitalization, days rehospitalized, level of social interaction outside the home, employment, level of dangerousness, and number of arrests were found between persons committed to out-patient treatment who began treatment, persons involuntarily hospitalized and later released and persons released instead of being involuntarily hospitalized. Patients on OPC who began treatment showed significantly improved compliance with medication and other treatment, increased visits to the community mental health centre, and higher retention in treatment six months after their hearings, even after expiration of their OPC orders. OPC was more likely to influence treatment compliance than social, clinical and systems outcomes. A similar analysis conducted among individuals with SMI showed comparable outcomes, except that differences in compliance with medication and other treatments were not significant, probably because of limitations in sample size (Hiday and Scheid-Cook 1989).

A more recent study in North Carolina found that OPC dramatically reduces rehospitalization rates. Fernandez and Nygard (1990) studied all patients in the state who had a first OPC in the three-year period after the less restrictive commitment statute was enacted. The patients' average number of involuntary hospitalizations declined from 3.7 before their initial OPC to 0.7 after the order and mean standardized total length of stay declined from 57.6 days before the OPC order to 38.4 days after. These findings represent decreases in readmission and lengths of stay of 82% and 33%, respectively.

In contrast to the above studies, a study by Bursten (1986) found no differences in readmission rates between patients ordered to mandatory treatment after involuntary hospitalization and patients in a control group. He concluded that mandatory out-patient treatment had no effect on hospital readmissions. This conclusion should be qualified, however, because of evidence that the out-patient law was not enforced. A more recent study by Munetz et al. (1996) examined community tenure and social functioning in a group of high recidivist patients placed on OPC. In a 12-month follow-up period, out-patient committed patients demonstrated reduced emergency room visits, hospital readmission, and lengths of stay. They also found a higher number of visits with psychiatrists.

Taken together findings from these studies of selected samples suggest that OPC decreases hospital readmission rates and lengths of stay (Hiday and Scheid-Cook 1987, 1989; Fernandez and Nygard, 1990; Keilitz, 1990; Hiday and Scheid-Cook 1991; Moloy 1992). These studies are limited because criteria used to select patients for OPC are largely unspecified. Unspecified treatment characteristics, including patients' access to and availability of services may also influence study outcomes. In fact, in some studies patients under OPC received no treatment. The next step in evaluating OPC would require better specification and control of potential confounding factors, most readily addressed in an RCT.

Randomized controlled trials of out-patient commitment

The Duke Mental Health Study (DMHS) was the first RCT of the effectiveness of OPC combined with community-based case management and examines the impact of legal coercion on outcomes in community treatment for persons with SMI (see Swartz et al. 1995, 1997, 1999b; Swanson et al. 2000). Between 1993 and 1996, the DMHS enrolled 331 subjects who had been involuntarily hospitalized and given a court order for a period of mandatory treatment in the community after discharge. Thus subjects initially received a form of OPC akin to conditional release. A control group was randomly assigned to be released from OPC, and received case management alone. Respondents with a recent history of serious assaultive behaviour were placed in a non-randomized comparison group, remaining on OPC for at least the initial period up to 90 days. Outcomes were assessed by means of follow-up interviews with subjects, family members and case managers every four months for a period of 16 months, and with retrieval and matching of service records, hospital admissions and arrest data for two years. Multi-variate statistical models were used to examine the impact of OPC—interacting with out-patient services—on a range of outcomes, including: hospital readmissions, violent behaviour, criminal victimization, substance abuse, homelessness, medication adherence, symptoms and quality of life.

Subjects were screened sequentially from a population of involuntarily hospitalized patients who had been ordered to undergo a period of OPC upon discharge. Eligibility criteria were: (1) age 18 years or older; (2) diagnosis of schizophrenia, schizoaffective disorder, other psychotic disorder or major affective disorder; (3) duration of disorder of one year or more; (4) significant functional impairment in activities of daily living; (5) intensive treatment within the past two years; (6) resident of one of nine counties participating in the study; (7) awaiting a period of court-ordered OPC. Key legal criteria for OPC in North Carolina include an SMI diagnosis, a mental status limiting a person's ability to seek or comply voluntarily with treatment, and the likelihood that without treatment the person will predictably relapse to the point of compromised personal safety.

Subjects randomly assigned to a control group were released from OPC. Subjects in the experimental group, by law, received an initial period of OPC not longer than 90 days. Thereafter, the commitment order could be renewed for up to 180 days if a psychiatrist and the court determined that the subject continued to meet legal criteria for OPC. Treatment personnel could not be and were not blinded to the study assignment of subjects. Subjects in the control group received immunity from any OPC during the year of the study. All subjects received case management and other out-patient treatment at one of four participating area mental health programmes representing nine contiguous urban and rural counties. An exception to the randomization procedure was necessary for ethical reasons in the cases of subjects with a recent history of serious assault involving weapon use or physical injury to another person within the preceding year. These subjects (the serious violent group) were required to undergo at least the initial period of OPC as ordered. Renewals were left to the discretion of the clinician and court.

Hospital readmissions findings

In bivariate analyses of group differences, comparing control and OPC group assignment alone, groups did not differ significantly in hospital outcomes; repeated measures multivariate analysis did, however, demonstrate that OPC subjects had lower odds of re-hospitalisation (Swartz *et al.* 1999b). Subjects who underwent sustained periods of OPC beyond the initial court order had approximately 57% fewer readmissions and 20 fewer hospital days compared to control subjects. Sustained OPC was shown to be particularly effective for individuals with psychotic disorders, reducing hospital readmissions approximately 72% and requiring 28 fewer hospital days compared to controls. In subsequent repeated measures analyses examining the role of out-patient treatment it was also found that sustained OPC reduced hospital readmissions only when combined with a higher intensity of out-patient services, above a median of more than three service events a month and averaging approximately seven services per month. These findings appear to demonstrate that OPC can work to reduce hospital readmissions when the court order is sustained and combined with regular treatment, particularly for individuals with psychotic disorders.

Violent behaviour outcome findings

Additional analyses from the DMHS examines violence as a longitudinal outcome (Swanson *et al.* 2000). The effect of OPC and MH services utilization on violence risk is similar to the findings for hospitalization as described above. Incidence of any violence during the year of follow-up in the RCT was significantly lower among respondents receiving extended OPC compared to controls and those with shorter periods of OPC (22.7% versus 36.8% and 39.7% respectively). Moreover, controlling for frequency of out-patient service events, OPC was shown to be effective only among those averaging 3 or more visits per month; OPC showed no effect on violence risk in respondents with fewer than 3 service events per month. Significant bivariate predictors of violence included: younger age (under age 40), being single, with low social support, urban residence, homelessness, greater functional impairment (Global Assessment of Functioning (GAF) score under 45), substance abuse, paranoid symptoms and having more than two hospital admission in the prior year. Staged multi-variable logistic regression analysis with stepwise selection yielded a reduced model with the following significant predictors of lower violence risk at follow-up (controlling for baseline violence history): (1) extended OPC and regular services utilization, (2) high change scores (improvement) on substance abuse and medication adherence, (3) social support and (4) age over 40. In this model, the predicted probability of any violent behaviour was cut in half, from 48% to 24%, as a result of extended OPC and regular out-patient service provision (see Fig. 9.2). Subjects who received the high intervention (sustained OPC and regular services), who concurrently remained free of substance abuse, and who took medications as prescribed during the year of the study had the lowest likelihood of any violence (13% predicted probability). By comparison, those who did not receive the high intervention, who continued to abuse substances, and who stopped taking their medications had a 53% predicted probability of violent behaviour during the year.

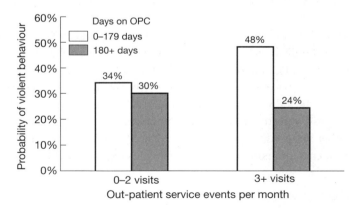

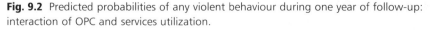

Fig. 9.2 Predicted probabilities of any violent behaviour during one year of follow-up: interaction of OPC and services utilization.

Perceived coercion

The DMHS also examined predictors of perceived coercion under OPC (Swartz *et al.* 1999*a*). Subjects' responses were compared using a modified version of the MacArthur Admission Experience Survey (MAES) which measures objective and subjective dimensions of coercion. Bivariate analyses indicated that significantly higher levels of coercion on the MAES were reported by several subject sub-groups, although potential confounding made interpretation of these findings uncertain. Multi-variate analyses showed higher levels of coercion among individuals neither married or cohabiting, with lower educational levels, those who did not view themselves as mentally ill, those with lower levels of global functioning, subjects with longer periods of OPC and subjects more frequently reminded about the consequences of treatment non-adherence by case managers. These and related analyses indicate that perceived coercion is significantly related to the duration of OPC, although other social-contextual and treatment factors, such as case manager behaviour, is also important. Additionally, while coercion is increased in the OPC group these results do not shed light on whether coercion is detrimental to co-operative engagement and long-term treatment retention.

Despite these findings of decreased readmission and violence under OPC, some limitations should be acknowledged. Length of time on OPC was a key variable in the intervention but could not be randomly assigned. If lower risk subjects were selected for longer periods of commitment, positive findings could be overstated. Legal criteria for renewal of OPC would seem to prevent selection of lower risk subjects for longer exposure to court-ordered treatment and indeed higher risk subjects appeared, in preliminary analyses, to receive longer periods of commitment. Still, unknown selection factors may have affected duration of OPC. In addition, out-patient service intensity was not controlled by the study, but varied according to clinical need and other unknown factors. As a result, selective provision of services could have influenced outcomes, although other preliminary analyses argue that this was not an important factor.

It appears that OPC can improve certain treatment outcomes when the court order is targeted toward individuals with psychotic disorders, sustained and combined with intensive treatment. OPC cannot substitute for intensity of treatment. It appears OPC influences both the service providers, perhaps by conveying a legal directive to prioritize treatment for the individual under the order, and acts on the individual by helping to motivate improved treatment adherence. Future analyses from this RCT are expected to examine other important outcomes such as family and care giver burden, criminal justice involvement, and more fully elucidate the mechanism of OPC's effectiveness.

New York OPC evaluation

In 1994, the New York State legislature passed a bill to establish a three-year pilot program to test and evaluate OPC in Bellevue Hospital as a first step toward considering permanent OPC legislation for the state (Policy Research Associates 1998; Steadman *et al.* 1999). The evaluation study compared a range of outcomes in a court-ordered group ($N = 78$) and a control group ($N = 64$) over a one-year follow-up period after hospital discharge. By design both groups received a package of enhanced services including intensive community treatment and priority eligibility for supportive housing. The study found no significant statistical differences between the control and experimental groups in follow-up hospitalizations, arrests, quality of life, symptoms, homelessness or other outcomes. The lack of significant differences between study groups seems to suggest that enhanced services—and not coercion *per se*—are the appropriate system response to the community-care needs of persons with SMI prone to relapse. However, the study's findings were weakened by a few methodological shortcomings. At least during the start-up phase of the pilot program, implementation and enforcement of OPC was haphazard. Non-compliance, for instance, was not routinely met with police pick-up orders and medication was not administered involuntarily. Participants and providers often did not clearly distinguish between having a court order and merely being part of the 'Bellevue Program' irrespective of study group assignment. In spite of randomization procedures, persons with co-occurring substance abuse were selected significantly more often for the court-ordered group (56% versus 39%), and this pre-existing risk factor, while controlled in study analyses, is likely to have diminished the statistical power to detect better outcomes for OPC respondents. Further, the study did not have a large enough sample size to test relevant interaction effects and excluded two categories of subjects who may be particularly appropriate candidates for OPC: those with history of serious violent behaviour, and those incompetent to make treatment decisions. Nevertheless, the findings from this study suggest that OPC may have no particular benefit, particularly if an enhanced range of services is available to SMI patients.

While these studies appear to provide contrary findings, both demonstrate wide variability in the implementation and practice of OPC. These differences render findings across all studies difficult to compare and interpret. Even within North Carolina, where the most consistent findings of OPC's effectiveness have been demonstrated, the 'dose' of OPC varied widely as did the services provided to patients. Given that most states in the USA explicitly permit OPC, attempts to better standardize the practice of OPC through practice improvement efforts or the establishment of practice guidelines is warranted if OPC is to be utilized appropriately.

While OPC is one form of coercion applied in mental health treatment, others are in use but little researched. For example, the use of representative payeeship—in which a patient's disability funds are held by an individual trusted by the patient and used contingently to reinforce behaviours such as medication compliance—may be equally effective to OPC. Other informal sanctions applied by families and care givers, such as insistence on medication compliance as a condition of financial support, have also been inadequately studied and may also be equal or more effective than OPC. Research is needed to compare the costs and benefits of a range of coercive interventions in treatment.

Future directions

Practice guidelines represent one approach to practice improvement, among others (e.g continuous quality improvement, formal training, modelling, standards/regulations and fiscal incentives—see Burns 1998). The US Institute of Medicine (1990) defined practice guidelines as systematically developed statements that could be used to assist clinician and consumer decision making about appropriate health care for specific clinical circumstances. Such guidelines are intended to improve the quality, appropriateness and effectiveness of care, and have been used to assist clinicians, consumers, payors and other stakeholders in making decisions about a range of health care decisions (Edmunds 1996). Practice guidelines are seen by federal and state policy makers as well as other payors in the USA as key activities in rationalizing decision making about the delivery of health care (Institute of Medicine 1997). Derived either from an evidence base and/or consensus, these guidelines function as a tool to improve clinical and functional outcomes by aligning clinical practice with the evidence base. A recent paper by Gilbert et al. (1998) summarized the benefits of algorithm-driven care: (1) reduction in unnecessary variation in clinical practice patterns, (2) facilitation of strategic clinical decision making, (3) making clinical decisions explicit, (4) improving the quality of treatment, (5) increasing the cost efficiency of treatment, (6) providing a metric to compare patient progress, (7) providing self-correcting feedback to improve the algorithm, and (8) providing a metric for evaluating when and whether to incorporate new medications into the algorithm. However, published research in the mental health field on guideline-driven care is limited to a study by Lin et al. (1997) in Seattle, Washington, on the treatment of depression in primary health care. In this study, achievement of guideline-driven practice occurred with consistent instruction and psychiatric consultation, but the benefits achieved did not persist when these resources were removed. Since the preceding study, recognition of the need to utilize a range of strategies to improve practice is apparent.

A multi-stage model for practice improvement research provides a logical method for pursuing this work. Samsa et al. (1998 and see Matchar et al. in press) outlined a seven-step model for practice improvement research which fits well with the needed practice improvement agenda for OPC:

Step 1: Identify a potential target of opportunity. In OPC, the opportunity to reduce rehospitalization, relapse and other negative outcomes among individuals with serious mental illness is potentially negated by negative effects of coercion under OPC.

Step 2: Synthesize information about optimal practice. Synthesis of existing and disparate empirical evidence about the effectiveness of OPC is needed.

Step 3: Synthesize information about current practice. The actual practice of OPC has been poorly characterized. Little is known about provider decision making about OPC, or about key steps in implementation of OPC orders. Interviews with key stakeholders in OPC—e.g. providers, patients, families and court officials, are needed to better understand barriers to the use of OPC.

Step 4: Identify reasons for discrepancies between current practice and optimal practice. Data from stakeholder interviews are needed to identify barriers between current and optimal practice.

Step 5: Develop a strategy for practice improvement. A strategy for practice improvement should explicitly address the barriers to optimal practice; define the OPC intervention functionally; recommend implementation options and include an implementation plan.

Step 6: Assess effectiveness and cost-effectiveness of the practice improvement strategy. A logical subsequent step in OPC research is the study of the cost-effectiveness of the intervention.

Step 7: Determine whether or not the practice improvement strategy should be implemented. Given the availability of practice guidelines for OPC, accompanying specific manuals for implementation and data on cost-effectiveness, policymakers should be in a better position to evaluate the value of an operationalized approach to OPC.

Conclusions

Out-patient commitment will continue to be a controversial treatment intervention regardless of empirical findings about its effectiveness or lack thereof. Advocates and opponents of OPC often use data about OPC's benefits or detriments as a 'straw man' to argue strongly held views about autonomy and paternalism in mental health treatment. Many opponents of OPC believe that it may serve as a barrier to improving services because policy makers will seize upon it as a 'cheap fix' to remedy a paucity of community-based services. However, data to date suggest that OPC, if it is effective, can only be so when more intensive services are provided, obviating use of OPC as an inexpensive remedy. More careful specification of the effects of OPC on sub-populations of concern under specific treatment conditions, combined with clear practice guidelines, could improve the practice of OPC.

Acknowledgements

From the Services Effectiveness Research Program in the Department of Psychiatry & Behavioral Sciences, Duke University Medical Center and the UNC·Duke Program in Services Research for People with Severe Mental Disorders. This work was supported by NIMH Grant MH 48103 and MH 51410. Portions of this chapter are adapted from Swartz *et al.* (2001).

References

Appelbaum, P. S. (1986) Out-patient commitment: the problems and the promise (editorial). *American Journal of Psychiatry*, **143**(10), 1270–2.

Borum, R., Swanson, J. W., Swartz, M. S. *et al.* (1997) Substance abuse, violent behavior, and police encounters among persons with severe mental disorders. *Journal of Contemporary Criminal Justice*, **13**(3), 236–49.

Borum, R., Swartz, M. S., Riley, S. *et al.* (1999) Consumer perceptions of involuntary out-patient commitment. *Psychiatric Services*, **50**, 1489–91.

Buchanan, A. and David, A. (1994) Compliance and the reduction of dangerousness. *Journal of Mental Health*, **3**, 427–9.

Burns, B. J. (1998) Services effectiveness research: relevance, challenges, and future directions. Frontiers of Science Lecture, Presentation at the American Psychiatric Association Annual Meeting, Toronto, Ontario, Canada, June 1, 1998.

Bursten, B. (1986) Posthospital mandatory out-patient treatment. *American Journal of Psychiatry*, **43**, 1255–8.

Campbell, J. and Schraiber, R. (1989) *In pursuit of wellness: The well-being project.* Sacramento: California Department of Mental Health.

Dixon, L., Adler, D., Berlant, J. *et al.* (1998) Confronting violence. *Psychiatric Services*, **49**, 865.

Edmunds, M. (1996) Clinical practice guidelines: Opportunities and implications. *Annals of Behavioral Medicine*, **18**, 126–32.

Fernandez, G. A. and Nygard, S. (1990) Impact of involuntary out-patient commitment on the revolving-door syndrome in North Carolina. *Hospital and Community Psychiatry*, **41**(9), 1001–4.

Fulop, N. J. (1995) Involuntary out-patient civil commitment. *International Journal of Law and Psychiatry*, **18**(3), 291–303.

Geller, J. L. (1992) Clinical encounters with out-patient coercion at the CMHC: Questions of implementation and efficacy. *Community Mental Health Journal*, **28**(2), 81–94.

Geller, J., Grudzinskas, A. J., Jr, McDermeit, M. *et al.* (1998) The efficacy of involuntary out-patient treatment in Massachusetts. *Administration and Policy in Mental Health*, **25**(3), 271–85.

Gilbert, D. A., Altshuler, K. Z., Rago, W. V. *et al.* (1998) Texas Medication Algorithm Project: Definitions, rationale and methods to develop medication algorithms. *Journal of Clinical Psychiatry*, **59**, 345–51.

Greeman, M. and McClellan, T. A. (1985) The impact of a more stringent commitment code in Minnesota. *Hospital and Community Psychiatry*, **36**, 990–2.

Hiday, V. A. (1992) Coercion in civil commitment: Process, preferences, and outcome. *International Journal of Law and Psychiatry*, **15**(4), 359–77.

Hiday, V. A. and Goodman, R. R. (1982) The least restrictive alternative to involuntary hospitalization, out-patient commitment: Its use and effectiveness. *Journal of Psychiatry and Law*, **10**, 81–96.

Hiday, V. A. and Scheid-Cook, T. L. (1987) The North Carolina experience with out-patient commitment: a critical appraisal. *International Journal of Law and Psychiatry*, **10**(3), 215–32.

Hiday, V. A. and Scheid-Cook, T. L. (1989) A follow-up of chronic patients committed to out-patient treatment. *Hospital and Community Psychiatry*, **40**(1), 52–9.

Hiday, V. A. and Scheid-Cook, T. L. (1991) Out-patient commitment for revolving door patients: Compliance and treatment. *Journal of Nervous and Mental Disorders*, **179**(2), 83–8.

Institute of Medicine (1990) *Broadening the base of treatment for alcohol problems.* Washington DC: National Academy Press.

Institute of Medicine (1997) *Managing managed care: quality improvement in behavioral health.* Washington DC: National Academy Press.

Jaffe, D. J. (1998) Treatment Advocacy Center, testimony at NYC Department of Mental Health hearing on the effectiveness of out-patient commitment, December 16, 1998, TAC website—www.psychlaws.org.

Keilitz, I. (1990) Empirical studies of involuntary out-patient civil commitment: is it working? *Mental and Physical Disability Law Reporter*, **14**, 368–79.

Kent, S., Fogarty, M. and Yellowlees, P. (1995) A review of studies of heavy users of psychiatric services. *Psychiatric Services*, **46**(12), 1247–53.

Lin, E. H. B., Katon, W. J., Simon, G. E. *et al.* (1997) Achieving guidelines for the treatment of depression in primary care: Is physician education enough? *Medical Care*, **35**, 831–42.

Mancuso, L. L. (1997) Involuntary intervention and coerced treatment of people with mental health disorders, Executive Summary: Center for Mental Health Services Meeting US Department of Health and Human Services, Sustance Abuse and Mental Health Administration, Center for Mental Health Services (CMHS).

Matchar, D. B., Samsa, G. P., Cohen, S. J. *et al.* (in press) A practice improvement trial implemented within managed care organizations: Rationale and design of the Managing Anticoagulation Services Trial (MAST). *Medical Care.*

McCafferty, G. and Dooley, J. (1990) Involuntary out-patient commitment: an update. *Mental and Physical Disability Law Reporter*, **14**, 277–87.

Miller, R. D. and Fiddleman, P. (1984) Out-patient commitment: Treatment in the least restrictive environment? *Hospital and Community Psychiatry*, **35**, 147–51.

Moloy, K. A. (1992) *Analysis: Critiquing the empirical evidence: Does involuntary out-patient commitment work?* Washington DC: Mental Health Policy Resource Center.

Monahan, J., Hoge, S. K., Lidz, C. W. *et al.* (1994) *Violence and mental disorder: Developments in risk assessment.* Chicago: The University of Chicago Press.

Mullen, P.E. (1997) A reassessment of the link between mental disorder and violent behavior, and its implications for clinical practice. *Australian and New Zealand Journal of Psychiatry*, **31**(1), 3–11.

Mulvey E. V. (1994) Assessing the evidence of a link between mental illness and violence. *Hospital and Community Psychiatry*, **45**, 663–8.

Mulvey, E. P., Geller, J. L. and Roth, L. H. (1987) The promise and peril of involuntary out-patient commitment. *American Psychologist*, **42**(6), 571–84.

Munetz, M. R., Grande, T., Kleist, J. *et al.* (1996) The effectiveness of out-patient civil commitment. *Psychiatric Services*, **47**, 1251–3

NAMI (1995) NAMI statement on involuntary out-patient commitment. *NAMI Advocate*, Sept./Oct. 20.

O'Keefe, C., Potensa D. P. and Mueser, K. T. (1997) Treatment outcomes for severely mentally ill patient on conditional discharge to community-based treatment. *Journal of Nervous and Mental Diseases*, **185**, 409–11.

Osher, F. C. and Drake, R. E. (1996) Reversing a history of unmet needs: Approaches to care for persons with co-occurring addictive and mental disorders. *American Journal of Orthopsychiatry*, **66**, 4–11.

Pescosolido, B. A., Monahan, J., Link, B. G. *et al.* (1999) The public's view of the competence, dangerousness and need for legal coercion among persons with mental illness. *American Journal of Public Health*, **89**, 1339–45

Policy Research Associates (1998) Final report: Research study of the New York City involuntary out-patient commitment pilot program. Prepared for New York City Department of Mental Health, Mental Retardation, and Alcoholism Services.

Samsa, G. P., Matchar D. B., Cohen, S. J. *et al.* (1998) A seven-step model for practice improvement research: Description and application to the managing anticoagulation services trial. *New Medicine*, **2**, 139–46.

Schalock, R. L., Touchstone, F., Nelson, G. *et al.* (1995) A multivariate analysis of mental hospital recidivism. *The Journal of Mental Health Administration*, **22**(4), 358–67.

Schwartz, S. J. and Costanzo, C. E. (1987) Compelling treatment in the community: distorted doctrines and violated values. *Loyola of Los Angeles Law Review*, **20**, 1329–1429.

Steadman, H. J., Dennis D. L., Gounis K. *et al.* (1999) Assessing the operation of a New York City program for involuntary out-patient commitment. In *Research in community and mental health: Coercion in mental health services* (ed. J. Morrissey and J. Monahan), Vol. 10, pp. 13–30. Stamford, CT: JAI Press.

Stefan, S. (1987) Preventive commitment: the concept and its pitfalls. *Mental and Physical Disability Law Reporter*, **11**, 288–302.

Swanson, J. W., Swartz, M. S., George, L. K. *et al.* (1997) Interpreting the effectiveness of involuntary out-patient commitment: A conceptual model. *Journal of the American Academy of Psychiatry and the Law*, **25**(1), 5–16.

Swanson, J. W., Swartz, M. S., Borum, R., Hiday, V. A., Wagner, H. R. and Burns, B. J. (2000) Involuntary outpatient commitment and reduction of violent behaviour in persons with severe mental illness. *British Journal of Psychiatry*. **176**, 324–331.

Swartz, M. S., Burns, B. J., Hiday, V. A. *et al.*(1995) New directions in research on involuntary out-patient commitment. *Psychiatric Services*; **46**(4), 381–5.

Swartz, M. S., Burns, B. J., George, L. K. *et al.* (1997) The ethical challenges of a randomized controlled trial of involuntary out-patient commitment. *Journal of Mental Health Administration*, **24**(1), 35–43.

Swartz, M. S., Hiday, V. A., Swanson J. W. *et al.* (1999*a*) Measuring coercion under involuntary out-patient commitment: Initial findings from a randomized controlled trial. In *Research in community and mental health: Coercion in mental health services* (ed. J. Morrissey and J. Monahan), Vol. 10, pp. 31–56. Stamford, CT: JAI Press.

Swartz, M. S., Swanson, J. W., Wagner, R. R. *et al.* (1999*b*) Can involuntary out-patient commitment reduce hospital recidivism? Findings from a randomized trial in severely mentally ill individuals. *American Journal of Psychiatry*, **156**(11), 1968–75.

Swartz, M. S., Swanson, J. W., Hiday, V. A. *et al.* (2001) A randomized controlled trial of out-patient commitment in North Carolina. *Psychiatric Services*, **52**, 325–9.

Tavolaro, K. B. (1992) Preventive out-patient civil commitment and the right to refuse treatment: Can pragmatic realities and constitutional requirements be reconciled? *Medicine and Law* **11**(3–4), 249–67.

Thienhaus, O. and Piasecki, M. (1998) Assessment of psychiatric patients' risk of violence toward others. *Psychiatric Services*, **49**, 1129–47.

Torrey, E. F. (1994) Violent behavior by individuals with serious mental illness. Special Issue: Violent behavior and mental illness. *Hospital and Community Psychiatry*, **45**(7), 653–62.

Torrey, E. F. (**1998**) TAC press release on the MacArthur study, TAC website—www.psychlaws.org.

Torrey, E. F. and Kaplan, R. (1995) A national survey of the use of out-patient commitment. *Psychiatric Services*, **46**(8), 778–84.

E. F. Torrey and M. T. Zdanowicz (1999) How freedom punishes the severely mentally ill. *USA Today*, June 7.

Van Putten, R. A., Santiago, J. M. and Berren M. R. (1988) Involuntary out-patient commitment in Arizona: A retrospective study. *Hospital and Community Psychiatry*, **39**(9), 953–8.

Zanni, G. and deVeau, L. (1986) In-patient stays before and after out-patient commitment. *Hospital and Community Psychiatry*, **37**, 941–2.

Chapter 10

Mentally disordered offenders and the community mental health team

Frank Holloway

Introduction

The policy context

This chapter reviews the role of the Community Mental Health Team (CMHT) in the management of the 'mentally disordered offender' (MDO). It is written from the perspective of psychiatric practice within the UK, where mental health policy is peculiarly and increasingly dominated by a preoccupation with the risks that people with a mental illness present to themselves and others and a culture of blame (Holloway 1996). Successive governments have made it clear that the assessment and management of the risk of self-harm and harm to others is the core function of UK mental health services (Department of Health 1994, 1995, 1998). As a result of the extreme preoccupation of the UK government with the issue of homicides by people with a mental illness, any homicide by a patient with a history of contact with mental health services precipitates an independent inquiry. Inquiries have a remit to identify shortcomings in the patient's clinical care and the extent to which policy guidelines were followed (Buchanan 1999a). All suicides are reported to a government-funded 'National confidential inquiry into suicide and homicide by people with a mental illness' (Appleby et al. 1999a). In addition, there will be a coroner's inquest and an internal inquiry within the service provider, both of which may be seen as identifying whom to blame. Current UK mental health policy is predicated on the belief that 'care in the community has failed' (Department of Health 1998); hence the need to reinvent the services in a form that will be 'safe, sound and supportive' (with the emphasis on 'safe').'Moral panic' in relation to mental health care, discernible in the UK and the USA (see Chapters 1 and 4), is less obviously apparent in the rest of Europe.

The threat of violence, socially unacceptable behaviour and suicide by people under their care preoccupies and potentially distorts the work of mental health professionals in the UK (Deahl and Turner 1997). This concern must partly reflect the comprehensive role of the CMHT and associated in-patient units in the UK, which work within sectorized mental health services (Bindman et al. 1996). A CMHT will have full responsibility for the needs of all known or referred patients of working age living within a defined catchment area, unless the patient is specifically under the care of some other service, for example a forensic mental health team.

Resources

There are no UK norms for community services but the generic CMHT is unlikely to be generously resourced. As a reasonably representative example which equates to national data on staffing, the author's service is located in a suburban area of average social morbidity in the UK according to the Mental Illness Needs Index (MINI; Glover 1996) that has the average amount of total health care spend devoted to mental health (11%). Eight teams, serving a population of on average 40 000, each consist of one consultant and one or two non-consultant psychiatrists, three community mental health nurses, an occupational therapist and some clinical psychologist sessions. There is access to social workers (currently responsible to the Social Services Department, not the health provider), some specialist psychotherapy and day care. The psychiatrists on the team also have 24-h responsibility to the in-patient service, which will have perhaps 120 admissions per year, and responsibility for a specialist function. Other team members will be expected to retain contact with their patients or clients during an in-patient episode. Each CMHT receives approximately 350 new referrals per year (the bulk of whom do not suffer from a severe mental illness) and is in contact with 300–400 people at any one time. It is expected to operate under the 'care programme approach', providing named keyworkers, risk assessments, care planning and follow-up to all patients/clients accepted on the caseload (Department of Health 1994).

The CMHT will have varying contact with specialist forensic practitioners depending on local resources, policies and procedures. There will also be a range of local substance misuse services, but these are unlikely to be closely integrated with adult mental health services and will focus their work on very different patient/client populations. In exceptionally well-resourced catchment areas the CMHT will not be generic but differentiated into a number of teams carrying out different functions, for example assessment and immediate treatment, continuing care and assertive outreach (see Craig and Pathare 1997 for a description of such a service). This differentiated model is much favoured by policy makers (Sainsbury Centre for Mental Health 1998) but is not clearly favoured by what little empirical evidence is available in the UK (Thornicroft *et al.* 1998).

In the UK the CMHT has become established in parallel with the closure of traditional mental hospitals and a consequent steep decline in in-patient bed numbers, particularly 'long-stay' beds (Thornicroft and Goldberg 1998). When carried out well, hospital closure has undoubtedly been successful for existing residents and is not associated with a significant amount of offending behaviour by those discharged (see Leff 1997; Treiman *et al.* 1999). However the impact of closure on the wider mental health service system has as yet not been quantified. Failure to plan for the needs for in-patient care of former long-stay hospital residents may have contributed to the pressure on acute beds (Treiman *et al.* 1999). It has been asserted that poor conceptualization of the needs of disabled, behaviourally disturbed and socially unacceptable patients newly accumulating within the services has led to a growth in the population of 'new long stay' patients inappropriately contained within acute wards (Henderson *et al.* 1998). In-patient services throughout the UK are currently under enormous strain, a problem best documented in London (Johnson *et al.* 1997). There is extreme difficulty accessing specialist forensic in-patient beds. Where there is a local community forensic service, this will usually be admitting its patients acutely to the local general adult mental health services, even when medium security is the preferred long-term option. CMHTs therefore operate in an environment that makes in-patient admission in general and transfer to in-patient forensic care in particular highly problematical. The lack of per-meability between CMHTs and forensic services, of course, works both ways. In a position of shortage of resources, hard-pressed community teams will rationally attempt to avoid responsibility for patients who are perceived as difficult, dangerous and presenting clinical needs outside their range of competence and will be reluctant to accept referrals of patients identified with a 'forensic' label.

Perspectives on the mentally disordered offender

Definitional issues

This chapter seeks to take an evidence-based approach to the care of the MDO. One important definitional issue, central to the book as a whole, is how to characterize the MDO. For the purposes of this chapter the broad and unsatisfactory definition adopted within the Reed Report is used: 'A mentally disordered person who has broken the law. In identifying broad service needs, this term is sometimes loosely used to include mentally disordered people who are alleged to have broken the law' (Department of Health and Home Office 1992). The definition clearly begs the question of the mean-ing of the term 'mentally disordered', which is in legal as well as psychiatric use. In the current UK policy context, as outlined in a recent discussion document (Home Office 1999), the mentally disordered will undoubtedly include people with offending behav-iour that occurs in the context of 'severe personality disorder'. The generic CMHT will be very unlikely to have any relevant, evidence-based treatment expertise (other than the psychopharmacological management of comorbid depressive and psychotic dis-orders) for the person with 'severe personality disorder'. The term 'broken the law' is also problematical, given the general reluctance of the criminal justice authorities in the UK to proceed with the prosecution of people who are in contact with mental health services. Serious offending behaviour can, on occasion, be glossed over as charges are either not pressed or subsequently dropped (see for example the case of Christopher Clunis (Ritchie *et al.* 1994)). On the other hand arbitrary processes can result in someone with a psychosis appearing before the courts as a result of a trivial public order offence, and hence becoming an MDO by Reed's definition (Department of Health and Home Office 1992), without that individual presenting any significant risk.

Past offending is not, of course, synonymous with dangerousness or risk. However patients with a history of offending behaviour will be heavily represented amongst those whose management presents obvious risk issues to the psychiatrist working within a CMHT. Offending behaviour, which is common amongst unemployed males of low social status who live in deprived inner urban areas, can also be coincidental with mental illness. A further not uncommon clinical scenario is the patient whose offending and mental illness are linked by a common factor, substance misuse. (There is some evidence that substance misuse is the major explanatory variable in the higher incidence of violent behaviour found amongst people discharged from psychiatric hospitals (Steadman *et al.* 1998).) The acquisitive burglar who steals in order to subsidize his crack cocaine habit, which from time to time precipitates psychotic episodes, represents a particularly challenging problem for the CMHT.

The Reed Committee report stated that 'the majority [of MDOS] can be looked after within general mental health or learning disability services'. The boundary between generic and specialist services for the MDO, however defined, is fraught with conceptual complexity (Cohen and Eastman 1997). In practice the generic/specialist distinction is a matter for local negotiation. The boundary will depend on factors such as the configuration and capacity of local services and the vagaries of the individual's life history and history of contact with mental health services. Buchanan explores the potentially difficult relationship between generic and forensic psychiatric services in Chapter 11.

One major element of UK policy has been the diversion of people from the criminal justice system to mental health services. There has been a rapid expansion of court and prison-based schemes for diversion (James and Hamilton 1991; Blumenthal and Wessely 1992; Joseph and Potter 1993; Exworthy and Parrott 1997; Weaver *et al.* 1997). This expansion has coincided with the acceleration of the mental hospital closure programme and an increasing policy emphasis on risk assessment and risk avoidance within mental health services. Increased demand on CMHTs to manage MDOs has therefore occurred at a time when the historic resource base for institutional care has been diminishing whilst popular and political expectations on mental health services to ensure public safety and manage people with socially unacceptable behaviour have been increasing.

The size of the problem

There is some useful epidemiological evidence about the size of the problem of offending behaviour, violence and suicide as experienced by CMHTs. At the extreme end of the spectrum, in England and Wales approximately 40 individuals per year commit a homicide and have been in psychiatric contact within the previous year (Shaw *et al.* 1999). This is from a total of approximately 600 individuals, the majority of whom are young men who are unemployed and/or unmarried (Appleby *et al.* 1999*b*). Substance misuse is common amongst perpetrators of homicide. Although rare as an occurrence, a homicide by a current or recent patient would afflict a CMHT in England and Wales serving a population of 40 000 once every 34 years (and possibly more frequently if one considers the peripatetic nature of disorganized psychiatric patients). This figure, although only illustrative, raises questions about the reality of the suggestion (Shaw *et al.* 1999) that mental health practitioners could have a conscious and direct impact on homicide rates (Geddes 1999). It does however confirm that certain professional groups (notably consultant psychiatrists working within CMHTs, particularly within inner urban areas characterized by high background levels of violence and deprivation) are at high risk of treating a patient during their professional lives who commits a homicide. A patient homicide leaves the professional exposed to the attendant personal and professional consequences, which will include being identified in a blanket fashion as incompetent (Morrall 1999). Professional fear of being caught up in a homicide inquiry in the UK is therefore not irrational.

The average CMHT will experience just under one patient suicide per year (extrapolating from Appleby *et al.* 1999*b*). A quarter of the total number of suicides occurring within the team catchment area will have been in recent contact with secondary mental health services. Studies in the UK and the USA have found suicide, which is increasingly prevalent amongst young men, to be associated with separation and bereavement, relationship difficulties, previous criminal charges, previous deliberate self-harm, psychotropic medication (Boardman *et al.* 1999) and access to firearms and substance misuse (Mosciki 1997). More accessible services in deprived inner urban areas are likely to have much higher rates of suicide, patient homicide and other offending behaviour by persons with psychiatric contact than inaccessible services working in rural or affluent suburban areas.

The work of the 'MacArthur violence risk assessment study' provides data on violence perpetrated by patients discharged from an episode of acute in-patient care (mean duration 9 days) in several sites in the USA (Steadman *et al.* 1998). The overall prevalence of violent acts in the following year by the sample was 27.5%, with a higher prevalence in patients with adjustment disorders or personality disorders and comorbid substance misuse (43%) and major mental illness and comorbid substance misuse (31.1%) than those with major mental disorders alone (17.9%). Interestingly the group without major mental disorder who were also without a substance misuse disorder who gained admission was too small to be included in the analysis, presumably reflecting a high threshold for admission into public mental health services in the USA. There was evidence in this study, which included a control group of non-patients living within one catchment area, that comorbid substance misuse rather than patient status was the most important determinant of future violent acts. Further analysis has also found that violent acts by the patient sample were associated with the particular sociodemographic characteristics of their neighbourhood independently of patient characteristics (Silver *et al.* 1999).

Evidence about violence and offending behaviour by people in contact with UK mental health services is limited. A study of patients with a psychotic illness in contact with a community mental health team focusing on the association between offending, imprisonment and aggression and comorbid substance misuse, carried out in an inner London catchment area, found a high lifetime prevalence of offending behaviour in the sample as a whole (46%) (Scott *et al.* 1998). There was a very low prevalence of recent imprisonment (3%) and a surprisingly high prevalence of recent hostile or aggressive behaviour as rated by community keyworkers (27%) but a low prevalence of assaultative behaviour in the past two years (4%). The study also found much higher levels of offending behaviour of all kinds amongst people with comorbid substance misuse (who comprised 29% of the total sample of psychotic patients in contact with the CMHT). An epidemiologically based study of people with a psychotic illness living in two inner urban areas in London found a much lower prevalence of violence or threatening behaviour over a two-year follow-up period. Nine per cent were violent (Johnson *et al.* 1998), although 38% of the sample had a lifetime history of violence and 26% had a criminal conviction. This study identified a previous history of violence, previous convictions and disability as measured by the GAF scale (American Psychiatric Association 1994) as predictors of subsequent violent acts: the influence of comorbid substance misuse was not explored. The discrepancies between these two studies reflect methodological differences in the ascertainment and definition of violence and offending behaviour. What is more striking is the commonality—past offending behaviour and violence is common amongst patients with a diagnosis of psychotic illness living in inner London (as is substance misuse (Menezes *et al.* 1996)) whilst significant violence in the near future is infrequent but by no means rare.

Previous offending behaviour, substance misuse, personality disorder, poor impulse control, adverse life events and recent aggression are common features of patients recently discharged from in-patient units to the care of CMHT staff, as are male sex, unemployment and unmarried status. All are robust 'actuarial' risk factors for future violence and/or self-harm (Buchanan 1999*b*; Appleby *et al.* 1999*b*). Mental health professionals, particularly those working in inner urban areas with high background levels of offending behaviour and social morbidity, are therefore seeking to provide care for substantial numbers of 'risky' individuals. This is even before one considers the presence of particular psychopathological features that are a specific cause of concern (such as delusions of control, thought insertion and persecutory delusions, which together form the 'threat/control override' complex identified in the risk literature (Link and Steuve 1994)).

Staff, user and carer perceptions

Community mental health staff experience a high degree of workplace stress (Carson and Fagin 1996). There is good evidence that the MDO patient or client will be perceived as contributing disproportionately to this stress. Feeling responsible for the welfare of their patients, patient relapses and fears of violence or aggression by patients were the three major patient related stressors identified by a mixed group of community mental health staff, whilst time pressure was a major non-patient related factor (Reid *et al.* 1999). Themes identified in a study of consultant psychiatrist who retired prematurely include both the generic stress associated with the job and a range of specific concerns. These included fear of failing their patients (with negative consequences to the patient), fears for personal safety, the level of violence committed by patients and fear of being 'crucified' in a future hospital inquiry into a patient suicide or homicide (Kendell and Pearce 1997). CMHT staff will often find themselves under extreme time pressure in making assessments of the risks that their patients present to themselves and others and will generally be carrying high caseloads.

Community mental health staff in the UK have been vociferous in their opposition to compulsory community treatment of the mentally ill. This might be formulated as either an admirable concern for their clients' civil liberties or an understandable worry over the consequences of being held to be responsible for the behaviour of their clients. Anecdotally CMHT staff are particularly unhappy to manage problematical behaviours which they either cannot understand (such as sexual offending and abnormal behaviour in the context of a severe personality disorder) or for which they lack clear treatment strategies (such as inappropriate anger and substance misuse, particularly abuse of stimulants).

There is little or no evidence on the perspective of either users or carers on the community care of the MDO although one high profile offender, Christopher Clunis, tried unsuccessfully to sue the authorities for lack of care in failing to prevent his offending behaviour. Families may experience extreme difficulty in accessing help for a mentally ill relative who is violent or threatening within the family home. This in part stems from a reluctance by the patient, carers and services to acknowledge the nature of the problem, as reflected in the prolonged average duration of untreated psychosis of first presentation patients (Lincoln and McGorry 1999). Problems in obtaining help may persist after the diagnosis is clear. In some jurisdictions families may make use of restraining orders, which they predict the patient will break, in order to ensure that violent behaviour or threats will result in their relative's incarceration and subsequent treatment (Solomon *et al.* 1995).

It is clear that patients in general commonly experience mental health services as coercive (Brown 1981; Pescosolido *et al.* 1998). This is likely to undermine adherence with treatment and the development of a therapeutic relationship with mental health services and may lead to worse clinical outcomes (Kaltiala-Heino *et al.* 1997). The perception of coercion on admission to a psychiatric hospital, which tends to be enduring, is not simplistically associated with compulsory treatment but is also determined by certain staff behaviours such as the use of force, threats and giving orders to patients (Lidz *et al.* 1998). On the other hand coercion is less likely to be experienced when the patient is subject to persuasion, respectfully included in a fair decision-making process, allowed a 'voice' in the process and has been treated with respect, concern and good faith (in a manner which has been termed 'procedural justice' (Lidz *et al.* 1995)). The MDO might be both particularly vulnerable to experiencing coercion, an objective fact for many if not most, and potentially be able to be treated with 'procedural justice' by the mental health and criminal justice systems. The USA experience of coercive community treatment is discussed in detail by Swartz and Swanson in Chapter 9.

The inquiry literature

The UK homicide inquiries have produced a rich body of independent reports that document the functioning of mental health services as they grapple with patients who go on to kill. There is also an impressive secondary literature (e.g. Petch and Bradley 1997; Peay 1997). Inquiries have been characterized as inefficient and methodologically inadequate for making general recommendations about the future of UK mental health services (Geddes 1999) and do not infrequently fall into the error of hindsight bias in ascribing causative status to the actions of caring professionals (Prins 1999). However, the literature does identify a range of issues that deserve attention by CMHT staff. Inquiries frequently reveal a lack of multi-disciplinary working and poor communication between agencies (such as the health service, social services and the police) and between staff within an agency (for example between nurses and doctors). Inexperienced staff, working in isolation, may be left to tackle highly complex clinical and social situations without adequate support and supervision. Even experienced staff may lack relevant basic skills. Failure to ensure that relevant information, particularly about dangerous behaviour, is communicated to key people is a common feature.

A recurring theme in the inquiry literature is the failure to understand the inner world of the patient, the details of their experiences and their social context (Holloway 1998). A major element in the management of 'risky' people is a detailed understanding of the person's life history and the context of past offending behaviour. Failure to take adequate account of the social context of patients who go on to kill has been blamed on the dominance of doctors within mental health services (Prins 1999). More realistically it stems from an inability of services, due to lack of resources, staff attitudes and inadequacies in training, to carry out the detailed information-gathering and assessment that characterizes a good quality risk assessment (Holloway 1998). Lack of detail and a cross-sectional approach inevitably characterizes even the best-resourced scheme for court diversion. It was perhaps therefore inevitable that a patient who went on to kill would not be admitted, despite being psychotic at the time, following an assessment by a court diversion service which would appear (with the very possibly faulty) benefit of hindsight to have been erroneous (Dixon *et al.* 1999).

Ethical issues for community mental health services

A set of four principles has been put forward as providing a framework for biomedical ethics (Beauchamp 1999). These are: respect for the autonomy of the individual;

non-maleficence (not causing harm); beneficence (doing good and balancing benefits against risks); and justice (fairness in the allocation of resources, benefits and risks). Practitioners within community mental health services face numerous ethical challenges (Szmukler 1999; Szmukler and Holloway 1998). Some reflect dilemmas long inherent within psychiatry. There is, for example, a clear tension between respecting the autonomy of the individual and forcible therapeutic intervention, justified by the principle of beneficence. Excessive emphasis on the former may lead to neglect, unmet need for services and other harms to the individual and society ('rotting with your rights on'). In contrast, the latter may be experienced as coercive and result in rejection of services (with potentially disastrous consequences later in the individual's psychiatric career) or alternatively may lead to a loss of human dignity and skills in an institutionalized patient.

Other ethical challenges are novel. There is a human right to privacy (enshrined in Article 8 of the European Convention on Human Rights, which is being incorporated into UK law). Assertive community treatment assumes that intrusion into the service user's privacy is ethically justified, since being assertive requires not taking 'no' as a reason for disengaging from active follow-up. UK policies now mandate follow-up for patients falling under the 'care programme approach' and 'supervised discharge', under which selected patients are placed under specific 'requirements' (for example to live in a certain place and attend an out-patient clinic (Eastman 1995)). Even more intrusive are procedures for out-patient commitment in the USA (see Swartz and Swanson Chapter 9). These interventions are generally justified on paternalistic grounds (the principle of beneficence being seen to trump autonomy in these cases).

There are important and largely unresolved issues about the ethics of information exchange between community care agencies (including the police), which undoubtedly erode the individual's rights to privacy and the traditional profound strictures surrounding medical confidentiality (Szmukler and Holloway 2001). As an example, one recommendation from the UK homicide inquiry literature is that: 'If an application is made for ordinary housing for mentally disordered offenders the forensic history and risk assessment must be disclosed, ideally with the patient's consent, but where there is a risk to others, disclosure may be necessary without such consent.' (Petch and Bradley 1997, emphasis added). It would seem that once one has fallen into the class of 'mentally disordered offender' traditional rights to confidentiality should be waived, a potentially disturbing and destructive development. Users of psychiatric services rightly expect confidentiality but an increasing range of 'stakeholders' in the mental health care system have been identified as having a legitimate right to know about the most intimate details of an individual's life. It is becoming increasingly difficult for professionals to promote the autonomy of their patients/clients and their privacy in the face of the therapeutic gaze of the state.

However a too conservative view of confidentiality, which does not encourage the involvement of the family or other carers in the treatment process, may deny the patient a vital source of effective community support (and cause carers untold distress). Szmukler and Bloch (1997) put forward practical suggestions for ensuring that carers are fully engaged in the treatment process. Treatment teams may have to consider disclosing information to carers, even when forbidden by the patient, in the patient's own best interests (consider the potentially suicidal person who has begun refusing medication). On occasion information must be disclosed in the relatives' interests. In US jurisdictions there is, of course, a positive 'duty to warn', within which the therapist is required to communicate a threat of violence made by a patient to the intended victim and law enforcement agencies (Binder and McNeil 1996). No such positive duty has been defined in UK law, as yet, but in circumstances of perceived risk to others traditional duties of medical confidentiality do not apply, providing the risk of harm is substantial.

Since much treatment by CMHT staff occurs in the community, there is also an increased likelihood that it becomes public. The curiosity of neighbours may be aroused, particularly with repeated visits to a reluctant patient/client, and especially if attempts to gain entry are noisily refused. Neighbours and other members of the public may come in time to recognize CMHT members, and thus that those visited are likely to be patients. Accessible CMHTs are also frequently contacted to intervene in situations identified by the public or non-statutory organizations where the referred client or patient does not perceive a problem, presents no obvious risk to themselves or others but is behaving in a socially unacceptable or distressing manner. People who are known to have had contact with the police and mental health services can, in certain areas, become victimized by elements of the local population. Well-intentioned attempts to carry out assertive community treatment may, on occasion, result in significant harms to the patient/client.

The MDO frequently presents the CMHT practitioner with conflicts of duty. The traditional focus of health care on the perceived welfare of the autonomous individual is already compromised within mental health services by the necessary practice of intervening to provide compulsory treatment in the patient's best interests. It is further eroded by the requirement within the field of forensic psychiatry to serve multiple masters, including the courts and the expectations of the public (see Gutheil 1999 and Fennell and Yeates Chapter 13). Within an increasingly risk-avoidant and litigious society, employing authorities will also have expectations on staff to minimize risk and public outcry on the one hand and to contain health care costs on the other. This represents a peculiar kind of double jeopardy for mental health providers. In a further twist to the ethical conundrums presented by the MDO, a decision by the treatment team to recommend costly long-term detention in hospital may minimize the potential risk the patient presents to themselves or others and hence be justified on paternalistic grounds. However this expenditure may also deprive many people within the local community of effective mental health care interventions as the mental health budget is exhausted.

Practical management of the mentally disordered offender

Philosophy of care

Managing the MDO requires the CMHT member to adopt a philosophy of care that is significantly at odds with the traditional focus of the mental health professional on fostering patient autonomy and respect for the individual's rights. One authority, commenting on the homicide inquiry literature, noted: 'Workers need to develop what I would call a more "robust" approach to dealing with offenders and offender-patients. Concern for civil liberties has sometimes obscured the need to place public protection at the forefront' (Prins 1999). Successful treatment of the MDO requires staff to have 'a clear conception of the clinical uses and therapeutic value of authority' (Lamb *et al.* 1999). Staff need to be prepared to work within a framework of court-imposed conditions of treatment, to monitor treatment compliance and substance misuse and to be directive about the offender patient's daily routine and living conditions. Practices outside the normal repertoire of the CMHT, such as routine urine testing of patients for substance misuse, are commonplace within MDO services. Workers may need rapidly to readmit a deteriorating or non-complaint patient (where there has been a clearly identified pattern of risk) or alternatively present the MDO who is failing to comply with probation conditions to the court, in the expectation that they will be imprisoned again.

The MDO who is diverted from the criminal justice system to the mental health services is inevitably subject to a degree of coercion by the treatment team. The inevitable negative effects upon the therapeutic relationship may be minimized by an open acknowledgement of the situation, clarity over the reasons for the offender patient's MDO status and honesty about the current and future behaviour of the treatment team. Consequences of particular actions, such as non-compliance, repeated substance misuse or further offending should be spelt out. Actions by the team when authoritative intervention is required should be carried out with clarity of purpose and courtesy towards the patient. There should be particular emphasis on making coercive treatment decisions as comprehensible as possible to the patient in order to meet criteria for 'procedural justice' (Lidz *et al.* 1995).

Working with the criminal justice system

It is vital for treatment teams and patients to be clear about the expectations upon them held by the criminal justice system. The courts 'place a greater emphasis on the potential dangerousness of the mentally ill offender than on the individual's rights' (Lamb *et al.* 1999). Courts may expect those working with the MDO to be concentrating on minimizing risk to the public and decreasing offending behaviour rather than the traditional psychiatric goals of controlling symptoms and maximizing social functioning. The court and probation service may also have naïve expectations of the capacity of mental health services to intervene in certain kinds of clinical problem, such as offending behaviour related to substance misuse and enduring personality traits. The court may indeed presume that the MDO managed as an out-patient 'will not be dangerous to others whilst under supervision and treatment in the community' (Lamb *et al.* 1999), an expectation that in many clinical situations is not clearly and obviously achievable.

The preparation of reports to the court represents an opportunity for effective liaison between key actors. In England and Wales these will generally consist of the court itself, the treatment team, the Crown Prosecution Service, the probation service, the patient/offender and their lawyer and the police service—a similar range of agencies can be generated in other jurisdictions. The treatment team will need to carry out an assessment of the clinical state and needs of the MDO. A psychiatric disposal under Section 37 of the 1983 Mental Health Act does not require there to be a link between the offending behaviour and mental disorder. However, in practice the court will expect a psychiatric report to address this issue and will additionally be particularly concerned to identify the ability of a mental health disposal to reduce future risk to the public. In any case the treatment team will have to make a formulation of the relationship between the offending and the mental disorder if there is to be effective care planning and risk management. The level of detail required for a good quality assessment is potentially daunting for the mainstream CMHT and difficult, complex or worrying cases may require specialist expertise (where this is available). Professionals preparing reports may need to be particularly assertive in obtaining details of the patient's past history of offending and witness statements relating to the current offence.

Community Mental Health Team staff treating MDOs need to understand how the criminal justice system works and the range of options available to the court in relation to the MDO. This will include knowledge about local mental health legislation in relation to the MDO (in England and Wales Part III of the 1983 Mental Health Act). Generic services will require readily accessible sources of expert advice about medicolegal issues that are rarely encountered in ordinary clinical practice (such as, for example, the disposal options available for the patient who is incompetent or unfit to plead). Advice may also be required about the drafting of realistic and appropriate recommendations to the court.

Management of risk

It is an uncomfortable fact that quite rationally when faced with overwhelming demand, health care professionals adopt a variety of well-worn pragmatic strategies (New 1996). These include *deterrence* (characterized by service charges, gate-keeping by primary care, unfriendly staff, inconvenient appointment times, poor quality care environments and prolonged duration between appointments); *deflection* (passing referrals to other agencies, shifting between 'health' and 'social' care or between generic, forensic and learning disability mental health services); *dilution* (thinly spreading service provision, adopting minimal standards of care, reducing skill-mix in a nursing team); *delay* (waiting lists, which for psychological treatments can become infinitely long); and *denial* (which involves not providing a treatment or service at all for more or less justifiable reasons). Most community mental health professionals will recognize these strategies operating within their day-to-day work. The less obviously desirable patient, such as the MDO, will be particularly likely to experience at least three of these five 'd's' when referred to a generic mental health service: deterrence, deflection and denial. Similar behaviour occurs within dedicated forensic mental health services, which to survive must be particularly effective in selecting those cases for whom they do take on responsibility (a luxury denied by the generic CMHT operating within a sectorized service). Service managers and key professionals need to be aware of the covert strategies adopted by staff (including themselves) in controlling workload and at the very least ensure that CMHTs are treating MDOs with fairness *vis-à-vis* the case-load as a whole. Hostile or rejecting attitudes should be avoided. Purchasers and crim-inal justice authorities need to be informed of the sorts of problems that cannot be tackled by a team given its resource and skills base (e.g. sexual offending, domestic violence not associated with a mental illness, severe personality disorder *per se*). Teams need to be aware of and make use of alternative options within the overall care system for dealing with particular issues, for example programmes targeted at anger manage-ment offered by the local probation service.

The importance of adequate assessment of the patient and formulation of the prob-lems that the patient presents has already been emphasized. Although the courts may expect the focus to be on risk (an issue discussed in detail by Skeem and Mulvey in Chapter 6) it is vital that assessment is as holistic as possible. Assessment should encompass a wide range of need domains (Phelan *et al.* 1995). The complex clinical pre-sentation of the socially chaotic offending individual should be broken down into com-ponent areas, which will include but not be restricted to mental state issues, socially unacceptable or self-harming behaviours, substance misuse, interpersonal relationships, living setting, income, daytime activities and educational and training needs. Outstand-ing criminal justice issues will obviously need to be highlighted. Effective assessment of the MDO above all requires access to informants, a longitudinal perspective on the indi-vidual's functioning, problems and strengths and attention to significant contextual issues. (The latter are usefully summarized in the violence risk assessment tool, the HCR-20 (Belfrage 1998): unrealistic future plans; exposure to destabliziers; lack of personal support; non-compliance with caring agencies; and psychosocial stress.)

Once the patient's needs have been disaggregated into bite-size chunks, a manage-ment plan (or in contemporary UK jargon a care plan) can be elaborated. This should not simply focus on the most obvious problem, such as the individual's 'personality disorder', 'psychosis' or 'risk', but set out in a reasonably logical and hierarchical fash-ion how the range of problems the patient personally experiences and presents to others should be tackled. The plan needs to be clear about who should be doing what by when and should be regularly reviewed. In complex situations individual CMHT members will need to have access to a network of care and sources of supervision, consultation and support. The individual professional should be acutely aware of the importance of communication in relation to the management of the 'risky' individual, lack of communication being the one clear and consistent message from the homicide inquiry literature (Petch and Bradley 1997). Keyworkers and responsible medical staff working with 'risky' individuals are well advised to engage in exhaustive communication with the patient, carers, CMHT colleagues and other involved services (subject, of course, to local rules of confidentiality). Local service managers and if necessary purchasers must be informed when resources are inadequate to meet the patient's needs in respect of critical issues of concern. It is particularly important to work with the family and informal carers who may, of course, be victims of the MDO as well as offering a potentially vital source of support for the individual (Lamb *et al.* 1999). The homicide inquiry literature contains a significant number of haunting statements of concern by carers about the risks the person is presenting which were not acted upon effectively by the professionals and which describe a pattern of failure by services to take the needs of carers seriously (see Prins 1999 for a series of examples).

A key aspect of risk management is to set out clear plans for intervention if things are going wrong. Clinicians should always be sensitive to the consequences of their assessments and predictions being incorrect (Holloway 1997). Staff should be prepared to reassess, reappraise and alter treatment plans. Relapse planning is now an established element in the treatment of psychosis. An individual 'relapse signature' can be elaborated (Birchwood 1996). Ideally early signs of relapse are identified with the patient and carers within a consensual process and a plan is developed for early intervention, which may include a small supply of extra medication, clear guidelines about how to contact the services and recommendations for how the services should respond if a crisis occurs (Sutherby *et al.* 1999). Care planning for the MDO may also be required for non-consensual interventions. A detailed risk assessment may also throw up very person-specific indicators for concern relating to the individual contextual factors associated with dangerous behaviour for that person: these will have to be incorporated within the treatment plan. In addition, the consequences for the patient of not adhering to the treatment plan need to be spelt out and acted upon by the team in a clear and consistent fashion. A risk management corollary to this statement is not to put into a care plan elements that cannot clearly be achieved (for example fortnightly assessments by the consultant psychiatrist and weekly contact with a CMHT keyworker in a 'risky' individual known to be reluctant to maintain contact with services) unless one is very confident that failure to adhere to the care plan will be identified and assertively acted upon.

Service models for working with the mentally disordered offender

Given the high profile of the MDO and the costs associated with their in-patient management, which is often in secure settings, the lack of research into models of community care for the offender patient is striking and surprising. Four logically distinct but practically overlapping patterns of community support for the MDO are in current operation. The first is the generic CMHT model, within which the offender/patient is managed by non-specialist local services. The second approach is a consultation/liaison model, within which specialist forensic practitioners offer advice, support and coworking with generic CMHT staff in relation to MDOs (Whittle and Scally 1998). Thirdly, a separate specialist team can provide a comprehensive intensive case management service for selected forensic clients (Solomon and Draine 1995). A final possible approach to the MDO is the forensic psychiatrist working independently from an institutional base to provide community management for 'risky' discharged individuals with *ad hoc* involvement of community and criminal justice professionals.

Although the majority of MDOs will always be managed by generic services, pure genericism is unfeasible for the community management of highly 'risky' individuals once a speciality of forensic psychiatry has been delineated. Consultation/liaison models will only prosper if the consultee finds their mentors to be credible and to give useful advice and practical assistance. There are particular difficulties in relation to the advisory role of forensic psychiatrists to CMHTs, at least in the UK, given their lack of experience and training in relation to the realities of community mental health care (and, more technically, the inapplicability of the conceptual tools they have been trained to use with institutionalized populations to the wider realm of the non-institutionalized mentally ill (Duggan 1997)). The only service model to date to have been empirically evaluated is the separate community forensic team. Surprisingly, the single reported controlled study into this approach, despite the face validity of the model, showed no evidence of efficacy (Solomon and Draine 1995). The (unreliable) homicide inquiry literature has produced one case where the single practitioner model was deemed to have failed badly (Scotland *et al.* 1998).

In England and Wales a Crown Court can make a 'restriction order' on a convicted offender/patient (Section 41 of the 1983 Mental Health Act) if, following conviction, 'it appears to the court, having regard to the nature of the offence, the antecedents of the offender and the risk of his committing further offences if set at large, that it is necessary for the protection of the public from serious harm'. The sub-group of MDOs subject to 'restriction orders' is characterized by extremely serious offending behaviour, detailed and continuing risk assessment, slow reintroduction into the community following a prolonged in-patient stay (often in conditions of high security) and long-term oversight by the authorities (through the Home Office Mental Health Unit (Potts 1995)). Experience of the community care of 'restricted' patients (who are technically 'conditionally discharged') has largely been positive. In practice, supervision of the 'conditionally discharged' patient involves a continuum of specialist forensic community care, consultation/liaison to the generic CMHTs and sole follow-up by the generic CMHT for the least risky patients.

Practical management problems

The mentally disordered offender presents a range of management problems that may lie outside the core competencies of the generic CMHT. Teams should consider refusing to take on some clinical problems that require specialist expertise, such as the management of sex offenders and certain kinds of severe personality disorder. The role of psychotherapy in the treatment of the MDO is discussed by Norton and Vince in Chapter 8. Equally important is a structure of supervision and support for staff working with the troubling and troubled patient, which can usefully include a psychotherapy component to allow staff to reflect on the feelings that the patients are engendering within them (notably fear, hostility and rejection). The MDO often presents with poor impulse control, threatening behaviour and comorbid substance misuse. Services should provide interventions aimed at these issues. Anger management can be offered in individual or group settings (Towl and Crighton 1996). Despite the clear epidemiological evidence that identifies substance misuse comorbidity as a key factor in self-harming and dangerous behaviour by people with a mental illness (Steadman *et al.* 1998), the research literature does not support a particular service model for working with dual diagnosis patients (Ley *et al.* 1999). Community Mental Health Teams managing MDOs will require at the very least close links with their colleagues within the substance misuse services. One study of discharged psychotic patients found that lack of treatment was more common amongst patients who went on to be violent, but the apparent protective effect of treatment all but disappeared when there was comorbid substance misuse (Swanson *et al.* 1997).

Conclusion

There are many pitfalls facing CMHTs in their work with the MDO within a risk-averse and blame-prone culture. MDOs represent a specially stigmatized sub-group of the mentally ill, and this stigma can readily attach itself to the treating staff. Clinicians face blame for the anti-social and self-harming acts of their patients as well as potential legal jeopardy from the patients themselves and notoriety if things go wrong (Lamb *et al.* 1999). Short-term risk management can unhealthily dominate decision making which, for people characterized by enduring maladaptive patterns of behaviour and/or severe and recurrent mental illnesses, should always have a strategic dimension. Successful management of the MDO requires clarity of purpose and the development of realistic and achievable treatment goals. Resources need to be adequate to the demands on the service and senior management should ensure a culture that is open and accountable but not seek to allocate blame to individuals when things go wrong. Staff should be sensitive to the ethical dilemmas they face in their work, which will continually require them to balance the promotion of the autonomy of the offender patient against the potential harms to the patient or others flowing from non-intervention. There should be opportunity for reflection and discussion over difficult ethical and clinical issues with colleagues. Above all, staff will require appropriate supervision, support and training for the many and complex tasks they undertake with the MDO.

References

American Psychiatric Association (1994) *Diagnostic and statistical manual of mental disorders* (4th edn). Washington DC: American Psychiatric Association Press.

Appleby, L., Shaw, J., Amos, T. *et al.* (1999*a*) Mental disorder and clinical care in people convicted of homicide: national clinical survey. *British Medical Journal*, 318, 1235–9.

Appleby, L., Shaw, J., Amos, T. *et al.* (1999*b*) *Safer services. Report of the national confidential inquiry into suicide and homicide by people with mental illness.* London: Stationery Office.

Beauchamp, T. L. (1999) The philosophical basis of psychiatric ethics. In *Psychiatric ethics* (ed. S. Bloch, P. Chodoff and S. A. Green), pp. 25–48. Oxford: Oxford University Press.

Belfrage, H. (1998) Implementing the HCR-20 scheme for risk assessment in a forensic psychiatric hospital setting: integrating research and clinical practice. *Journal of Forensic Psychiatry*, 9, 328–38.

Binder, R. L. and McNeil, D. E. (1996) Application of the Tarasoff ruling and its effect on the victim and the therapeutic relationship. *Psychiatric Services*, 47, 1212–15.

Bindman, J., Davies, S., Taylor, R. *et al.* (1996) Developments in mental health policy in the United Kingdom. *Epidemiologia e Psichiatria Sociale*, 5, 87–91.

Birchwood, M. (1996) Early intervention in psychotic relapse: cognitive approaches to detection and management. In *Cognitive–behavioural interventions with psychotic disorders* (ed. G. Haddock and P. D. Slade), pp. 171–211. London: Routledge.

Blumenthal, S. and Wessely, S. (1992) National survey of current arrangements for diversion from custody in England and Wales. *British Medical Journal*, 305, 1322–5.

Boardman, A. P., Grimbaldeston, A. H., Handley, C. (1999) The North Staffordshire Suicide Study: a case-control study of suicide in one health district. *Psychological Medicine*, 29, 27–33.

Brown, P. (1981) The mental patients' rights movement and mental health institutional change. *International Journal of Health Services*, 11, 523–40.

Buchanan, A. (1999*a*) Independent inquiries into homicide. *British Medical Journal*, 318, 1089–90.

Buchanan, A. (1999*b*) Risk and dangerousness. *Psychological Medicine*, 29, 465–73.

Carson, J. and Fagin, L. (1996) Stress in mental health professionals: cause for concern or an inevitable part of the job? *International Journal of Social Psychiatry*, 42, 79–81.

Cohen, A. and Eastman, N. (1997) Needs assessment for mentally disordered offenders and others requiring similar services. *British Journal of Psychiatry*, 171, 412–16.

Craig, P. and Pathare, S. (1997) Assertive community treatment for the severely mentally ill in West Lambeth. *Advances in Psychiatric Treatment*, 3, 111–18.

Deahl, M. and Turner T. (1997) General psychiatry in no-man's land. *British Journal of Psychiatry*, 171, 6–8.

Department of Health (1994) Guidance on the discharge of mentally disordered people and their continuing care in the community. HSG(94)27.

Department of Health (1995) *Building bridges: A guide to arrangements for inter-agency working in the care and protection of severely mentally ill people.* London: HMSO.

Department of Health (1998) *Modernising mental health services. Safe, Sound and Supportive.* London: Department of Health.

Department of Health and Home Office (1992) Review of health and social services for mentally disordered offenders and others requiring similar services: Final summary report. Cmnd 2088 (Chairman Dr John Reed, CB). London: HMSO.

Dixon, K., Herbert, P., Marshall, S. *et al.* (1999) The Dixon Team inquiry report. London: Kensington and Chelsea and Westminster Health Authority.

Duggan, C. (1997) Introduction. Assessing risk in the mentally disordered (ed. C. Duggan). *British Journal of Psychiatry*, **170**, Suppl. 32, 1–3.

Eastman, N. (1995) Anti-therapeutic community mental health law. *British Medical Journal*, **310**, 1081–2.

Exworthy, T. and Parrott, J. (1997) Comparative evaluation of a diversion from custody scheme. *Journal of Forensic Psychiatry*, **8**, 406–16.

Geddes, J. (1999) Suicide and homicide by people with mental illness. *British Medical Journal*, **318**, 1225–6.

Glover, G. (1996) Mental Illness Needs Index (MINI). In *Commissioning Mental Health Services* (ed. G. Thornicroft and G. Strathdee). London: HMSO.

Gutheil, T. G. (1999) Ethics and forensic psychiatry. In *Psychiatric Ethics* (ed. S. Bloch, P. Chodoff and S. A. Green), pp. 345–362. Oxford: Oxford University Press.

Henderson, C., Bindman, J. and Thornicroft, G. (1998) Can deinstitutionalised care be provided for those at risk of violent offending? *Epidemiologia e Psichiatria Sociale*, **7**, 42–51.

Holloway, F. (1996) Community psychiatric care: from libertarianism to coercion. 'Moral Panic' and mental health policy in Britain. *Hhealth Care Analysis*, **4**, 235–43.

Holloway, F. (1997) The assessment and management of risk in psychiatry: can we do better? *Psychiatric Bulletin*, **21**, 283–5.

Holloway, F. (1998) Reading about: risk assessment. *British Journal of Psychiatry*, **173**, 540–3.

Home Office (1999) *Managing dangerous people with severe personality disorder. Proposals for policy development*. London: Home Office.

James, D. V. and Hamilton, L. W. (1991) The Clerkenwell scheme: assessing efficacy and cost of a psychiatric court liaison service to a magistrates' court. *British Medical Journal*, **303**, 282–5.

Johnson, S., Leese, M., Brooks, L., Clarkson, P., Guite, H., Thornicroft, G., Holloway, F. and Wykes, T. (1998) Frequency And Predictors Of Adverse Events: the PriSM Psychosis Study (3) *British Journal of Psychiatry*, **173**, 376–384.

Johnson, S., Ramsay, R., Thornicroft, G. *et al.* (1997) London's Mental Health. The Report of the King's Fund for London Commission. London: Kings Fund.

Joseph, P. L. A. and Potter, M. (1993) Diversion from custody, I: Psychiatric assessment at the magistrates' court. *British Journal of Psychiatry*, **162**, 325–30.

Kaltiala-Heino, R., Laippala, P. and Salokangas, R. K. (1997) Impact of coercion on treatment outcome. *International Journal of Law and Psychiatry*, **20**, 311–22.

Kendell, R. and Pearce, A. (1997) Consultant psychiatrist who retired prematurely in 1995 and 1996. *Psychiatric Bulletin*, **21**, 741–5.

Lamb, H. R., Weinberger, L. E. and Goss, B. H. (1999) Community treatment of severely mentally ill offenders under the jurisdiction of the criminal justice system: a review. *Psychaitric Services*, **7**, 907–13.

Leff, J. (ed.) (1997) *Community care—illusion or reality*. Chichester: John Wiley.

Ley, A., Jeffrey, D. P. and Siegfried, N. (1999) Treatment programmes for people with both severe mental illness and substance misuse. In *The Cochrane Library* (Issue 3). Oxford: Update Software.

Lidz, C. W., Hoge, S., Gardner, W. *et al.* (1995) Perceived coercion in mental hospital admission: pressures and process. *Archives of General Psychiatry*, **52**, 1034–9.

Lidz, C. W., Mulvey, E. P., Hoge, S. P. *et al.* (1998) Factual sources of psychiatric patients' perceptions of coercion in the hospital admission process. *American Journal of Psychiatry*, **155**, 1254–60.

Lincoln, C. and McGorry, P. (1999) Pathways to care in early psychosis; clinical and consumer perspectives. In *The recognition and management of early psychosis. A preventive approach* (ed. P. D. McGorry and H. J. Jackson), pp. 51–80. Cambridge: Cambridge University Press.

Link, B. G. and Steuve, A. (1994) Psychotic symptoms and the violent/illegal behaviour of mental patients compared to controls. In *Violence and mental disorder. Developments in risk assessment* (ed. J. Monahan and H. Steadman), pp. 137–159. Chicago, IL: Chicago University Press.

Menezes, P. R., Johnson, S., Thornicroft, G., Marshall, J., Prosser, D., Bebbington, P. and Kuipers, E. (1996) Drug and alcohol problems among individuals with severe mental illness in South London. *British Journal of Psychiatry*, **168**, 612–19.

Morrall, P. (1999) Homicides committed by the mentally ill and the role of the psychiatric disciplines. *Science, Discourse and Mind*, **1**, 1–11.

Mosciki, E. K. (1997) Identification of suicide risk factors using epidemiologic studies. *Psychiatric Clinics of North America*, **20**, 499–517.

New, B. (1996) The rationing agenda in the NHS. *British Medical Journal*, **312**, 1593–1601.

Peay, J. (1997) Clinicians and inquiries: Demons, drones or demigods? *International Review of Psychiatry*, **9**, 171–7.

Pescosolido, B. A., Gardner, C. B. and Lubell, K. M. (1998) How people get into mental health services: stories of choice, coercion and 'muddling through' from 'first-timers'. *Social Science and Medicine*, **46**, 275–86.

Petch, E. and Bradley, C. (1997) Learning the lessons from homicide inquires: Adding insult to injury? *Journal of Forensic Psychiatry*, **8**, 161–184.

Phelan, M., Slade, M., Thornicroft, G. *et al.* (1995) The Camberwell Assessment of Need (CAN): the validity and reliability of an instrument to assess the needs of the seriously mentally ill. *British Journal of Psychiatry*, **167**, 589–95.

Potts, J. (1995) Risk assessment and management: A Home Office perspective. In *Psychiatric patient violence—risk and response* (ed. J. Crichton), pp. 35–48. London: Duckworth.

Prins, H. (1999) *Will they do it again?* London: Routledge.

Reid, Y., Johnson, S., Morant, N. *et al.* (1999) Explanations for stress and satisfaction in mental health professionals: a qualitative study. *Social Psychiatry and Psychiatric Epidemiology*, **34**, 301–8.

Ritchie, J. H., Dick, D. and Lingham, R. (1994) The report of the inquiry into the care and treatment of Christopher Clunis. London: HMSO.

Sainsbury Centre for Mental Health (1998). *Keys to engagement*. London: Sainsbury Centre for Mental Health.

Scotland, Baronness, Kelly, H and Devaux, M. (1998) The report of luke warm luke mental health inquiry. London: Lambeth, Southwark and Lewisham Health Authority.

Scott, H., Johnson, S., Menezes, P. *et al.* (1998) Substance misuse and risk of aggression and offending among the severely mentally ill. *British Journal of Psychiatry*, **172**, 345–50.

Shaw, J., Appleby, L., Amos, T. (1999) Mental disorder and clinical care in people convicted of homicide: national clinical survey. *British Medical Journal*, **318**, 1240–4.

Silver, E., Mulvey, E. P. and Monahan, J. (1999) Assessing violence risk among discharged psychiatric patients: toward an ecological approach. *Law and Human Behavior*, **22**. 237–55.

Solomon, P. and Draine, J. (1995) One year outcomes of a randomised trial of case management with seriously mentally ill clients leaving jail. *Evaluation Review*, **19**, 256–73.

Solomon, P., Draine, J. and Delaney, M. A. (1995) The use of restraining orders by families of severely mentally ill adults. *Administration and Policy in Mental Health*, **23**, 157–61.

Steadman, H. J., Mulvey, E. P., Monahan, J. *et al.* (1998) Violence by people discharged from acute psychiatric inpatient facilities and by others in the same neighborhoods. *Archives of General Psychiatry*, 55, 393–401.

Sutherby, K., Szmukler, G. I., Halpern, A. *et al.* (1999) A study of 'crisis cards' in a community psychiatric service. *Acta Psychiatrica Scandinavica*, 100, 56.

Swanson, J., Estroff, S., Swartz, M. (1997) Violence and severe mental disorder in clinical and community populations: The effects of psychotic symptoms, comorbidity, and lack of treatment. *Psychiatry*, 60, 1–22.

Szmukler, G. (1999) Ethics in community psychiatry. In Psychiatric ethics (ed. S. Bloch, P. Chodoff and S. A. Green), pp. 363–82. Oxford: Oxford University Press.

Szmukler, G. I. and Bloch, S. (1997) Family involvement in the care of people with psychoses: an ethical argument. *British Journal of Psychiatry*, 171, 401–5.

Szmukler, G. and Holloway, F. (1998) Ethics in community psychiatry. *Current Opinion in Psychiatry*, 11, 549–53.

Szmukler, G. and Holloway, F. (2001) Confidentiality in community psychiatric practice. In *Confidentiality* (ed. C. Cordess) London: Jessica Kingsley. pp. 53–70.

Thornicroft G. and Goldberg, D. (1998) Has community care failed? Maudlsey Discussion Paper No. 5. London: Institute of Psychiatry.

Thornicroft, G., Wykes, T., Holloway, F., Johnson S. and Szmukler, G. (1998) From efficacy to effectiveness in community mental health services: the PRiSM psychosis study (10). *British Journal of Psychiatry*, 173, 423–6.

Towl, G. J. and Crighton, D. A. (1996) *The Handbook of Psychology for Forensic Practitioners*. London: Routledge.

Treiman, N., Leff, J. and Glover, G. (1999) Outcome of long stay psychiatric patients resettled in the community: prospective cohort study. *British Medical Journal*, 319, 13–16.

Weaver, T., Taylor, F., Cunningham, B. *et al.* (1997) The Bentham Unit: a pilot remand and assessment service for male mentally disordered remand prisoners. II: Report of an independent evaluation. *British Journal of Psychiatry*, 170, 462–6.

Whittle, M. C. and Scally, M. D. (1998) Model of forensic psychiatric community care. *Psychiatric Bulletin*, 22, 748–50.

Part 3

The relationship between psychiatric services for mentally disordered offenders and other agencies

Who does what? The relationships between generic and forensic psychiatric services

Alec Buchanan

Introduction

In 1991 the Royal College of Psychiatrists published a council report, 'Good medical practice in the aftercare of potentially violent or vulnerable patients discharged from in-patient psychiatric treatment'. In 2000 the College revised the report. The intervening years had seen a number of changes affecting the care of mentally disordered offenders living in the community. The College attributed these changes to a widely held view that community care was failing.

First among the changes affecting care was a requirement, in England and Wales, that an inquiry be held whenever a homicide was committed by someone recently in contact with psychiatric services (Department of Health 1994a; see also Buchanan 1999a). The reports of these inquiries were usually published. Second, government circulars had placed increasing emphasis on structure in psychiatric care by introducing administrative devices such as the care programme approach and the supervision register (Department of Health 1990 1994b).

Third, the law and its related guidance had changed. The 1995 Mental Health (Patients in the Community) Act introduced supervised discharge (see Department of Health 1996) whereby, without the involvement of a court, discharged patients could be required to live where directed and to attend for appointments. The 1983 Mental Health Act had been amended by the 1997 Crime (Sentences) Act so that offenders in the 'psychopathic disorder' category could be placed in hospital but still receive a prison sentence. The Mental Health Act's code of practice had been revised (see Horne 2000).

The report which the Royal College of Psychiatrists made available in 2000 differed in several respects from its predecessor. The name had changed to indicate that it concerned not the violent or vulnerable but simply the violent. Its length had doubled. It drew attention to some of the difficulties facing those working with mentally disordered offenders in the community including lack of resources, lack of familiarity with patients and pressures from other staff. Finally, a quarter of its length was taken up with a new section entitled 'Risk assessment and management'.

The context in which care is provided to the mentally disordered offender in the community

Bennett reflected on the process whereby large mental hospitals were being replaced by community provision in 1973:

> There is, and always has been, a tendency in psychiatry to divide patients into those we want to treat and those we do not ... this distinction ... reflects, perhaps, an intolerance rooted in the inability of doctors and other professionals to deal with feelings of hostility or repugnance ... the psychiatry we have to bring back to the community from the mental hospital is the "undesirable" psychiatry (Bennett 1973:61)

Bennett argued that while proper planning could facilitate the delivery of services, it could not govern the quality of those services. The wider issue which he addressed was how best to provide care to all of those who suffered from mental disorders, not simply those deemed desirable by clinicians.

This distinction made by psychiatric services, between desirable patients and others, had been noted earlier (Rudolph and Cumming 1962; Mesnikoff 1969). Bennett considered it unique to the care of the mentally disordered. Its origins may lie in the increased levels of responsibility which some psychiatric patents are seen as having for the manifestations of their conditions. The conclusion that they are less deserving of help may follow from this. The risk of contracting a number of degenerative and inflammatory and neoplastic conditions may be increased by choices which people make in the course of their lives. But, once present, the symptoms of those conditions are not seen as under the same degree of voluntary control as the behaviour of some psychiatric patients.

Cumming (1971) identified three steps necessary to prevent this and other forms of discrimination from interfering with the delivery of care. First, the fee-for-service system, by which doctors and services were remunerated, had to end. Second, the right to refuse to make or accept referrals had to be abolished. And, third, geographical responsibility had to replace the right of services to choose their patients. While the fee-for-service has largely been abolished outside general practice, and while areas of geographical responsibility have been created under the rubric of 'catchment areas', the right to refuse to accept a referral has remained. No one has found a way of making a doctor or, indeed, a service look after a patient who has been deemed, disingenuously or otherwise, 'inappropriate' or 'in need of services which we are unable to provide'.

Permeating the changes which ensued was a devaluation of the subjective. Medical care had traditionally been based on a voluntary agreement between someone needing help and someone believing that they could provide it. In the latter years of the twentieth century this emphasis on the voluntary contract, on the alleviation of distress and the improvement of function at the request of the sufferer, was less evident. More emphasis came to be placed on the 'management' of patients, on their 'allocation' to appropriate services (see Chapter 1). The word 'care' itself came to be used, as here, not in its empathic verbal form but as a noun, standing for something to be dispensed.

How is psychiatric care provided to mentally disordered offenders in community in the UK?

Commissioning services for mentally disordered offenders

Services for mentally disordered offenders in the UK, like services for other groups, are purchased on behalf of the Department of Health by health authorities. The process was reviewed by the Mental Heath Foundation in 1997. The reviewers pointed to the broad range of needs, from substance abuse to housing to mental illness, with which mentally disordered offenders presented. As services became increasingly specialized, they argued, these patients were disproportionately likely to fall between the referral criteria of the different specialities.

They did not add that this is often no accident. Whether they are establishing specialist services or working in them, practitioners like to be able to choose their client group. Sometimes that client group will be defined in terms of anti-social behaviour. More often it will be defined according to the usual medical criteria of symptoms, signs and diagnosis. Exclusion criteria may then be invoked to 'preserve' or 'protect' the service. Especially where the service operates on limited resources, a case can usually be made for excluding those patients whose use of services in the past has interfered with their own care or that of other patients.

The Mental Health Foundation then reviewed the problems of matching supply and demand, concluding that the supply of offenders with mental health problems was largely dictated by the criminal justice system. This is a complicated area. A substantial minority of patients in the special (high security) hospitals of the UK are detained under the provisions of Part 2 of the 1983 Mental Health Act and their detention has therefore not been ordered by a court. In addition, the number of special hospital and regional secure unit beds is fixed and, at least in the case of secure units, inadequate (Department of Health and Home Office 1992). It is likely that the resulting pressure on resources has some limiting effect on the number of hospital disposals made at court. In these circumstances the degree to which the criminal justice system determines 'supply' may be less marked than the Mental Health Foundation concluded.

The task of establishing how best to match supply to demand is further complicated when a backlog of 'difficult to place' cases means that it is difficult to anticipate the effect of providing resources. Patients are never perfectly placed, and the system in which they live is to some extent dynamic. A reduction in the pressure for beds which follows the making of provision to meet a particular need can have unpredictable effects elsewhere as services operating under reduced pressure change their admission criteria. A similar effect occurs in the community, perhaps most noticeably when the number of acute beds diminishes and the level of psychiatric pathology which is deemed compatible with existence in the community rises. It also affects the provision of specialist accommodation. Charities and other organizations which administer sheltered accommodation have to react to the requirements of those on whose funds they depend for their existence. When the perception of purchasers in respect of need changes, the services and client groups catered for by these agencies will change also.

Finally, the Mental Health Foundation reviewers reflected on what they called the 'interface' between forensic and general psychiatry. They concluded that community mental health teams would continue to be the main sources of psychiatric care for the majority of mentally disordered offenders. They concluded also, however, that there was a need for community teams to have access to forensic psychiatric expertise in managing patients and in assessing their needs and risks.

The components of a service

These were reviewed by Reed (1984) in respect of community psychiatric care. The range of needs demonstrated by mentally disordered offenders means that it is not appropriate to provide a separate service for them unless each of the components is available.

Hospital beds. Inner city psychiatry lacks sufficient in-patient facilities (see Johnson *et al.* 1997). The consequent problems are more pressing in the management of the mentally disordered offender because the perceived risks attendant upon delayed admission are greater. Management of patients who may present a risk when their mental state changes, whether that risk is to others or the self, is impossible without good access to a range of in-patient facilities. These facilities have to include provision of intensive care and the ability to admit both voluntary and involuntary patients.

Out patient clinics. These will include out-patient clinics where patients see doctors or nurses and, in many cases, specialist clinics where patients receive medication. They have to include the provision of facilities for the haematological monitoring of people who are receiving treatment with atypical anti-psychotics and the provision of blood level monitoring either for reasons of assessing compliance or dose adjustment.

Emergencies. An effective system for managing emergencies may be life saving and may also avoid the need for admission to hospital. There needs to be provision for patients to be seen urgently out of hours or without anticipated appointment times. The behaviour of many mentally disordered offenders when unwell means that general hospital casualty departments have difficulty in meeting their needs. Much preferable are specialist psychiatric emergency departments.

Day hospitals and facilities for out-patient rehabilitation. Day hospital and rehabilitation services already 'sub-specialize' to the extent that separate services are provided for some groups, for instance, the elderly. They tend to provide rehabilitation with a different emphasis from that adopted by hospital-based occupational therapy, more attention being paid to learning social skills and handling social relationships. Many of the treatments are provided in group settings with obvious implications for their continuing viability if their target populations are reduced in size as a result of sub-specialization.

In other respects, however, out-patient treatment facilities for groups of offender patients can benefit from specialization by virtue of that specialization leading to the concentration of particular types of clinical problem within their client groups. The most obvious examples are services for sex offenders and people with difficulties in managing anger. Psychology services for problems such as these are also most commonly provided in group settings and can have difficulty in recruiting sufficient numbers in general psychiatric populations.

Provision for longer term care. Early plans to close the great majority of long-stay beds were partially shelved with the recognition of the emergence of a group of 'new long stay' patients (Wing 1982; Bewley *et al.* 1981). How new this group was must be questionable. Most of the descriptions of these populations reveal people suffering from mental illnesses which have not completely responded to treatment and who remain in need of higher levels of support than can comfortably be provided by community services. Patients fulfilling this description have never been uncommon. Alternative housing and hostel provision are crucial additional community resources (David 1988). This need has become more apparent in the UK since the 1996 Housing Act reduced the duties on local authorities to continue to house tenants whose mental disorders render them difficult neighbours (Burney 2000).

Throughout, there needs to be a recognition that the provision of care is a physical business. Psychiatrists may have become 'knowledge workers', to use the phrase of Rose (see Chapter 1), and discussions of services can often seem abstract. But looking after someone implies seeing them, giving them medicine or listening to them speak. It implies communicating with other members of a team. It implies writing in records and seeing what others have written. The corollary is that the physical environment is crucial. Working from more than one site, for instance, can work only if the infrastructure allows staff to overcome the difficulties which physical separation causes.

The ethical and legal context

The 'European rules on community sanctions and measures' (Council of Europe 1994) describe a set of standards to enable national legislators and practitioners to ensure that community sanctions are applied in a just and effective manner. The rules state:

> The nature, content and methods of implementation of community sanctions and measures shall not jeopardise the privacy or the dignity of the offenders or their families, nor lead to their harassment. Nor shall self-respect, family relationships, links with the community and ability to function in society be jeopardised. Safeguards shall be adopted to protect the offender from insult and improper curiosity or publicity

The rules do not distinguish mentally disordered from other offenders.

In the UK until the end of the 1980s, with the exception of legal provision relating to the conditional discharge of restriction orders made under Section 41 of the 1983 Mental Health Act, there was little official guidance relating to the care of mentally disordered offenders in the community. In the 1990s the volume of advice and guidance increased. The relevant documents were reviewed by the Mental Health Foundation in 1997. An updated list appears as Table 11.1. Many of the documents contain considered discussion of the problems of providing care to mentally disordered offenders in the community.

Such advice can be of help to professionals and there is a widespread perception in the UK that the care programme approach has helped to prevent some of the worst examples of inappropriate care for people at risk to themselves or who present a risk to others. The advice has also bred a suspicion, however, that what is being sought is less an improvement in public safety and more a politically expedient placement of blame. With regard to probation circulars issued during the same period, Shaw noted:

> The precise purpose of these Circulars as instruments of public protection is not always accepted by field staff, since some of the assumptions are seen as unsubstantiated or as having little scientific validity. Discussions with practitioners engaged in the supervision of dangerous offenders disclose that the principal purpose of these Circulars is seen as the protection of government departments and the avoidance of embarrassment to ministers when disasters occur ... When instructions are given, blame can be levelled at staff if elements within them are not followed (Shaw 1996:160–161)

Similar conclusions have been reached by psychiatrists in relation to guidance in respect of health care (Deahl and Turner 1997). In an era when therapeutic interventions are increasingly expected to be evidence based, the introduction of regulatory procedures such as the supervision register seems to have been immune to such strictures.

The incorporation of the European Convention on Human Rights into UK legislation will change the legal context in which care is provided to mentally disordered offenders in the community. Statute law makes only occasional reference to confidentiality. The 1995 Mental Health (Patients in the Community) Act makes separate provision, in respect of the release of information to third parties, for patients who have, 'a propensity to violent or dangerous behaviour towards others' (Section 25E, Subsection 7). The only other legal device to bolster confidentiality is the, little used, application of 'breach of confidence' at common law. Once the 1998 Human Rights

Act comes into force, however, Article 8 of the European Convention of Human Rights, which safeguards the privacy of personal information as well as home and family life, will become binding on English courts. The implications for the exchange of information essential to multi-disciplinary care and risk management may be substantial (McHale 2000).

Models of care and supervision for mentally disordered offenders in the UK

Forensic psychiatric out-patient services in the UK evolved in the 1990s to meet two sets of perceived needs. Those perceived needs derived from similar ones in generic services. The first was that of meeting the requirements of sequential administrative changes in the UK, described in the introduction, which resulted from government initiatives including the care programme approach and the supervision register. The second was the assumption that by providing more assertive supervision the chances of patients dropping out of services or of having changes in their mental states go unrecognized would be minimized.

Most services demonstrate elements of the 'assertive outreach' approach, particularly that whereby the persistence of health workers is used as a substitute for active compliance on the part of the patient (see Gauntlett *et al.* 1996; also Chapter 5). The term was coined in the USA in the 1980s (Stein and Test 1980) and British (Burns and Guest 1999) and Australian (Hoult 1986) models have also been described. Other principles of assertive outreach include the targeting of patients often screened out by other services, the assumption of ongoing responsibility for patients through admissions to hospital and periods of imprisonment, providing advocacy for clients seeking help from other agencies, crisis management, domiciliary visiting, team working, the involvement of clients' families and indefinite treatment (see McGrew and Bond 1995).

Services designed along these lines have been shown to reduce drop-out rates but not consistently to improve patients' quality of life or levels of functioning. When resources permit them to offer a comprehensive service they may also have a role in preventing admission. It has also been shown, however, that where the amount of therapeutic input is limited the effect of such services can be increased bed use, presumably through increased detection of need (see Tyrer *et al.* 1995).

By contrast, there are few research findings relating to what supervision comprises or what it can realistically be expected to achieve. Coker and Martin (1985), studying life sentenced prisoners released on parole and without seeking to describe psychiatric provision, distinguished two elements, oversight and assistance. They found that although there was no evidence that supervision prevented recidivism, a probation officer could forestall some offences by activating recall or initiating another form of intervention. They concluded that the belief that supervision allowed the prevention of serious crime was 'justification for a social institution that is also a politically indis-

Table 11.1 Central guidance on mentally disordered offenders since 1990
(see also Mental Health Foundation 1997)

Year	Title	Notes	Source
1990	Circular 66/90—Provision for mentally disordered offenders	Advice to police, courts, psychiatric services and social services on diversion of mentally disordered from criminal justice system	Home Office
1990	Circular HC(90)23/LASSL(90)11— Caring for people. The care programme approach (CPA) for people with a mental illness referred to the specialist psychiatric services	Required health authorities to implement CPA, described policy background, emphasis on systematic arrangements, multi-agency approach and continuity of care	Department of Health
1992	Circular EL(92)24—Assessment of need for services for mentally disordered offenders and patients with similar needs	Required regional health authorities to ensure regular assessments of need for secure provision	Department of Health
1993	*Mental illness key area handbook*	Advice to managers on achieving improvements in mental health through health promotion, alliances between agencies, targeting and local purchasing	HMSO
1993	Circular EL(93)54—Priorities and planning guidance	Health authority purchasing plans to include range of secure and non-secure provision	Department of Health
1994	*Mental illness key area handbook* (2nd edn)	See above. Introduced field trials version of the Health of the Nation Outcome Scales	HMSO
1994	HSG(94)5—Introduction of supervision registers for mentally ill people from 1 April 1994	Health authorities to identify patients 'significantly' at risk and maintain a register. All reviews under CPA to consider whether patient should be included	NHS Management Executive
1994	HSG(94)27—Guidance on the discharge of mentally disordered people and their continuing care in the community	Recommended practice for patients being discharged from in-patient facilities based on application of CPA. Requirement for independent inquiry in cases of homicide	NHS Executive
1995	Circular 12/95—Mentally disordered offenders: inter-agency working	Clarification of existing guidance, incorporation of findings of independent inquiries into homicide, describes recommended practice, emphasizes importance of inter-agency co-operation	Home Office and Department of Health

1995	Care programme approach implementation package	Documentation covering assessment and care conforming with national and local requirements	Quality Development Unit
1996	Circular LASSL 96/16—The spectrum of care: summary of mental health services	Provides audit pack for CPA. Emphasizes that 24 h nursed beds are essential to comprehensive service	NHS Executive
1996	Building bridges. a guide to arrangements for inter-agency working for the care and protection of severely mentally ill people	Describes principles of inter-agency working, recommends targeting of severe mental illness, advises on application of CPA and patient confidentiality	Department of Health
1996	Circular HSG(96)11/LAC(96)8— guidance on supervised discharge (after-care under supervision) and related provisions	Explains provision of Mental Health (Patients in the Community) Act 1995 in relation to supervised discharge	Department of Health
1997	Circular HOC 52/1997—Crime (Sentences) Act 1997	Introduces amendments to Mental Health Act 1983 including hospital and limitation directions and extended maximum duration of interim hospital orders	Home Office
1997	Circular HOC 39/1997—Sex Offenders Act 1997	Requires sex offenders to register with the police within 14 days of release from detention (or going on leave from hospital)	Home Office
1997	Circular HSG(97)37—Guidance to hospital managers and local authority social services departments on the Sex Offenders Act 1997	States that hospital managers are expected to support effective implementation of the act. Specific guidance in relation to young sex offenders and hospital patients	NHS Executive
1998	Modernizing mental health services: safe, sound and supportive	Emphasis on minimizing risks of harm to self or others, needs assessment, primary care base and new information systems	Department of Health
1999	National service framework for mental health	Introduces standards set by the National Institute on Clinical Excellence to be delivered by clinical governance and monitored by the Commission for Health Improvement	Department of Health
1999	Safer services. National confidential inquiry into suicide and homicide by people with mental illness. Report	Recommends patient passports, assertive outreach, changes to legislation to extend compulsion, central dissemination of policies on clinical management of personality disorder	Department of Health

pensable part of the strategy for the release of lifers'. Coker and Martin noted that most probation officers did not share a definition of 'strict' when applied to supervision. They considered more frequent contact and a more controlling approach likely to be counterproductive, bringing with them resentment on the part of the life licensee which in turn adversely affected the relationship between him and the probation officer. They considered this relationship the source of the majority of the benefits which supervision had to offer.

Supervision in psychiatry cannot be seen as primarily a surveillance and crime control process. Limits on resources, the current legal and administrative framework in which psychiatric care in the community is provided in the UK and the voluntary nature of the therapeutic relationship combine to ensure that this will remain the case. Psychiatric writers emphasize the provision of support. Even this depends on an open and co-operative relationship with the patient (Grounds 1995). Grounds was concerned that those responsible for purchasing health care seemed to make a distinction between health and social care and required health authorities to fund only the former. He was concerned also that only 'health gains' were used to assess outcome. He concluded that the good delivered by supervision was in many instances better measured in terms of social consequences than medical ones and that stability was a more appropriate outcome than any measurable improvement in health.

Joint and separate care by general and forensic psychiatric services

There is no consensus in the UK as to the extent to which the care of mentally disordered offenders should be integrated with that of other patients (see Chapter 5). The advantages of specialized provision were discussed with regard to ethnic issues by Bhui *et al.* (2000). Specialist services allow the development of specialized skills. These skills may include the recognition of unusual clinical needs and the introduction of forms of treatment that might otherwise be overlooked. Drawbacks include the marginalization of the specialist service and the adverse effects on staff morale and recruitment which follow. There is likely also to be a loss of skills in general services consequent on the removal of one group of patients.

Separate, sometimes called 'parallel', systems of care for mentally disordered offenders in the UK are usually provided by forensic psychiatric services. They have the advantage of corresponding to a widespread view that there is a group of patients who, while not fully responsible when they commit crimes and therefore not suitable for punishment, are sufficiently 'different' from other psychiatric patients to warrant being treated separately (Gunn 1977). Smaller specialized units and correspondingly smaller numbers of staff are more easily administered. And it may no longer be possible for every hospital to offer, among its range of services, specialist provision for mentally disordered offenders.

Among the disadvantages which Gunn identified in 1997 were the increased stigmatization of mentally disordered offenders and the development of 'banishment pressure', a vicious circle whereby the existence of a service for unpopular patients, particularly when that service removes them from other patients and staff, increases the pressure for patients to be referred to that service. Gunn attributed banishment pressure to stigma and fear, the latter in turn the consequence of a lack of skills and resources.

Gunn's concerns have largely been borne out. Along with stigma comes a reduction in the duty of care which general services see themselves as owing offender patients. In the 1990s the development of forensic 'outreach' teams was accompanied by concern that their advantages, for instance in terms of a shortening of admissions to secure wards, were outweighed by the disadvantages of separate services. Burns (2001) argued that those services should reflect the natural history of the disorders they treat, not the criminal histories of their patients. Integration of offender and non-offender patients would serve to remove some of the myths which surround forensic patients and the treatment they receive and would improve understanding of the full range of consequences of the disorders from which they and other patients suffer.

This has not prevented others from advocating the development of specialist provision. The 'Inquiry into the care and treatment of Christopher Clunis' (Ritchie *et al.* 1994) suggested that psychiatric services identify a 'special supervision group' comprising patients who met two out of four criteria: (1) having been compulsorily detained more than once, (2) having a history of violence or persistent offending, (3) having failed to respond to treatment from general services and (4) being homeless. They wished to see these patients cared for by a specialist multi-disciplinary team with a limited and protected case load. These patients required, the inquiry team thought, assertive follow-up with close supervision.

In order to achieve the level of supervision required the team suggested a maximum of 15 patients per keyworker. A similar ratio was suggested by the Sainsbury Centre for Mental Health (1998) in their review of care for people with severe mental illness who are hard to engage with services.

Unresolved questions in the care provided to mentally disordered offenders in the community in the UK

What is the most suitable model of care for mentally disordered offenders in the community?

The case loads of services offering assertive community treatment (ACT) and other of Witheridge's (1991) 'overlapping abstractions' resemble those of some forensic psychiatric out-patient clinics. And the principles according to which the two types of services operate are similar (Whittle and Scally 1998; see Snowden *et al.* 1999 for a review). The ACT approach may confer particular advantages on mentally disordered offenders in terms of reduced in-patient stays (Burns 2001). In some respects, however, the scope of the service offered to mentally disordered offenders has to be broader than that implied by most descriptions of ACT.

First, services need to be able to offer services to patients some of whose difficulties are more closely related to their personality than to mental illness. The administrative definition of forensic psychiatry (see below) and the development of catchment areas jointly mean that, whatever the preferences of individual clinicians, some such patients will stay in the forensic psychiatric system and be unable to leave hospital unless a service is able to be provided to them in the community. A number of practical problems, such as anger, impulsiveness and unwanted sexual behaviour may require to be addressed specifically. Their treatment, or at least their treatment in cases where the person has acted violently, is likely to lie outside what psychologists and other therapists in general psychiatry regard as their remit.

Second, the duration of treatment is likely to be longer. The disabilities of many patients who are in contact with forensic psychiatric out-patient services are often such that they require extended treatment. In many other cases they remain in follow-up after chemotherapeutic and psychological interventions have been exhausted. Sometimes this is because remaining in follow-up offers the patient access to practical help which is not available elsewhere. In other cases, however, continued contact can be justified by reference to the risks which attend relapse and the increased opportunity of detecting any such relapse if the patient continues to be seen. Such cases are likely to be more frequent in forensic psychiatry. Out-patient services need to be able to offer this form of extended contact.

Third, the importance of the multi-disciplinary team is greater where the range of problems which the patient poses extend to include contact with the criminal justice system. Issues of confidentiality, for instance, become more complicated. Social workers, in particular, can find themselves appraised of information which those responsible for housing their client might expect them to pass on. One suggestion is that social workers should not make undertakings to receive confidences they cannot keep and should negotiate explicit 'confidentiality contracts' with their clients (Thompson 1984). While measures such as these may help, they cannot ensure that the social worker will be able to control the information to which he becomes privy and cannot resolve his difficulty over what to then do with it. Dilemmas such as these cannot be resolved except in an environment where the range of a patient's problems can be discussed by all of those engaged in his or her care.

What criteria should govern entry into a specialist service for mentally disordered offenders?

Despite the development, in some areas, of parallel out-patient services for forensic patients, there is no accepted definition of 'forensic' other than that whereby it is taken, tautologically and administratively, to refer to a patient who has previously been looked after by forensic services. Attempts to make a distinction between forensic and other patients on the basis of diagnosis or history of violence reveal only that psychiatric diagnostic categories are insufficiently robust and, in areas of socio-economic deprivation, a history of violence too common, for these to serve as criteria for the making of a distinction in all cases.

The criterion referred to most frequently is that of risk to others (see Chapter 5). For psychiatric services caught between the scylla of failing to maximize patients' independence and the charybdis of providing inadequate public protection, distinguishing a 'high risk group' holds obvious attractions. Politicians and health planners are also likely to find attractive a technology which offers the theoretical possibility of separating those most likely to act violently from other patients and of providing them with separate services and, perhaps, legal sanctions (see Grounds 1995). In these circumstances risk has come to be an (often informal) criterion for access to forensic psychiatric or other services for mentally disordered offenders in the community.

There is little evidence, however, that the actuarial means of prediction currently available can be used in routine clinical practice to separate, to a useful degree, those who will act violently from those who will not (Buchanan 1999b). Predictions made by clinicians, the only alternative to an actuarial measure, are no better and probably worse (Monahan 1997). The difficulties are compounded because the information available to services when patients first present is always incomplete. And risk takes various forms. Some of these can only be managed properly by a comprehensive general psychiatry service and some cannot be managed by community psychiatric services at all.

It is more likely that any successful attempt to distinguish a group of mentally disordered offenders who will be offered parallel care at community level will be based on clinical needs. These needs will be defined locally. Several components may be important, however. First, the clinical backgrounds of some patients indicate a need for observation of a quantity and quality which is sufficiently different from the norm to warrant their being offered a separate service. Their monitoring may involve improving the quality of the information available through the development of long-term relationships with the patient. It may require more frequent visits and the collation of information from a number of different sources.

Second, the risks to themselves and others which many people looked after in general psychiatry present when unwell are not sufficient to warrant their admission to hospital. Care is then routinely provided to them in the community. If this is to be done safely it requires a degree of resource, in terms of physical structure such as day centres and personnel, and a degree of flexibility which is greatly in excess of that required for observation. Even when a critical mass exists to justify the observation and monitoring functions described above, it may not exist to justify the separate provision of resources to allow the care of sick people in the community.

Third, the risks attendant on looking after some patients in the community mean that access to senior staff and multidisciplinary discussion needs to be regular and flexible. Patient numbers and resource limitations, particularly when psychiatry is practised in inner city areas, make this difficult to achieve in generic services (see Holloway 1997).

How might general and forensic services apply these criteria?

Stretched services and administrative devices such as the care programme approach and the supervision register have combined with political, public and press concerns over violent acts by the mentally disordered to increase the potential costs which clinicians perceive as attaching to clinical responsibility. Clinicians are understandably reluctant to take responsibility for cases where they perceive a risk and where they doubt their ability to intervene to reduce that risk. This is particularly the case for Mapother's 'objecting or objectionable' patients (Mapother 1929). The effect, at times, has been to reduce what should be an integrated system of provision in the UK to its constitutive elements.

Even when a critical mass exists to justify a separate service for mentally disordered offenders, cases where input from forensic out-patient services will be appropriate will not always be identified at the point of referral and not all cases initially so identified will, in fact, appropriately be keyworked by forensic services. Psychiatric services cannot control the quality of information which they receive from referrers. Considerations of efficiency, clarity to referrers and clinical responsibility would seem to suggest a single point of contact for referrers to mental health services. In view of the likely needs of most patients referred it seems most appropriate that this should be the community mental health team for the area in which the patient lives.

It some cases, however, it will be appropriate for forensic services to undertake the assessment or ongoing treatment. At present community forensic services do this with many referrals from the probation service, some from GPs, some from prisons and with most from regional secure units and secure hospitals. These are areas where specialist skills are likely to be of most benefit. The difficulty of establishing referral criteria to specialist services which are reliable and valid means that whatever system generic and specialist services develop has to be flexible enough for decisions to change in the light of new information. It also requires that relationships between services be allowed to develop over time in an atmosphere which encourages co-operation.

Conclusion

Differing local needs render hazardous any conclusions regarding appropriate provision for mentally disordered offenders in the community which are intended for general application. Some tentative conclusions seem possible.

(1) Treatment for mentally disordered offenders in the community is seen by some as, at best, peripheral to the proper practice of psychiatry, nursing and psychology. Clinicians note that the threat of harm to others distorts care (Deahl and Turner

1997). Managers recognize that forensic psychiatric input increases in-patient stays and therefore costs (see Chapter 10). In some instances the reaction to providing treatment can be overtly hostile, as unpopular patients are seen as affecting adversely the care of others and as using the resources expended upon them inappropriately.

It is in this light that the enthusiasm of advocates of expanding services, some of whom are obliged by their own service guidelines to have as their primary aim public protection (see Harding and Cameron 1999), should be seen. In view of the need to provide long-term care to some patients and the problems of transferring that care, it is not appropriate for any service to be established unless there is reliable evidence of commitment in this regard both from those responsible for purchasing care and from those responsible for managing its provision.

(2) Not all tragedies can be avoided. Perhaps few can be. It is unlikely that the culture of blaming services for the activities of some of their clients will significantly diminish in the UK in the foreseeable future. This is one reason why all of those responsible for providing care have to be willing to support those services in adverse critical climates. It is also a reason why services for mentally abnormal offenders have to develop systems which adhere to the relevant guidelines and attempt to learn the, often vague and sometimes contradictory (Petch and Bradley 1997), lessons of inquiries into tragedies elsewhere.

(3) Where considerations of critical mass permit the establishment of a dedicated service for mentally disorder offenders, that service should be run according to standards of good quality community care, with multi-disciplinary input provided flexibly in location and time. The service needs to be consistent with the requirements of the care programme approach and relevant legislation. Such services will always have less resources than their generic counterparts and this, combined with the nature of their work, should lead to their regulating their own case loads, subject to their meeting expectations couched in terms of their clinical output.

(4) Even when considerations of critical mass permit the establishment of a specialist service, however, there will be a need for access to the wider range of resources, including immediate admission to an intensive care ward and day-centre provision, which only general psychiatry can provide. Unless the relative resource allocation to general and forensic services changes radically, it will not be appropriate to attempt to provide, for forensic psychiatry patients in the UK, a parallel service which offers the same range of provision as that which is already provided in general psychiatry.

(5) Where local needs, including those relating to critical mass, warrant the provision of separate services to mentally disordered offenders in the community, allocation to respective services should be according to clinical need. In particular, it has been suggested here, it may be appropriate for specialist forensic psychiatric out-patient

services to meet a need for increased levels of supervision over a sustained period combined with regular access to an experienced multi-disciplinary team in circumstances where clinical deterioration will usually result in admission to hospital. Services thus configured and adequately resourced should not restrict their remit by excluding those with personality disorders, should be able to provide long-term care and should develop multi-disciplinary working in order to deal with the complex ethical and legal problems, such as those relating to confidentiality, which such cases can present.

(6) Whatever system of integration is adopted, there will be a need to identify the correct first point of referral, be it general or forensic psychiatry and, on occasions, to transfer patients from one service to the other. The characteristics and reputations of some offender patients, combined with the perceived consequences of being responsible for providing treatment when something goes wrong, can make professionals reluctant to take responsibility for their care, even in situations where the same professionals are sure that somebody ought to.

It seems unlikely that protocols or algorithms designed to assist decision making will help in this regard (but see Cohen and Eastman 1997). Relationships between services have to develop over time. The quality of those relationships will in part reflect the willingness of the respective staff members to co-operate with one another and the degree to which they share a view of who should, and who should not, be provided with a service.

One theoretical advantage of protocols is that, when combined with standardized assessments of an entire patient group, they should be able to establish what proportion of patients will go where and hence provide a means of allocating resources. There is, as yet, no evidence that such a system of allocating resources can work, although it may be possible in future. If resource allocation is to be tailored to demand this may best be done, in forensic and other sub-specialities of psychiatry, by means of an expectation couched in terms of output.

(7) The administrative and regulatory atmosphere under which services develop should change in order that clinicians are encouraged to take people on for treatment. Professional responsibility, it was argued above, can generate a disincentive to clinicians taking on patients when it is seen as entailing clinical responsibility for someone else's illegal acts. Psychology services in the UK seem to have less difficulty in this regard, perhaps because the relationship between a psychologist and a client is based less on the provision of ongoing care than is the case for doctors and nurses. It may be relevant also that because psychology places less emphasis on disease and illness the client is seen as more of an active participant in his or her care and hence as a responsible agent in other respects. If other forms of care provision in mental health were able to generate the same atmosphere, the frequency with which help was offered would increase.

There remains the question of whether the latter years of the twentieth century have seen, through its increasing links with social services and other agencies, the engagement of British psychiatry with a population with which it previously had only superficial contact. Among the ways in which this new population differs may be the extent to which its members regard themselves, and are regarded by others, as 'sick' or as requiring to be looked after, yet psychiatry will attempt to 'treat' or 'manage' them using traditional, often paternalistic and patronising, models of care. The question of whether such a change has occurred is an empirical one. If it has, it will imply a more radical change in the way help is provided than anything which has so far been proposed.

Acknowledgement

The author thanks Dr Paul Bowden and the Revolving Doors Agency for their help.

References

Bennett, D. (1973) Community psychiatry. *Community Health*, **5**, 58–64.

Bewley, T., Bland, M., Mechen, D. *et al.* (1981) "New chronic" patients. *British Medical Journal*, **283**, 1161–4.

Bhui, K., Bhugra, D. and McKenzie, K. (2000) Specialist services for minority ethnic groups? Maudsley Discussion Paper No. 8. London: Institute of Psychiatry.

Buchanan, A. (1999*a*) Independent inquiries into homicide. *British Medical Journal*, **318**, 1089–90.

Buchanan, A. (1999*b*) Risk and dangerousness *Psychological Medicine*, **29**, 465–73.

Burney, E. (2000) Ruling out trouble: anti-social behaviour and housing management. *Journal of Forensic Psychiatry*, **11**, 268–73.

Burns, T. (2001) To outreach or not to outreach. *Journal of Forensic Psychiatry*, **12**, 13–17.

Burns, T. and Guest, L. (1999) Running an assertive community treatment team. *Advances in Psychiatric Treatment*, **5**, 348–56.

Cohen, A. and Eastman, N. (1997) Needs assessment for mentally disordered offenders and others requiring similar services. *British Journal of Psychiatry*, **171**, 412–16.

Coker, J. and Martin, J. (1985) *Licensed to live*. Oxford: Basil Blackwell.

Council of Europe (1994) *European rules on community sanctions and measures*. Strasbourg: Council of Europe.

Cumming, E. (1971) Three issues affecting partnership among mental health agencies. *Hospital and Community Psychiatry*, **22**, 33–7.

David, A. (1988) On the street in America. *British Medical Journal*, **296**, 1016.

Deahl, M. and Turner, T. (1997) General psychiatry in no-man's land. *British Journal of Psychiatry*, **171**, 6–8

Department of Health (1990) Joint Health/ Social Services Circular. HC(90)23/LASSL(90)11. London: Department of Health.

Department of Health (1994*a*) HSG(94)27 Guidance on the discharge of mentally disordered people and their continuing care in the community. London: Department of Health.

Department of Health (1994*b*) Introduction of supervision registers for mentally ill people from 1 April 1994. London: Department of Health.

Department of Health (1996) LAC(96)8 Guidance on supervised discharge (after-care under supervision) and related provisions. London: Department of Health.

Department of Health and Home Office (1992) Review of health and social services for mentally disordered offenders and others requiring similar services: final summary Report. Cmnd 2088. London: HMSO.

Gauntlett, N., Ford, R. and Muijen, M. (1996) *Teamwork: models of outreach in an urban multi-cultural setting*. London: Sainsbury Centre: London.

Grounds, A (1995) Risk assessment and management in clinical context. In *Psychiatric patient violence: risk and response* (ed. J. Crichton), pp. 43–9. London: Duckworth.

Gunn, J. (1977) Management of the mentally abnormal offender: integrated or parallel. *Proceedings of the Royal Society of Medicine*,**70,** 877–80.

Harding, J. and Cameron, A. (1999) What the probation officer expects of the psychiatrist. *Advances in Psychiatric Treatment*, **5,** 463–70.

Holloway, F. (1997) The assessment and management of risk in psychiatry: could we do better? *Psychiatric Bulletin*, **21,** 283–5.

Horne, J (2000) The Mental Health Act code of practice. *Journal of Forensic Psychiatry*, **11,** 485–8.

Hoult, J. (1986) Community care of the acutely mentally ill. *British Journal of Psychiatry*, **149,** 137–44.

Johnson, S., Ramsay, R., Thornicroft, G. *et al.* (1997) *London's Mental Health*. London: King's Fund.

Mapother, E. (1929) Mental hygiene in adults. *Journal of the Royal Sanitary Institute*, **50,** 165–75.

McGrew, J. and Bond, G. (1995) Critical ingredients of assertive community treatment: judgement of the experts. *The Journal of Mental Health Administration*, **22,** 113–25.

McHale, J. (2000) Confidentiality and psychiatry: dilemmas of disclosure *Journal of Forensic Psychiatry*, **11,** 255–9.

Mental Health Foundation (1997) *Commissioning services for offenders with mental health problems*. London: Mental health Foundation.

Mesnikoff, A. (1969) Urban psychiatry—effects on the psychiatric institute: some comments on the dynamics of institutional change. In *Urban challenges to psychiatry* (ed. L. Kolb, V. Bernard and B. Dohrenwend), pp. 293–318. Boston: Little Brown.

Monahan, J. (1997) Actuarial support for the clinical assessment of violence risk. *International Review of Psychiatry*, **9,** 167–9.

Petch E. and Bradley C. (1997) Learning the lessons from homicide enquiries: adding insult to injury? *Journal of Forensic Psychiatry*, **8,** 161–84.

Reed, J. (1984) The elements of an ideal service: the clinical view. In *Psychiatric services in the community* (ed. J. Reed and G. Lomas), pp. 77–85. London: Croom Helm.

Ritchie, J., Dick, D., Lingham, R. (1994) The report of the inquiry into the care and treatment of Christopher Clunis. London: HMSO.

Royal College of Psychiatrists (1991) Good medical practice in the aftercare of potentially violent or vulnerable patents discharged from in-patient psychiatric treatment. Council Report CR12. London: Royal College of Psychiatrists.

Royal College of Psychiatrists (2000) Good medical practice in the aftercare of potentially violent patents in the community. Council Report to Replace CR12. London: Royal College of Psychiatrists.

Rudolph, C. and Cumming, J. (1962) Where are additional psychiatric services most needed? *Social Work*, **7,** 15–20.

Sainsbury Centre for Mental Health (1998) *Keys to engagement*. London: Sainsbury Centre.

Shaw, R. (1996) Supervising the dangerous in the community. In *Dangerous People* (ed. N. Walker), pp. 154–178. London: Blackstone.

Snowden, P., McKenna, J. and Jasper, A. (1999) Management of conditionally discharged patients and others who present similar risks in the community: integrated or parallel? *Journal of Forensic Psychiatry*, **10**, 583–96.

Stein, L. and Test, M. (1980) Alternative to mental hospital treatment. 1: Conceptual model, treatment program and clinical evaluation. *Archives of General Psychiatry*, **37**, 392–7.

Thompson, I. (1984) Ethical issues in community-based psychiatry. In *Psychiatric services in the community* (ed. J. Reed and G. Lomas), pp. 44–54. London: Croom Helm.

Tyrer, P., Morgan, J., Van Horn, E., Jayakody, M., Evans, K., Brummell, R., White, T., Baldwin, D., Harrison-Read, P. and Johnson, T. (1995) A randomised controlled study of close monitoring of vulnerable psychiatric patients. *Lancet*, **345**, 756–9.

Whittle, M. and Scally, M. (1998) Model of forensic psychiatric community care. *Psychiatric Bulletin*, **22**, 748–50.

Wing, J. (1982) Long term community care: experience in a London borough. *Psychological Medicine Monograph Supplement 2*. Cambridge: Cambridge University Press.

Witheridge, T. (1991) The "active ingredients" of assertive outreach. *New Directions for Mental Health Services*, **52**, 47–64.

Chapter 12

Multiple agencies with diverse goals

James McGuire

Introduction

Considering the complexity of the questions, it is hardly surprising that work in the field of forensic mental health services is sporadically confusing. This is all the more so given the divergence of the perspectives and contexts within which its questions are addressed. Metaphorically speaking, such work is done in a kind of 'seismic zone', an unstable and sometimes disputed territory where large domains of professional and practical shareholdings intersect. While charged with an overall common goal, the respective contributors are often uncertain, and intermittently at loggerheads, over how to achieve it. This chapter is about some of the sources of the perplexity and misunderstanding that pervade this field, their manifestation on different levels, and their impact on joint delivery of effective services for mentally disordered offenders.

The field of activity in which we are interested here currently carries the label 'forensic'. While this term has been enthusiastically embraced by many practitioners and in numerous service settings, application of the word has in itself led to some disgruntlement, and a few authors have voiced criticism of the ways in which its original meaning has gradually become expanded and distorted. As has been pointed out by Blackburn (1996), the traditional definition of the word makes a clear link with the provision of evidence to facilitate some type of legal decision making. Over approximately the last decade or so it has fallen into common usage to refer to a whole gamut of activities associated with persons who have broken the law. This has included an array of agencies and staff groups whose services are called into play thereby, *after* all the legal decisions have been made. Most of these services and their practitioners rarely if ever have any direct contact with legal personnel or with courts of law. Amongst the more outlandish phrases thrown up as a result of this etymological elasticity have been references to 'forensic behaviour' (when the intended meaning was 'violence') and discussion of the 'forensic individual' (when the party so designated was a compulsorily detained patient).

This extension of meaning has now however become so firmly entrenched as to make it probably futile to resist. In what follows, an attempt will be made to delineate some of the reasons why collaborative working in this area appears to continue to pose problems. Difficulties are encountered on several levels, and four of them will be considered in turn. The first derives from the theoretical models and empirical bases of the disciplines involved. The second arises in the application of these models within a legal context. The third relates to the manner of training of the multifarious practitioner groups which, some directly, others more tangentially, play a part in this field. The fourth relates to organizational aspects of service provision in a multi-agency context.

Theories and models of mental disorder

Confusion exists first at the level of theory and basic science. While on a routine daily basis most practitioners probably give little thought to such issues, their underlying assumptions concerning the causes of what they are dealing with guide many other aspects of their actions. It will be useful first, therefore, to examine some of the fundamental concepts put forward which illuminate the thinking of professionals at work in 'forensic' services.

Whatever the theoretical orientation adopted, causal pathways are universally acknowledged to be complex and multi-factorial. To add further to these intricacies, there are numerous conceptual overlaps, and in some cases a lack of clarity or of focus, amongst the potentially relevant explanatory models. They can therefore be categorized in various ways. Mechanic (1999), as an example, enumerates biological, epidemiological, developmental and sociological perspectives. Eastman (1992, 2000) classifies psychiatric–phenomenological, psycho-understanding and psychometric approaches. Three main collections of models will be briefly surveyed here, successively from (1) biomedical, (2) psychological and (3) sociological viewpoints. One fundamental distinction that underlies many others is between an expectation that disorders represent discrete categories and one whereby they are considered as points on a continuum.

Biomedical

The biomedical view, which is an example of the former type, is probably the dominant one in western healthcare systems. It is rooted in a conceptualization of mental disorders as a form of brain disease (Schwartz 1999). According to this view otherwise intact physiological processes, such as central nervous system functioning, are disrupted by a *pathogen*; this may be a neurochemical or metabolic imbalance, a toxic substance or an invading micro-organism. For example, schizophrenia has been considered to be a result of breakdown in the normal functioning of neurotransmitters such as dopamine and serotonin (McKenna 1997; Schwartz 1999). A related element of this type of model is a search for possible genetic markers of mental illness, and a proportion of research on psychotic and other severe disorders has been focused upon the question of the extent to which there is evidence of heritability of specific syndromes.

The application of the biomedical model is pivoted upon the use of diagnostic classifications systems such as the Diagnostic and Statistical Manual (DSM-IV; American

Psychiatric Association 1994) or the International Classification of Diseases (ICD-10; World Health Organization 1992). In this respect it mirrors the form of algorithmic process underpinning physical medicine. As in that field, the purposes of diagnosis are generally regarded as four-fold: (1) description, classification and taxonomy; (2) provision of a causal model for understanding a disorder; (3) prognosis, or the prediction of the likely progress and outcome of an illness; and (4) decision making with regard to therapeutic interventions.

Undoubtedly, some types of mental disorder have a clear and well-established underlying organic pathology (see Lishman 1997). However, it has frequently been pointed out that in many other cases, and especially with reference to the more prevalent 'functional' disorders, this is not so and that classification systems such as the DSM are not founded on a theoretical model of the disorders they subsume (Mechanic 1999). Indeed for the majority of the conditions identified under DSM, there is simply no known organic aetiology (Pilgrim and Rogers 1993). To such an objection, Wing *et al.* (1998) have retorted that description and classification are merely the first stages of scientific investigation of mental disorders, which will in due course yield findings concerning the causal factors responsible for the disease, at least for some kinds of disorder. Other objections to DSM-IV as a nosological system have been lodged by Clark *et al.* (1995), who surveyed research noting a high degree of comorbidity of different diagnoses, alongside considerable heterogeneity within some DSM headings.

On a different note, Blashfield and Fuller (1996) have criticized the political and economic context within which the DSM approach has been framed. In a somewhat ironic departure these authors attempted to predict some key characteristics of the presumed next version of the system, 'DSM-V'. Employing 'clinical empiricism' and extrapolating from previous DSM manuals, they predicted that it will contain 1026 pages and run to 415 000 words. It will define 390 disorders, encompassing 1800 diagnostic criteria. Its cover will be brown, and it will yield a net revenue for the American Psychiatric Association of US$80 million. Kutchins and Kirk (1997) have cast the utilization of DSM as a form of imperialist or expansionist exercise, in which virtually any behaviour might at some stage be classifiable as a form of mental disorder. Some psychiatrists, such as Breggin (1991), have adduced evidence of links between the biomedical understanding of individual distress and the prescription of inappropriate somatic treatments, giving rise to major professional and ethical concerns.

Psychological

A second approach to the understanding of mental disorder draws upon psychologically based research and places more emphasis on the concept of continuity between 'normal' and 'abnormal' phenomena. Thus the same learning and developmental processes which produce relatively well-adjusted individuals, when operating in different combinations or separate pathways, may lead to distress and disorder. An important distinction must be made within this framework. One approach relies upon a 'trait' or personality-based approach in which certain relatively stable 'charactero-logical' features are thought to be associated with greater risk for development of prob-lems. This dimensional or 'axial' approach can coexist with the types of diagnostic classification systems just mentioned. Counterposed to it, behavioural or 'situational' approaches place firmer emphasis on the roles of learning processes, on the circum-stances in which actions occur, and on their patterning over time. Within this broad framework there are numerous specific causal mechanisms; the most widely favoured at present, given converging empirical support, are 'cognitive social learning' models. Over the past two decades a certain degree of rapprochement has occurred between trait and situationist views in the form of an *interactionism* in which both personal and environmental factors are held to contribute to the topography of behaviour in any given context (Endler and Magnusson 1976). There are many more specific theoretical models within this: Peterson (1999) outlines psychodynamic, cognitive–behavioural, humanistic–phenomenological and family-systems approaches, whilst other authors have attempted to propose coherent, integrative approaches employing elements from all of these. Thus, for example, with reference to depression, Gilbert (1992) has enun-ciated a model which places psychological propensities within an evolutionary frame-work. This model acknowledges the reciprocal roles of brain chemistry and reported experience and takes into account both cognitive information processing and personal vulnerability factors alongside an examination of the role of environmental stressors, life events and levels of social support. Similarly, in examining available evidence concerning the development of adolescent aggression, which if persistent may be a precursor to adult criminality, psycho-social processes emerge as the most powerful contributory factors (McGuire 1997a). However, they interact with underlying tem-peramental features which can be described as psychophysiological in nature, and which may be the result of individual differences that are inherited.

Psychological models, though ostensibly focused on 'the mind', are not founded on a neglect or disregard of biological processes. It is assumed that neural events underlie psychological phenomena; however, there may be a gross difference in the kinds of processes emphasized. Most existing biomedical models focus on events at the synapse and on the action of neurotransmitters. This is also the site of action of most psycho-pharmacological agents. Learning and memory however are encoded in neural net-works which in many respects can be understood in terms of 'Hebbian' principles. The repeated joint firing of sets of neurons strengthens the synaptic links between them, and facilitates future activity amongst the connections so laid down.[1] Examples of this are given by Robertson (1999), who reviews evidence concerning the plasticity of neuronal systems and the processes by which certain inter connections become established.

These developments are underscored by the emergence in recent years of the hybrid discipline known as 'neurophilosophy' (Churchland 1988; Dennett 1993). This is a

----

[1] This process is known as *long-term potentiation*. See Kandel *et al.* (1995).

branch of the philosophy of mind in which an attempt is made to converge with ideas and findings from the neurosciences. While many proposals within this remain highly speculative and controversial, the field as a whole may be on the verge of a new epoch in building realistic models of the relationship between 'hard-wired' physiological circuitry, evidence concerning neuronal plasticity, and psychological experience and behaviour. There is a two-way transactional process between human information processing, or 'computational' capacities, and the environment.

Psychological models are also open to criticism: they are often perceived from a sociological standpoint as individualist, positivist and deterministic, taking insufficient account of social and cultural factors. From a medical viewpoint they are sometimes seen as divorced from biological reality and ultimately redundant, if the underlying neurochemical causes of disorder can be tracked down.

Sociological

In a sociological perspective, as might be expected, there is a move away from focusing on individuals as the 'unit of analysis' in understanding disorder and breakdown. At the very minimum, it is argued that a disorder or cluster of symptoms cannot be assumed to be the result of individual pathology alone. Social factors, such as material deprivation, oppressive environments or life stresses, may have played an important part in its aetiology (Thoits 1999). The causal mechanisms therefore lie at least in part not within individuals but in the social milieu. Hence, for example, while the pattern of symptoms associated with 'schizophrenia' is found in many cultures, the ways in which this is manifested and the social behaviour of individuals varies according to cultural expectations (Mechanic 1999). Similarly, when the course of schizophrenia was mapped longitudinally in a study by the World Health Organization, comparing evidence from 10 different countries and cultures, sizeable differences in continuity of symptoms and rates of recovery were found. In countries such as Sri Lanka and Mauritius, progress was considerably better than in the UK, the Netherlands or Russia (Warner 1985). A more recent study in Madras, India found 77% of patients to be asymptomatic at 10-year follow-up (Thara and Eaton 1996).

Added to this, the process of 'labelling' individuals as suffering from mental disorders is itself a factor in the equation, and the impact of this upon persons so labelled can be substantial. In early versions of this concept, it was held that such labels were more powerful determinants of the severity and duration of an illness than any underlying disorder in itself. However, in recent revisions of this model it has been contested that labelling can have positive as well as negative consequences (Link and Phelan 1999).

But at another level, this entire set of concepts can itself be made subject to scrutiny, and the procedures by which various terms have been allotted to certain kinds of reported experience or behaviour become part of the inquiry. Thus, the concept of mental illness is itself a construct and must be understood in the social, cultural and professional context within which it arose (Szasz 1961). At a more elaborate level, then, the meanings of all the elements in this interplay must be examined as phenomena in themselves, as they have been subject to a process of social construction.

Sociological models too may be subject to some limitations. Social constructionist perspectives have illuminated the processes through which individuals and groups come to create a culturally shared representation of reality; the social world as we encounter it is a product of human interaction itself (Searle 1995). But extreme forms of constructionism and relativism which incorporate denials of the validity of any claims concerning the nature of external 'reality' place obstacles in the way of building conceptually integrative links. And whereas a sociologically informed perspective is invaluable for envisioning the wider context in which actions occur and decisions are made, it does not easily generate recommendations that are feasible and practicable in the individual case.

Integrative models

Of course, as with many other problems, no single conceptual model is adequate to the task of explaining the panoply of observations and available data. It is essential to view both mental disorder and other problems such as persistent criminality within a multi-layered, integrative framework. As Mechanic (1999) has remarked ' . . . it is pointless to argue whether illnesses are biological or social. They all represent interactions among biological potentialities, individual vulnerabilities, environmental conditions, social stressors, social networks and supports, psychological orientations, and learned behavior'. In moments of considered thought, most clinicians and other practitioners would probably subscribe to such an integrative view. That, at least, is the consensus on a superficial level. It is less obvious whether so many bear this complexity in mind when considering individual cases or making decisions in regard to them. The tendency to prefer neat, simplistic solutions to any problem we confront is fairly ubiquitous; and it is difficult to avoid the suspicion that many practitioners all too often resort to such thinking.

Thus one difficulty that emerges from this brief survey is as follows. The professional groups who work with individuals suffering from mental disorders and whose role it is to provide services to them are trained in different ways. Most will be much more familiar with one of the aforementioned perspectives, and are perhaps likely to have absorbed that basic orientation to the exclusion of others. In ordinary interaction, when discussing individual cases they are unlikely to address openly their contrasting, indeed sometimes conflicting, acquired assumptions.

An initial source of confusion therefore may derive from the background training and qualifications of individuals working in forensic psychiatry and allied fields. In many instances they have been nurtured in different theories and 'basic science'. Further, there are ongoing uncertainties, unresolved issues and continuing disputes in all of this terrain. Many variables are poorly specified and their mutual impact is unknown. Is it any wonder that divergences exist when these far from satisfactory states of knowledge are applied to 'real-world' problems?

The legal context

However complex the above differences appear to be, they become even more so when placed in a legal context. The modes of thinking on which legal decision making is based are in essence very different from those involved in a scientific approach to events. Such notions as causation are employed in both: but at the centre of most legal systems notions of 'fully voluntary action' ('free will') and capacity to make informed choices play paramount roles. This stance lies at the heart of most penal philosophies, and is conjoined with other fundamental concepts concerning individual responsibility for actions.

So, for example, in most circumstances when giving an account of a criminal act for which a *mens rea* must be established a person is deemed responsible if, in general terms, he or she could have chosen whether or not to commit that act and aspects of the circumstances were not such as to impede the making of a free choice between those alternatives. The law of course recognizes situations where certain constraints operate upon persons. These may then constitute mitigating factors, affecting the sentence imposed, or may amount to full defences which can be taken into account by courts in arriving at findings of guilt.

The prime difficulty is that this conceptualization of human behaviour is in some crucial respects at odds with the scientific approach adopted within most of the models represented earlier. Legalistic notions of causation (Hart and Honoré 1985) make little allowance for the possibility that actions may be other than fully voluntary. A sequence of events, only the last segment of which was deliberate in the ordinary-language meaning of that term, might be considered in law to be the cause of an event, so leading to a finding of guilt. Similarly, in law a person may be convicted of an offence where the mental element consisted of negligence. He or she may have considered whether or not there was a certain risk, and concluded wrongly and unreasonably that there was not (Smith and Hogan 1992).

The cardinal area upon which this has the most powerful impact is the crucial issue of responsibility or culpability for criminal acts. From a psychologically informed standpoint this is likely to be on some continuum. From a legal perspective it is constrained into a very limited set of mutually exclusive choices. These are usually expressed in dichotomous terms (fit versus unfit to plead; guilty versus innocent; responsible versus of diminished responsibility). While specific provision for such debate is made in the 1957 Homicide Act, in principle the question of degrees of responsibility arises with reference to almost any type of behaviour. For the individual defendants or plaintiffs concerned, such decisions are likely to have dramatically divergent consequences. The psychological reality of apportioning responsibility for action is much more complex than current court decisions allow. It may be that a new type of legal discourse is required, informed by scientific thinking; and that a new dialogue should be embarked upon between mental health professionals, on the one hand, and judges, legal academics and philosophers of law, on the other, concerning the nature of responsibility for actions. The concept of therapeutic jurisprudence represents one potential avenue for embarking upon this (Wexler and Winick 1996).

One consequence of reconsidering the relationship between legal and psychological models of behaviour may be that a defence such as automatism could lose its validity as describing a form of involuntary conduct. It has been argued (McSherry 1998, 1999) that as the majority of actions fall on a continuum between involuntary and willed behaviour, apparently dissociative states or automatic acts may contain a partially planned component. On this basis it has been suggested that such defences be subsumed with a general defence of mental impairment.

But to consider an obverse example, there are circumstances in which persons are considered in legal terms to have been reckless as to consequences of their actions. The psycho-legal test for this resides in whether or not an abstractly constructed 'reasonable man' or 'prudent bystander' might have foreseen those consequences (Smith and Hogan 1992).[2] However, psychological research has shown that some individuals may not have the personal or cognitive capacity to appreciate the consequences of actions. This might be thought to be a component of those cognitive abilities generally believed to be captured in the concept of 'general intelligence', and which can be summarized in the intelligence quotient (IQ). However, many psychologists consider that IQ is only one type of measure of intellectual or cognitive capacity. The achievement of any given score on an intelligence test may be a poor indicator of, for example, an individual's ability to solve everyday practical problems, or to anticipate the repercussions of acting in a specific manner. Concepts such as 'bounded rationality' (the capacity to apply reason within a restricted frame of reference) are simply not admissible to contemporary legal thinking.

In the specific case of legal decision making with regard to mentally disordered offenders, there may be a yawning gap between legal decisions and the psychological reality of the factors at play when an 'index' anti-social act was perpetrated. An individual may be made subject to mental health legislation if he or she has been assessed by a psychiatrist approved under the 1983 Mental Health Act. However, there may be no necessary or demonstrable causal connection between the diagnosed mental disorder and the recorded anti-social behaviour. There is at present no systematic empirical basis concerning the multiplicity of possible inter-connections between

---

[2] This applies principally to recklessness decided under the 'Cunningham' test, where it must be shown that the defendant was aware of the existence of an unreasonable risk but still proceeded to act. But it might also apply to 'Caldwell/Lawrence' recklessness, where there was an obvious risk, but the defendant ' . . . failed to give any thought to the possibility of its existence' (Smith and Hogan 1992).

mental disorders and criminal acts. Some mental states, such as delusional beliefs or command hallucinations, or emotional states such as extreme anger, jealousy or rage, have been associated with increased risk of violence. Conversely some illegal behaviours, such as possession of and frequent use of proscribed drugs, may contribute to the development of a mental disorder (in DSM, they may *constitute* such a disorder). In other cases, an individual may have serious mental health problems and have committed serious anti-social acts, but the two may be causally unconnected. Indeed, the degree of connection between them may be close or distant. Both may be products of similar background and developmental processes yet still not be directly linked in a causal chain resulting in the actions which brought the individual to the attention of the legal system or mental health services. This may have crucial practical consequences. Despite the fact that in some circumstances there may not be a causal connection between an individual's mental disorder and his or her criminality, the persistence of the former can be adduced as adequate justification for continued detention even if in other respects the risk of repetition of the behaviour is judged to be low.

The core question of what type of relationship (if any) obtains between mental disorder and crime has been the subject of much research; however, the issue remains incompletely resolved. Several approaches have been adopted in attempting to clarify this issue, for example involving the application of epidemiological and criminological, as against psychiatric models (Wessely and Taylor 1991). One recent review suggests the underlying relationship is ' . . . small and easily obscured by more influential criminogenic factors' (Crichton 1999).

The most frequently used methodology for investigation of this has involved measuring the joint prevalence of mental health diagnoses and illegal acts. For example, how many people diagnosed as schizophrenic are also convicted of assaults (or have histories of aggressive behaviour)? Alternatively, how many persons with criminal convictions (say for assault) can be diagnosed as suffering from mental disorders? Over the past 20 years the consensus position on this has reversed, from a comparative scepticism concerning the degree of overlap (Monahan 1981) to a recognition that mental disorder represents increased risk for violence in certain circumstances (Monahan and Steadman 1994; Peay 1996a). Some reviews and studies have delineated more clearly the conditions under which psychiatric syndromes of certain types and in certain stages of development or crisis may pose increased risk of violent acts (Buchanan 1993; Monahan 1997; Taylor *et al.* 1994). A recurrent finding of other studies of this type is that of a further inflation of risk levels given the presence of concomitant substance abuse (Monahan 1997; Rice and Harris 1995).

Professional groups, training and status

If the roots of the 'forensic mental health services' tree are intertwined, its branches are even more so. We have seen that there are different scientific models underpinning approaches to the study of mental disorders. These have implications for the interpretation of research findings obtained, indeed for the types of research carried out. Placed in a psycho-legal setting, their ramifications become additionally difficult to discern. At the level of service provision, the multiple perspectives brought to bear on what are allegedly common problems has the potential to add still further to the bewilderment.

The forensic mental health field is one in which numerous professional groups work. The background and training of these groups is extremely diverse, and varies considerably even in such crude indices as its overall time-span. Police training is spread over a two-year period but covers a wide range of issues. While the police have certain powers under Sections 135 and 136 of the Mental Health Act, and their role in respect of these and in diversionary schemes has been increasing (Bean 1999), their training in respect of mental health issues remains fairly minimal. Legal personnel, though having in common degree qualifications in law and experience of legal practice, beyond this diverge into many specialisms and career pathways, and with varying degrees of status from solicitor to barrister, clerk, circuit judge, recorder and high court judge. Psychiatry requires six years of medical training, progression through various positions as registrar and the passing of collegiate membership examinations. Psychiatric nursing entails a three-year training to become a Registered Mental Nurse; this is usually followed by specialism, for example in community psychiatric nursing, or forensic psychiatric nursing which is concentrated in secure units and hospitals. Clinical psychologists must possess a first degree in psychology, applied experience usually in a clinical setting, and then pursue a three-year doctoral qualification; in many services they are supported by graduate assistants. While many social workers have university degrees, the requirements of the profession are a diploma or certificate qualification, and specific experience and training for 'approval' under the 1983 Mental Health Act. Probation officers complete an initial social work qualification which traditionally took two years to complete, then work in offender services. Given their different intensities and modes of training, there are not surprisingly other salient differences between these professional groups. These include the routine language and terminology employed customarily in their work and variations in underlying perspectives, explanatory models and ethos along some of the lines outlined above.

Psychiatrists, psychiatric nurses and clinical psychologists are employed by health service agencies (at the time of writing, National Health Service trusts). Social workers and probation staff are local government employees, but their agencies and those of the police are each organizationally separate and have their own management structures. Psychiatrists and psychiatric nurses have their theoretical roots in a similar biomedical ethos. While in recent years it may be that a majority of psychiatrists have become more firmly attached to that ethos, in psychiatric nursing there has been an increasing influence of sociological models (see Mason and Mercer 1998) (a strand of which has been present for some time in the thinking of some psychiatrists). Clinical psychologists, though often working alongside psychiatrists, adopt a different theoretical stance not surprisingly informed by psychological models, though those specializing in neuropsychology become more fully versed in organic explanations of disorder. Social work and probation staff have much more exposure to sociological thinking, often adopting criminological models that invoke large-scale societal explanations of deviance, of circumstances and conditions affecting it, and social constructions of it. In residential units, alongside all of these groups, there are other professionals to be found. They include occupational therapists and a range of other specialist staff, providing specific behavioural, cognitive, art, music, drama and other therapeutic activities, as well as counselling from a variety of theoretical orientations.

Status and power

These differences in position in the system of forensic mental health services are also characterized by significant differences in status, power and influence. Whilst this is infrequently discussed, there is a manifest hierarchy or 'pecking order' in the relationships between the groups just itemized (Pilgrim and Rogers 1993). This is embedded most clearly in the formalities of the 1983 Mental Health Act, which allocates differential statutory powers to various professions. The pre-eminent role is given to psychiatry, and embodied in the title 'Responsible Medical Officer'. This might be in part because treatment takes place in the settings we call hospitals where, traditionally, medical staff have hegemony. Whether this is the most appropriate way of doing things overall can of course be queried. This position remains, despite the fact, discussed earlier, that there is no known *medical* origin of most of the disorders and dysfunctions associated with the types of problem addressed by the Act.

Psychiatry is a branch of medicine and, given the status of the latter in society, it may not be surprising that it holds this position of hegemony in relation to mental health service provision. Yet the position of psychiatry in this respect is a product of historical forces, as the entire medical profession itself has evolved through internal struggles, for example in the eighteenth century between surgeon-apothecaries and physicians (Lawrence 1994). The ascendancy of medicine in respect of the management of those deemed 'mad' occurred primarily in the period between 1808 and 1845. During that epoch, a series of parliamentary acts created the conditions of segregation and confinement which became the model for the county lunatic asylums, alongside the requirement that these institutions should be under the custodianship of medical staff. As a result of these and other developments, the major patterns of modern medical practice that are familiar in the UK today were in place by 1920 (Lawrence 1994).

Psychiatrists are now seen in most countries as the primary providers of information on mental health status to courts. For example in France, whilst upwards of 70 psychiatrists are appointed to furnish testimony to the Supreme Court, the number of psychologists so appointed is a mere three. Given the scale of this discrepancy, such a position might seem immutable and incontestable. Yet a systematic comparison of psychiatric, psychological and social work reports by Petrella and Poythress (1983), in which reports were rated 'blind' by independent legal personnel, concluded that the latter two were of superior quality on a range of measurable characteristics. In preparing reports psychologists and social workers consulted with a wider range of sources of information, and were more methodical in linking the evidence they had gathered to the conclusions drawn and the recommendations made. Yet the status of 'forensic' psychiatrists has been such that in pursuit of enhanced status the same adjectival title has been appropriated by amongst others, psychiatric nurses, social workers and prison psychologists. This is in some cases a travesty, as the groups so described are often as far removed from locus of legal decisions as it is possible to be.

These amendments in job titles perhaps testify to an underlying friction, rooted in status discrepancies which many perceive to be unjustified. Some authors have questioned the usefulness of biomedical models when considering mental disorder from legal and ethical standpoints (Greenberg and Bailey 1994). If biomedical models are only part of a broader picture, and somatic treatments are no more efficacious than some other interventions, the question of why a particular profession remains in an overall commanding position perhaps warrants serious questioning. The position lends substance to the long-standing sociological critique that the primary role of psychiatry is the social control of deviance (Miller and Rose 1986). Perhaps more worryingly, the place of psychiatry in secure hospitals may complement the control-oriented ethos of some nursing groups as symbolized in their continued membership of the Prison Officers' Association. Indeed, that symbiosis may be a long-term endemic cause of recurrent abuses of power in such settings.

Systems of agencies and services

The fourth area of potential difficulty to be considered in the present chapter is the organizational context within which mental health services are provided. Individuals with severe and enduring mental health problems inevitably have multiple needs. Addressing these problems alone and providing adequate long-term support will require a full range of psychiatric rehabilitation services (Pickett et al. 1999). If their problems are compounded by a history of anti-social behaviour, and especially if this has involved personal violence or has resulted in a period of incarceration or hospitalization, their management in the community necessitates delivery, in a carefully co-ordinated fashion, of a range of interventions and services. Patterns of service provision in forensic psychiatry and allied services have been described in some detail by Eastman (1993) and more recently by Heywood (2000), who also uses a series of case vignettes to depict different modes of entry to these services and the variety of pathways through them.

Hence, service users will require access to housing; to social security payments including disability living allowances; to physical health services, to psychotropic medication where this has been prescribed; to services of community psychiatric nurses; in many cases, to family services; and to psychological therapies. The latter may not be provided by psychologists as such and may encompass individual therapy including behavioural, cognitive, interpersonal, cognitive-analytic or other approaches; and group therapies, such as anger management, social skills training, empathy training, problem-solving or sex offender treatment programmes. The mode of delivery of all of these may vary between localities. In some instances they will be organized through Community Mental Health Teams, elsewhere the process may be directed by 'case managers', in yet other instances it may be configured through some permutation of individual and team responsibilities.

The overall goal of these staff groups and the agencies they represent is a shared one. While this might be expressed in many different ways, broadly speaking it revolves around the provision of treatment and support to the individual service user and his or her family or other carers, whilst maintaining community safety. In every individual case there will be a host of specific objectives, dictated by the assessed needs of the client in question, and the realities of the local arrangements established to try to meet them. Not unnaturally, charged with providing a service of a particular kind to someone, staff in most agencies direct their efforts towards ensuring that such provision can be made.

The above describes only the community-based components of the system. On the custodial side, numerous research studies have shown the high levels of mental health problems amongst both convicted (Gunn *et al.* 1991) and remand prisoners (Brooke *et al.* 1996). Within health services, regional secure units and special hospitals currently provide in the region of 2500 beds in England and Wales. The latter have in recent years regrettably been sustained in a virtually continuous state of uncertainty punctuated by occasional crises (Bingley 1993).

Risk assessment, prediction and management

In forensic mental health services, the commonly agreed focus for much joint working is in the assessment, understanding and management of *risk factors*. There is now a copious volume of research material on risk assessment and prediction with reference to violent behaviour and other forms of anti-social conduct. Broadly speaking, risk assessment strategies are classified into two sorts: *actuarial* or empirically driven (involving measurement of a specified set of factors derived from a systematic research base, which are usually then statistically combined); and *clinical* or founded on the experience and subjective judgment of individual clinicians. A lengthy history of research clearly demonstrates the superiority of the former over the latter for purely predictive purposes; yet clinical judgment can still be shown to have a valuable contribution to make (Monahan 1997). To these two groups Melton *et al.* (1997) added a third, which they entitled *anamnestic* risk assessment. This entails compilation of a checklist of risk factors on an actuarial basis, supplemented by clinical judgment. That information is then conjoined to the assembly of an inventory of situations in which individuals may be at risk of manifesting the 'target' problem behaviour, together with a set of procedures for estimating the probabilities of such circumstances occurring.

The work of Monahan and Steadman (1994) amongst others has been taken as confirmation that the current generation of research studies in the field of risk assessment represents a major shift in our ability to recognize and assess key factors in this respect. Monahan (1993), in reviewing the profound and far-reaching implications of the 'Tarasoff' case, provided an invaluable framework for the establishment and implementation of risk assessment and risk communication procedures. One of the key recommendations was that information on risk variables should be collected from four broad domains: respectively *dispositional*, *historical*, *contextual* and *clinical*. Recent developments in the psychometric instrumentation of risk assessment are reviewed by Blackburn (2000*a*).

Given that states of prolonged or uncontrolled anger or psychotic symptoms such as delusions and hallucinations have been shown to elevate risks of engaging in violent or anti-social behaviour (O'Kane and Bentall 2000), it should be possible to draw on a wide range of psychological research on factors influencing these phenomena over time. I have argued elsewhere that it would obviously be beneficial if the study of relatively rare acts of extreme aggression were to be integrated with the study of assessment of risk levels across the field of offender treatment in general (McGuire 2000). These arguments are strengthened by a study reported by Bonta *et al.* (1998), who conducted a meta-analytic review of long-term follow-up studies, to examine which factors were the best predictors of criminal and violent recidivism amongst mentally disordered offenders. The set of studies identified incorporated 68 independent samples. Predictor variables were classed into four groups: *demographic*, *criminal history*, *deviant lifestyle* and *clinical* factors (including psychiatric diagnosis). The most accurate predictors proved to be criminal history variables: indeed the overall pattern obtained was a close parallel to that typically found with non-mentally-disordered-offender populations. Conversely, the poorest predictors of recidivism were clinical variables. Most notably, although a DSM diagnosis of anti-social personality disorder was associated with a greater risk of future criminality, no other diagnostic category emerged as significant, and diagnosed psychosis was negatively correlated with future recidivism. If these findings are correct, the intervention approaches adopted in work with offenders in general may be equally applicable to clients with mental disorders.

A focus on the distinction between static and dynamic risk factors and on the relation between statistical and clinical prediction could enhance our ability to conduct systematically informed risk assessments (Monahan 1997; Serin 1993). Of course, given any genuine improvement in the ability of clinicians to make accurate predictions of behaviour, a separate series of ethical issues is raised thereby, such as the legitimacy of making forecasts of risks of personal violence (Grisso and Appelbaum

1992). But if accuracy of prediction of violence can be substantially improved, then we may indeed be on the threshold of a new and potentially transformed clinical, ethical and organizational era. This is firmly implied in recent publications by Monahan (1996, 1997).

Treatments and outcomes

That a variety of different therapies can be effective for reduction of a range of mental health problems is now well supported by systematic evidence (Dobson and Craig 1998; Roth and Fonagy 1996; Nathan and Gorman 1998). However, problems remain concerning the process of translating research findings, usually gained from randomized controlled trials that are markedly dissimilar to most applied healthcare settings, into usable strategies or practice guidelines for deployment by active clinicians.

By comparison with the relatively large number of trials of treatments for mental health problems such as depression, anxiety or obsessive-compulsive disorder, well-designed studies of interventions with mentally disordered offenders are fairly rare. For example, in the review cited earlier by Bonta et al. (1998) only 14 studies were located that included treatment as an independent variable. No overall positive evidence of treatment effects could be discerned within these studies, but problems of design and methodology, for example the absence of appropriate comparison groups, made the findings difficult to interpret. The reasons for the relative paucity of treatment-outcome studies in this field reside partly in the difficulty of carrying out such research, given the legal constraints upon assigning individuals to artificially constructed groups, together with the need for much lengthier follow-ups.

A limited quantity of evidence is available concerning the treatment of individuals with personality disorders or classified as 'psychopaths' (Bateman and Fonagy 2000; Blackburn 2000b; Lösel 1998; Perry et al. 1999; Sanislow and McGlashan 1998). The majority of these studies were, not surprisingly, conducted in institutional settings, and indicate potential efficacy in respect of some behavioural therapies and therapeutic community approaches. But the findings so obtained contain a number of inconsistencies, and cannot be extrapolated with confidence to provision of treatment services in community-based settings.

However, some studies have been undertaken comparing out-patient samples containing mixed diagnostic categories, for example insanity acquittees, allocated to different levels of parole or intensity of supervision. Recently Heilburn and colleagues (Heilbrun and Griffin 1998; Heilbrun and Peters 2000) have reviewed a series of evaluative studies of community-based psychiatric treatment with mentally disordered offenders (patients found Not Guilty by Reason of Insanity) alongside other evaluations of supervision of clients with mental disorders who had been placed on probation or parole. The principal outcome criteria employed in these studies were rearrest for new offences and readmission to hospital. Other indicators were occasionally used, such as evidence of symptom reduction, clinical progress, community adjustment and rates of revocation of parole conditions. However few studies included comparison groups.

Some of the findings reported in these studies are once again difficult to interpret. For example, comparisons have been made between discharged patients allocated to different types of community supervision. However, samples may be assessed in different jurisdictions in which it is not clear whether staff practices regarding case management and recall have been standardized. If increased supervision simply means increased surveillance, there will be a higher rate of 'technical violations' of parole, leading to a higher failure rate in the supposedly better-supported group. Thus in some instances in which patients are allocated to an 'assertive case management' service, there has been evidence that the case managers are more likely to reincarcerate clients for less serious violations of their release conditions (Wiederanders *et al.* 1997). However, other studies have yielded supportive evidence of the value of assertive case management, which involves intensive work to build therapeutic alliances with clients, combined with increased levels of access to a range of community services (Bloom *et al.* 1992; Dvoskin and Steadman 1994; Wilson *et al.* 1995). Generally, rearrest rates on conditional release were found to be comparatively low (the highest rate reported was 16%).

The same authors (Heilbrun and Griffin 1998; Heilbrun and Peters 2000) have also forwarded a set of principles for effective community-based forensic services, combining guidelines for sound ethical practice with such recommendations as can be extracted from the limited research base. A properly run, high-quality service of this type would place a central emphasis on the need for good communications between agencies. There would be an explicit balance between individual rights, the need for treatment and public safety. There would be an awareness of the range of treatment needs of clients. Service managers would employ a 'demonstration model' in assessing risk of harm and treatability. This requires establishing a system of collecting and combining information in a way that can be directly used by practitioners and is validated by clinical research evidence. Efforts would be made to clarify legal requirements such as confidentiality and duty to protect. There would be application of sound risk management procedures. Finally, policies would be in place for acting upon principles for promoting healthcare adherence.

Service delivery problems

Even where comparative studies have been undertaken of individuals managed in different sectors of a service, there are difficulties in extrapolating these findings to the complex world of inter-agency liaison and collaborative case management. It is in this realm that it has frequently been thought some of the major obstacles lie to provision of adequate levels of treatment, support and risk management.

Where failures have occurred, and have led to tragic consequences such as homicides by mentally disordered offenders, the functioning of the entire system of services has been placed under scrutiny and practitioners and managers called to account. Events of this kind have repeatedly received considerable publicity, one impact being that in 1994 formal inquiries into such incidents were placed on a mandatory footing by the Department of Health. There are now numerous inquiry reports and reviews of cases such that their cumulative findings have themselves been subject to reappraisal and in-depth analysis (Boyd 1996; Peay 1996b; Reith 1998).[3]

It is vital to maintain a balanced perspective on the nature of these events and on the level of the associated risks as compared to others, connected for example with road deaths, which society appears to absorb and somehow accept (Taylor and Gunn 1999). It is likely that the alarm caused by such incidents has its roots in continuing stigmatization, and even demonization, of people with severe or enduring mental health problems (see Chapters 1 and 4). Nevertheless many serious issues have been raised by such inquiries, and many inter-agency communication problems noted, perhaps best illustrated in the findings of the Clunis Inquiry (Ritchie et al. 1994).

Possibly the dominant recurring theme in inquiry reports has been that of communication problems between services (Reith 1998). Various reasons have been adduced for such problems, but it is undoubtedly the case that multiple agencies with goals and responsibilities which sometimes diverge, but partially overlap, do not always have a shared vision of their common task, nor agreed or well-tested procedures for enacting it. Even where multi-disciplinary teams exist, inquiries into tragic incidents have suggested that often, they may not ' . . . operate in a meaningful way' (Reith 1998). It has been suggested in the present chapter that at least part of the failure of communication between agencies and professional groups is traceable to their different origins, models and philosophies of practice, tacitly inculcated through their respective experiences of professional training. It is hypothsized that this influences perspectives and modes of thinking at a level below that of specialist terminology or everyday discourse. This is a difficult proposition to test, but whether or not direct evidence could be obtained in support of it, there appear to be other ways in which barriers to communication between professionals are engendered.

In the past, there is no doubt that there have simply been limited amounts of contact between practitioners working in different sectors of the system. Research has illustrated this for example with regard to relationships between probation officers and psychiatrists (Hudson et al. 1993; Roberts et al. 1995). This has also emerged from the few studies conducted on probation orders with conditions of psychiatric treatment, which have fallen into declining usage in recent years (Rooney 1994). At the present

---

[3] Given the time, effort and expense involved, there have been calls for major reforms to the inquiry process (e.g. Crichton and Sheppard 1996). It has also been reported, but not at the time of writing officially confirmed, that in future such inquiries may be limited to those where major lessons might be learnt, or where there is significant public interest (Community Care, 'Independent inquiries into killings may end'. December 1999, p. 2).

moment new multi-agency efforts, in some instances placing probation staff in 'lead roles', have been reported to be working more beneficially (Bhui 1999; Grant 1999).

Several inquiries have noted the lack of a systematic method or a multi-professional approach to the conduct of risk assessments. Thus, for example, Kemshall (1998) has suggested that probation officers feel very ill equipped to carry out risk assessments and management of mentally disordered offenders; yet they are often in the 'front line' of regular contact with these clients. Concepts such as 'risk' are infamously elusive. It is difficult to arrive at clear and agreeable working definitions; there is a lack of an adequate empirical base for assessment and decision making and an absence of agreed procedures for collection and processing of relevant data. Even were such a task accomplished, a formula would be required for combining the end-product with clinical judgement and a means found for embedding such practices within different contexts in a range of agency settings.

Such a finding underlines the potentially immense importance of multi-disciplinary teams. Recently Tyrer et al. (1999) have reported on an extensive review of available literature on the impact of Community Mental Health Teams (CMHTs) on persons with comorbid severe mental illness and personality disorders. Though initially identifying a potential 1200 studies for review, only five satisfied inclusion criteria. However, there was tentative evidence of positive impact of teams in reducing suicide rates and hospital readmissions. By contrast, no conclusions were permissible regarding the effects of teams on clinical indicators such as mental state or social functioning of clients.

Full implementation of the Care Programme Approach is intended to avert many of the previously known problems of monitoring of risk and inter-agency communication (Mason 2000). Properly emplaced, it could enable agencies to work collaboratively to the maximum benefit of clients and the minimization of risk. Thus, it is widely felt amongst practitioners—and the findings of inquiries lend support to this expectation—that the key to rehabilitation or community maintenance resides not in individualized interventions, but in the assembly and delivery of well co-ordinated support services. Regrettably, this alone does not appear to be conducive to effectiveness in the absence of high-quality clinical interventions or treatment programmes which form the ingredients of an all-round service. There are some exceptionally well-documented studies of demonstration projects in which considerable extra resources were invested in services for clients with long-term mental health problems (Bickman 1996; Lehman et al. 1994). Most importantly, these services were designed such that significant changes were made in the targeted service systems, and these improvements in service functioning were monitored and demonstrably maintained. However, controlled comparisons failed to discover measurable improvements in the well-being, symptom levels or community adjustment of clients. Perhaps disappointingly then, integration may be necessary, but does not *in itself* appear to be a sufficient condition of effective service delivery. The constituent services or ingredients thereof must themselves also be of high quality (Morrissey 1999).

Confidentiality

Another possible reason for poor inter-agency communications which is identified in some of the reports collated by Reith (1998) reflects variant expectations and practices with regard to client confidentiality. Of the 28 reports surveyed by Reith, ten made recommendations concerning confidentiality; others also raised it as an issue of major concern.

In some instances potentially relevant information was withheld from certain personnel because to disclose it would have constituted a breach of confidence. In three cases, for example, information was not passed to housing departments for fear of jeopardizing the client's prospects of obtaining accommodation. In another case, relevant evidence concerning a person's history of assaults was not communicated to a consultant psychiatrist. In the case of Shaun Armstrong, at one point the patient was admitted to hospital following an overdose on the same day that a child protection investigation commenced but none of this information was passed on to his consultant. In yet another case important information was not passed on to a general practitioner. These were some of the 'breakdowns in communication' that are frequently mentioned in such calamities. Some staff were thought to have 'misguided beliefs' concerning the pre-eminent importance of confidentiality. In two cases, those of Frank Hampshire and Anthony Smith, crucial information was not shared with or obtained from the patients' closest relatives because principles of confidentiality were thought to be sacrosanct and to take precedence. In other cases, it was thought workers were 'hiding behind' confidentiality, enabling them for example to avoid the awkwardness of asking delicate questions of relatives. In most inquiry reports it was recommended that considerations of risk and safety should be understood to override confidentiality limits. In another instance the inquiry report recommended that an index of essential documentation be compiled.

It is difficult to resolve the question of how individuals negotiate dilemmas of confidentiality versus duty to protect, or other problems that may arise in circumstances where they may also have a dual role as therapeutic and forensically oriented practitioners. Some commentators have perceived irreconcilable conflicts in these roles and propose that they should never be combined (Strasburger *et al.* 1997). Others have remained more sanguine about the prospects of integrating them, provided certain strictures are followed (McGuire 1997*b*).

Resources

A final potential reason for the difficulties frequently encountered in community forensic mental health services may of course be that the entire system is significantly underresourced. There are numerous anecdotal reports of colossal workloads on the part of many practitioner groups. While this may be difficult to distinguish from an undercurrent of malaise which appears to infect many human service professions, there is no doubt that community care initiatives were from the outset placed under considerable financial strain. It may be no accident that per capita spending on health in the UK is one of the lowest in Europe (*Economist*, March 1996). In turn, that might be a sequela of a widespread aversion to levels of personal taxation sufficient to sustain broader community goals.

References

American Psychiatric Association (1994) *Diagnostic and statistical manual of mental disorders.* (4th edn). Washington DC: American Psychiatric Association.

Bateman, A. W. and Fonagy, P. (2000) Effectiveness of psychotherapeutic treatment of personality disorder. British Journal of Psychiatry, **177**, 138–143.

Bean, P. (1999) The police and the mentally disordered in the community. In *Mentally disordered offenders: Managing people nobody owns* (ed. D. Webb and R. Harris). London and New York: Routledge.

Bhui, H. S. (1999) Probation-led multi-agency working: A practice model. *Probation Journal*, **46**, 119–21.

Bickman, L. (1996) A continuum of care: more is not always better. *American Psychologist*, **51**, 689–701.

Bingley, W. (1993) Broadmoor, Rampton and Ashworth: Can good practice prevent potential future disasters in high-security hospitals? *Criminal Behaviour and Mental Health*, **3**, 465–71.

Blackburn, R. (1996) What is forensic psychology? *Legal and Criminological Psychology*, **1**, 3–16.

Blackburn, R. (2000a) Risk assessment and prediction. In *Behaviour, Crime and Legal Processes: A Sourcebook for Forensic Practitioners* (ed. J. McGuire, T. Mason and A. O'Kane). Chichester: John Wiley (in press).

Blackburn, R. (2000b) Treatment or incapacitation? Implications of research on personality disorders for the management of dangerous offenders. *Legal and Criminological Psychology*, **5**, 1–21.

Blashfield, R. K. and Fuller, A. K. (1996) Predicting the DSM-V. *Journal of Nervous and Mental Disease*, **184**, 4–7.

Bloom, J. D., Williams, M. H. and Bigelow, D. A. (1992) The involvement of schizophrenic insanity acquittees in the mental health and criminal justice systems. *Clinical Forensic Psychiatry*, **15**, 591–604.

Bonta, J., Law, M. and Hansen, K. (1998). The prediction of criminal and violent recidivism amongst mentally disordered offenders: A meta-analysis. *Psychological Bulletin*, **123**, 123–42.

Boyd, W. (ed.) (1996) *Report of the confidential inquiry into homicides and suicides by mentally ill people.* London: Royal College of Psychiatrists.

Breggin, P. R. (1991) *Toxic psychiatry.* London: Harper Collins.

Brooke, D., Taylor, C., Gunn, J. and Maden, A (1996) Point prevalence of mental disorder in unconvicted male prisoners in England and Wales. *British Medical Journal*, **313**, 18–21.

Buchanan, A. (1993) Acting on delusion: a review. *Psychological Medicine*, **23**, 123–34.

Cavadino, P. (1999) Diverting mentally disordered offenders from custody. In *Mentally disordered offenders: Managing people nobody owns* (ed. D. Webb and R. Harris). London and New York: Routledge.

Churchland, P. M. (1988) *Matter and Consciousness.* Cambridge, MA: MIT Press.

Clark, L. A., Watson, D. and Reynolds, S. (1995) Diagnosis and classification of psychopathology: Challenges to the current system and future directions. *Annual Review of Psychology*, **46**, 121–53.

Crichton, J. (1999) Mental disorder and crime: coincidence, correlation and cause. *Journal of Forensic*

Psychiatry, **10**, 659–77.

Crichton, J. and Sheppard, D. (1996) Psychiatric inquiries: learning the lessons. In *Inquiries after homicide* (ed. J. Peay). London: Duckworth,

Dennett, D. (1993) *Consciousness explained*. London: Penguin.,

Dobson, K. S. and Craig, K. D. (ed.) (1998) *Empirically supported therapies: best practice in professional psychology*. Thousand Oaks, CA: Sage.

Dvoskin, J. A. and Steadman, H. J. (1994) Using intensive case management to reduce violence by mentally ill persons in the community. *Hospital and Community Psychiatry*, **45**, 679–84.

Eastman, N. L. G. (1992) Psychiatric, psychological, and legal models of man. *International Journal of Law and Psychiatry*, **15**, 157–69.

Eastman, N. L. G. (1993) Forensic psychiatric services in Britain: A current review. *International Journal of Law and Psychiatry*, **16**, 1–26.

Eastman, N. L. G. (2000) Psycho-legal studies as an interface discipline. In *Behaviour, Crime and Legal Processes: A Sourcebook for Forensic Practitioners* (ed. J. McGuire, T. Mason and A. O'Kane). Chichester: John Wiley (in press).

Endler, N. S. and Magnusson, D. (ed.) (1976) *Interactional psychology and personality*. New York: John Wiley.

Gilbert, P. (1992) *Depression: the evolution of powerlessness*. Hove: Lawrence Erlbaum Associates.

Grant, D. (1999) Multi-agency risk management of mentally disordered sex offenders: a probation case study. In *Mentally disordered offenders: managing people nobody owns* (ed. D. Webb and R. Harris). London and New York: Routledge.

Greenberg, A. S. and Bailey, J. M. (1994) The irrelevance of the medical model of mental illness to law and ethics. *International Journal of Law and Psychiatry*, **17**, 153–73.

Grisso, T. and Appelbaum, P. S. (1992) Is it unethical to offer predictions of future violence? *Law and Human Behavior*, **16**, 621–33.

Gunn, J., Madden, A. and Swinton, M. (1991) Treatment needs of prisoners with psychiatric disorders. *British Medical Journal*, **303**, 338–341.

Hart, H. L. A. and Honoré, T. (1985) *Causation in the law* (2nd edn). Oxford: Clarendon Press.

Heilbrun, K. and Griffin, P. A. (1998) Community-based forensic treatment. In *Treatment of offenders with mental disorders* (ed. R. M. Wettstein). New York: The Guilford Press.

Heilbrun, K. and Peters, L. (2000) The efficacy of community treatment programmes in preventing crime and violence. In *Violence, crime and mentally disordered offenders: concepts and methods for effective treatment and prevention* (ed. S. Hodgins and R. Muller-Isberner). The Hague: Kluwer.

Heywood, D. (2000) Systems of services in forensic psychiatry. In *Behaviour, crime and legal processes: a sourcebook for forensic practitioners* (ed. J. McGuire, T. Mason and A. O'Kane). Chichester: John Wiley.

Hiday, V. A. (1999) Mental illness and the criminal justice system. In *A handbook for the study of mental health: social contexts, theories and systems* (ed. A. V. Horwitz and T. L. Scheid). Cambridge: Cambridge University Press.

Hudson, B. L., Cullen, R. and Roberts, C. (1993) *Training for work with mentally disordered offenders*. London: Central Council for Education and Training in Social Work.

Kandel, E. R., Schwartz, J. H. and Jessell, T. M. (1995) *Essentials of neural science and behavior*. Stamford, CT: Prentice-Hall.

Kemshall, H. (1998) The dangerous are always with us: dangerousness and the role of the probation service. *Vista: Perspectives on Probation*, **2**, 136–153.

Kutchins, H. A. and Kirk, S. A. (1997) *Making us crazy: DSM: The psychiatric bible and the creation of mental disorders.* Glencoe, IL: The Free Press.

Lawrence, C. (1994) *Medicine in the making of modern Britain 1700–1920.* London: Routledge.

Lehman, A., Postrado, L., Roth, D., McNary, S. and Goldman, H. (1994) An evaluation of the continuity of care, case management, and client outcomes in the Robert Wood Johnson program on chronic mental illness. *Milbank Quarterly,* **72,** 105–22.

Link, B. G. and Phelan, J. C. (1999) The labeling theory of mental disorder (II): the consequences of labeling. In *A handbook for the study of mental health: social contexts, theories and systems* (ed. A. V. Horwitz and T. L. Scheid). Cambridge: Cambridge University Press.

Lishman, W. A. (1997) *Organic psychiatry* (3rd edn). Oxford: Blackwell.

Lösel, F. (1998) Treatment and management of psychopaths. In *Psychopathy: theory, research and implications for society* (ed. D Cooke and R. A. Hare). The Hague: Kluwer.

Mason, T. (2000) Care and management in the community. In *Behaviour, crime and legal processes: a sourcebook for forensic practitioners* (ed. J. McGuire, T. Mason and A. O'Kane). Chichester: John Wiley (in press).

Mason, T. and Mercer, D. (ed.) (1998) *Critical perspective in forensic care: inside out.* Basingstoke: MacMillan.

McGuire, J. (1997*a*) Psycho-social approaches to the understanding and reduction of violence in young people. In *Violence in children and adolescents* (ed. V. Varma). London: Jessica Kingsley.

McGuire, J. (1997*b*) Ethical dilemmas in forensic clinical psychology. *Legal and Criminological Psychology,* **2,** 177–92.

McGuire, J. (2000) Commentary: Heilbrun and Peters, 'The efficacy and effectiveness of community treatment programmes in preventing crime and violence among those with severe mental illness in the community'. In *Violence among the Mentally Ill: Effective Treatments and Prevention Strategies* (ed. S. Hodgins). Dordrecht: Kluwer Academic Publishers.

McKenna, P. J. (1997) *Schizophrenia and related syndromes.* Hove: Psychology Press.

McSherry, B. (1998) Getting away with murder? Dissociative states and criminal responsibility. *International Journal of Law and Psychiatry,* **21,** 163–76.

McSherry, B. (1999) Criminal responsibility and voluntary conduct: legal versus psychological concepts. Paper delivered at the joint Conference of the American Psychology–Law Society and the European Association of Psychology and Law, Trinity College Dublin.

Mechanic, D. (1999) Mental health and mental illness: definitions and perspectives. In *A handbook for the study of mental health: social contexts, theories and systems* (ed. A. V. Horwitz and t. L. Scheid). Cambridge: Cambridge University Press.

Melton, G. B., Petrila, J., Poythress, N. G. *et al.* (1997) *Psychological evaluations for the courts: a handbook for mental health professionals and lawyers.* New York, NY: The Guilford Press.

Miller, P. and Rose, N. (ed.) (1986) *The power of psychiatry.* Cambridge: Polity Press.

Monahan, J. (1981) *Predicting violent behavior: an assessment of clinical techniques.* Beverley Hills, CA: Sage.

Monahan, J. (1993) Limiting therapist exposure to *Tarasoff* liability: Guidelines for risk containment. *American Psychologist,* **48,** 242–50.

Monahan. J. (1996) Violence prediction: The past twenty and the next twenty years. *Criminal Justice and Behavior,* **23,** 107–20.

Monahan, J. (1997) Clinical and actuarial predictions of violence. In *West's companion to scientific evidence* (ed. D. Faigman, D. Kaye, M. Saks and J. Sanders). St. Paul, MI: West Publishing Company.

Monahan, J. and Steadman, H. (ed.) (1994) *Mental disorder and violence: developments in risk assessment.* Chicago, IL: University of Chicago Press.

Morrissey, J. P. (1999) Integrating service delivery systems for persons with a severe mental illness. In *A handbook for the study of mental health: social contexts, theories and systems* (ed. A. V. Horwitz and T. L. Scheid). Cambridge: Cambridge University Press.

Morrissey, J. P., Calloway, M., Bartko *et al.* (1994) Local mental health authorities and service system change: Evidence from the Robert Wood Johnson program on chronic mental illness. *Milbank Quarterly*, **72**, 49–80.

Nathan, P. E. and Gorman, J. M. (ed.) (1998) *A guide to treatments that work.* New York, NY: Oxford University Press.

O'Kane, A. and Bentall, R. P. (2000) Psychosis and offending. In *Behaviour, crime and legal processes: a sourcebook for forensic practitioners* (ed. J. McGuire, T. Mason and A. O'Kane). Chichester: John Wiley.

Peay, J. (1996*a*) Themes and questions: the inquiry in context. In *Inquiries after homicide* (ed. J. Peay). London: Duckworth.

Peay, J. (ed.) (1996*b*) *Inquiries after homicide.* London: Duckworth.

Perry, J. C., Banon, E. and Ianni, F. (1999) Effectiveness of psychotherapy for personality disorders. *American Journal of Psychiatry*, **156**, 1312–21.

Peterson, C. (1999) Psychological approaches to mental illness. In *A handbook for the study of mental health: social contexts, theories and systems* (ed. A. V. Horwitz and T. L. Scheid). Cambridge: Cambridge University Press.

Petrella, R. C. and Poythress, N. G. (1983) The quality of forensic evaluations: An interdisciplinary study. *Journal of Consulting and Clinical Psychology*, **51**, 76–85.

Pickett, S. A., Cook, J. A. and Razzano, L. (1999) Psychiatric rehabilitation services and outcomes: an overview. In *A handbook for the study of mental health: social contexts, theories and systems* (ed. A. V. Horwitz and T. L. Scheid). Cambridge: Cambridge University Press.

Pilgrim, D. and Rogers, A. (1993) *A sociology of mental health and illness.* Buckingham: Open University Press.

Reith, M. (1998) *Community care tragedies: a practice guide to mental health inquiries.* Birmingham: Venture Press.

Rice, M. E. and Harris, G. T. (1995) Psychopathy, schizophrenia, alcohol abuse and violent recidivism. *International Journal of Law and Psychiatry*, **18**, 333–42.

Ritchie, J., Dick, D. and Lingham, R. (1994) *The report of the inquiry into the care and treatment of Christopher Clunis.* London: HMSO.

Roberts, C., Hudson, B. L. and Cullen, R. (1995) The supervision of mentally disordered offenders: the work of probation officers and their relationship with psychiatrists in England and Wales. *Criminal Behaviour and Mental Health*, **5**, 75–84.

Robertson. I. H. (1999) *Mind sculpture: your brain's untapped potential.* London: Bantam Books.

Rooney, H. (1994) Probation orders with conditions of psychiatric treatment. Unpublished MSc dissertation, University of Liverpool.

Roth, A. and Fonagy, P. (1996) *What works for whom: a critical review of psychotherapy research.* New York, NY: Guilford Press.

Sanislow, C. A. and McGlashan, T. H. (1998) Treatment outcome of personality disorders. *Canadian Journal of Psychiatry*, **43**, 237–50.

Schwartz, S. (1999) Biological approaches to psychiatric disorders. In *A handbook for the study of mental health: social contexts, theories and systems.* (ed. A. V. Horwitz and T. L. Scheid). Cambridge: Cambridge University Press.

Searle, J. R. (1995) *The construction of social reality.* London: Penguin.

Serin, R. C. (1993) Decision issues in risk assessment. *Forum on Corrections Research*, **5**, 22–5.

Smith, J. C. and Hogan, B. (1992) *Criminal Law* (7th edn) London: Butterworths.

Strasburger, L. H., Gutheil, T. G. and Brodsky, A. (1997) On wearing two hats: role conflict in serving as both psychotherapist and expert witness. *American Journal of Psychiatry*, **154**, 448–56.

Szasz, T. S. (1961) *The myth of mental illness: foundations of a theory of personal conduct.* New York, NY: Harper & Row.

Taylor, P. J. and Gunn, J. (1999) Homicides by people with mental illness: myth and reality. *British Journal of Psychiatry*, **174**, 9–14.

Taylor, P. J., Garety, P., Buchanan, A. *et al.* (1994) Delusions and violence. In *Mental disorder and violence: developments in risk assessment* (ed. J. Monahan and H. Steadman). Chicago, IL: University of Chicago Press.

Thara, R. and Eaton, W. W. (1996) Outcome of schizophrenia: the Madras longitudinal study. *Australian and New Zealand Journal of Psychiatry*, **30**, 516–22.

Thoits, P. A. (1999) Sociological approaches to mental illness. In *A handbook for the study of mental health: social contexts, theories and systems* (ed. A. V. Horwitz and T. L. Scheid). Cambridge: Cambridge University Press.

Tyrer, P., Coid, J., Simmonds, S. *et al.* (1999) Community mental health teams for people with severe mental illnesses and disordered personality. *The Cochrane Library* (Issue 2), 1–23.

Warner, R. (1985) *Recovery from schizophrenia: psychiatry and political economy.* London: Routledge and Kegan Paul.

Wessely, S. and Taylor, P. J. (1991) Madness and crime: criminology versus psychiatry. *Criminal Behaviour and Mental Health*, **1**, 193–228.

Wexler, D. B. and Winick, B. D. (ed.) (1996) *Law in a therapeutic key: developments in therapeutic jurisprudence.* Durham, NC: Carolina Academic Press.

Wiederanders, M., Bromley, D. L. and Choate, P. A. (1997) Forensic conditional release programs and outcomes in three states. *International Journal of Law and Psychiatry*, **20**, 249–57.

Wilson, D., Tien, G. and Eaves, D. (1995) Increasing the community tenure of mentally disordered offenders: An assertive case management program. *International Journal of Law and Psychiatry*, **18**, 61–70.

Wing, J. K., Sartorius, N. and Üstün, T. B. (1998) *Diagnosis and clinical measurement in psychiatry.* Cambridge: Cambridge University Press.

World Health Organization (WHO) (1992) *The international classification of mental and behavioural disorders (ICD-10)* (10th edn). Geneva: World Health Organization.

Chapter 13

'To serve which master?'—criminal justice policy, community care and the mentally disordered offender

Philip Fennell and Victoria Yeates

Introduction

'Which master?'—What is the balance between therapy for mental disorder, retribution in the sense of a period of detention proportionate to the severity of the offence ('just deserts'), and public protection from future offending? Is the mentally disordered offender primarily a prisoner or a patient? What is the balance in the psychiatrist's role between therapist, custodian and protector of society? This chapter focuses on England and Wales, where in terms of overall policy the key state authorities are the Home Office, the Department of Health, and the Welsh Office. In ideological terms the field is dominated by philosophies of risk management, populist retributivism and the protection of the rights of victims or potential victims. The major countervailing forces are the human rights of the offenders under the European Convention on Human Rights, and the reluctance of the psychiatric profession to be involved in preventive detention without the prospect of therapeutic intervention having some success. In terms of decision making about individual offenders, the key players are: (1) the Home Office Mental Health Unit, which oversees the management of the patients who are subject to restriction orders; (2) the psychiatrists who are in charge of the treatment of detained patients and patients in the community; and (3) the Mental Health Review Tribunal, which has the power to discharge offender patients.

The chapter examines the contradictory philosophies and policies at play in the system of care of mentally disordered offenders and the impact of the case law of the European Court of Human Rights on that system. We argue that a convergence is taking place between the values and legal structures of the hospital system, on the one hand, and the penal system on the other, a convergence with profound implications for the community care of mentally disordered offenders and the nature of the doctor/patient relationship. We trace how the Government's pursuit of radical risk management policies within the constraints of European Convention case law has affected and will continue to affect community care policies for mentally disordered offenders, and particularly how it has altered the balance between therapy, retribution and social defence.

Risk management

The social control of so-called 'risky populations' has always been a goal of criminal justice policy,[1] but lately it has become an increasingly overt pre-occupation.[2] Since the early 1990s mentally disordered people in general, let alone those who have committed criminal offences, are increasingly portrayed as a risky population. A steady procession of inquiries into homicides by former psychiatric in-patients has increased the association in the public mind between mental disorder and dangerousness, leading to increasing demands for protection not just from mentally disordered offenders, but from offenders generally. This in turn has resulted in a role redefinition whereby risk management has become a central part of the job of psychiatrists and other mental health professionals, and philosophies of risk management now permeate decision making in both the psychiatric system and the penal system.

Risk management may be defined as the identification, assessment, elimination or reduction of the possibility of incurring misfortune.[3] As Nikolas Rose has put it, risk management 'operates through transforming professional subjectivity':

> It is the individual professional who has to make the assessment and management of risk their central professional obligation They have to assess the individual client in terms of the riskiness they represent, to allocate each to a risk level, to put in place the appropriate administrative arrangements for the management of the individual in the light of the requirement to minimise risk and to take responsibility, indeed blame—if an untoward incident occurs. It appears that it is no longer good enough to say that behaviour is difficult to predict and 'accidents will happen'. Every unwelcome incident may be seen as a failure of professional expertise: someone must be held accountable.[4]

Detention is the ultimate risk management mechanism of both the penal and the psychiatric systems to protect society from dangerous offenders. Both the penal and the psychiatric systems provide for detention in different levels of security. In both sectors great reliance is placed on strategies of 'graduated relaxation of security'. Patients and prisoners who start in high security are gradually tested in conditions of lesser security before release to the community through probation or supervised aftercare. Both

---

[1] See, for example, Kellow Chesney's discussion of the Victorian pre-occupation with 'the dangerous classes', *The Victorian Underworld* (Pelican).

[2] The most obvious example being the Government's proposals in relation to 'dangerous people with severe personality disorder', discussed below.

[3] Castel, R. (1991) From dangerousness to risk. In *The Foucault Effect: Studies in Governmentality*. (ed. G. Bruchell, C. Gordon, C and P. Miller). Hemel Hempstead: Harvester Wheatsheaf.

[4] Rose, N. (1997) At risk of madness: law, politics and forensic psychiatry. Paper delivered at the *Cropwood Conference on The Future of Forensic Psychiatry*. St John's College, Cambridge 19–21 March 1997. See also Chapter 1.

sectors concern themselves with the management of risk to the public, and risk management becomes more difficult once a patient or prisoner leaves detention and is made subject to community supervision.

The reason why detention, or the power to detain indefinitely, is the bedrock of risk management is that the authorities can use recall to detention as the safety net for risk management in the community. A significant policy aim of the Home Office is to facilitate risk management by three main legal expedients: (1) extendable detention where a mentally disordered offender presents a serious risk to the public; (2) continued control over offenders who are discharged into the community; and (3) easy recall to detention in hospital or prison of those whose conduct in the community gives rise to concern. The main countervailing force to these developments is individual rights, particularly those conferred by Articles 3, 5, 6 and 8 of the European Convention on Human Rights (ECHR). The Human Rights Act 1998 requires all public authorities (including courts and tribunals) to act compatibly with convention rights, and requires ministers introducing legislation to certify to Parliament that the relevant Bill is compatible with Convention rights.

The ECHR has undoubtedly improved the situation for mentally disordered offenders in many respects, improving their due process safeguards, requiring the right to review of detention before a tribunal with the power to order (as opposed to recommend) discharge (established in *X v UK*[5]), protecting against arbitrary recall to hospital (as in *James Kay v UK*[6]), and in some cases even seeming to create positive rights to aftercare for patients who no longer meet the legal criteria for psychiatric detention (as in *Stanley Johnson v UK*[7]).

But the developing Strasbourg jurisprudence on detention on grounds of unsoundness of mind (Article 5(1)(e)), detention following conviction of a criminal offence (Article 5(1)(a)) and detention for the prevention of crime (Article 5(1)(c)) has led to more subtle responses by the Home Office in terms of its desire to manage the risk posed by mentally disordered offenders. The drive for 'Convention compliance' whilst pursuing policy goals in relation to preventive detention is leading to a convergence between the penal system and the hospital system. This convergence manifests itself in a number of ways. Once the great advantage of psychiatric detention over imprisonment was that it allowed for potentially indefinite detention. Life sentences have now become possible in relation to an increasing range of offences, with offenders not being released until they are deemed no longer to pose a risk. Increasingly, psychological treatment programmes are used in the prison system for personality disordered offenders subject to discretionary life sentences, and offenders released from prison are subject to supervision and recall.

---

[5] (1981) 4 EHRR 188.

[6] (1994) 40 BMLR 20.

[7] (1997) 40 BMLR 1.

The advantage of imprisonment over a hospital order was that the offender could be required to serve a minimum period in detention, whereas someone who was a patient would be entitled to discharge once they were no longer mentally disordered to the extent that they required detention. The hybrid order introduced by the Crime Sentences Act 1997 and the Government's proposals for 'dangerous people with severe personality disorder' both seek to ensure that personality disordered offenders serve a period of detention proportionate to the gravity of their offence, and there is a possibility that this will be extended to offenders with mental illness.

Juridically, the Government has realized that for Convention purposes it is easier to achieve its policy goals, allowing for indeterminate detention whilst at the same ensuring that the offender serves a minimum period of detention proportionate to the seriousness of the crime, if mentally disordered offenders have the legal status of prisoners first and patients second.

Prisoners and patients: legal status

The prison population is over 60 000. In 1991 Gunn and colleagues carried out a study of 5% of the male prison population and found that 1% were diagnosed schizophrenic and 10% personality disorder (74% of whom required psychiatric treatment).[8] Although the growth of forensic psychiatry as a specialism has been dramatic, from two consultants in 1962 to 70 consultants in 1992,[9] the capacity of the health service to absorb mentally disordered offenders is limited. There were 1305 patients detained in high security special hospitals on 31 March 1999. In addition, there were about 600 permanent medium secure beds. The Reed Committee, established in 1990 to review health and social services for mentally disordered offenders, reported in 1992 that 1500 medium secure beds were needed.[10] The number of court admissions increased from 1500 in 1988–9 to 2110 by 1994–5, but then fell back to 1900 in 1998–9.[11] A small but rapidly growing private sector has developed for patients who present difficult behaviour, where local health or social services authorities pay for the care of patients in the private sector because NHS trusts in their areas do not provide sufficient specialist provision. The numbers of admissions of detained patients to private hospitals has increased from 220 in 1988–9 to 1250 in 1998–9. Until 1998–9 approximately 100 patients per year were admitted to private hospitals under the offender provisions of the Mental Health Act. The total for 1998–9 was 205. Until

---

[8] Gunn, J., Maden, A. and Sinton, M. (1991) Treatment needs of prisoners with mental disorder. *British Medical Journal* **303**.

[9] *Review of Health and Social Services for Mentally Disordered Offenders and Others Requiring Similar Services*. (Chairman Dr John Reed) (The Reed Report) Cm 2088 1992, para. 2.8.

[10] *Ibid.*, para. 2.7 and 5.19.

[11] In-patients formally detained in hospitals under the Mental Health Act 1983 and other legislation, England: 1988–9 and 1994–5 to 1998–9. *DoH Statistical Bulletin* 1999/25, para. 3.5–6.

1998–9 somewhere between 150 and 160 offender patients were admitted annually to the special hospitals. The 1998 figure was down to 121, but this excluded transfers where there was no change in the patient's legal status. Between 1700 and 1800 offender patients annually are admitted to special hospitals and other NHS facilities, about a third of whom are transferred from prison. Local psychiatric hospitals may be hard pressed to cope with requests to provide for offender patients. Although many offenders may be able to be managed in open wards, some need more security and limited numbers of beds are available in lockable wards.[12] As for community care places, these are at a premium, and the move to the community is one of the crucial points of blockage of the system of graduated relaxation of security. Whilst the penal system has the capacity to absorb large numbers of offenders, the ability of the health service to do so is limited by three main constraints: the lack of facilities, the reluctance of the psychiatric profession to become involved in treating those whom they do not believe likely to respond to treatment, and competing demands for health and social services budgets.

Patients

Article 5 of the European Convention allows 'lawful' detention on grounds of unsoundness of mind provided that it is carried out in accordance with a procedure prescribed by law. To be lawful detention must not be arbitrary. Detention is not arbitrary if it is in conformity with the procedural and substantive requirements of domestic law and is carried out for the purpose allowed by the Convention. In *Winterwerp v the Netherlands*[13] the European Court of Human Rights laid down three conditions of lawful psychiatric detention. The government must be able to show by reliable evidence before a competent authority that (1) a true mental disorder has been established by objective medical expertise; (2) the mental disorder is of a kind or degree warranting compulsory confinement; and (3) if detention is to be prolonged, the government must be able to show that the continued confinement is based on the persistence of the disorder.

For Convention purposes offenders detained under the Mental Health Act system of hospital orders and restriction orders are patients detained on grounds of unsoundness of mind. Until the ruling of the European Court of Human Rights in *X v UK*,[14] the Home Secretary, a government minister, retained control over the discharge of restriction order patients. These patients could have their cases referred to a Mental Health Review Tribunal, which could advise the Home Secretary on suitability for discharge, but the Home Secretary was not bound by their advice. The European Court of Human Rights held that Article 5(4) entitles everyone detained on grounds of

---

[12] *Op. cit.*, note 8, para. 5.15–5.16.

[13] (1979) 2 EHRR 387.

[14] *X v UK* (1981) 4 EHRR 188.

unsoundness of mind to seek review of the lawfulness of their detention before a court or tribunal. In order to be a competent court for the purposes of Article 5(4) the Mental Health Review Tribunal had to be given the power to discharge restricted patients if the conditions which justified the initial detention were no longer met. The judicial body had to have the final say regardless of the minister's view.

In order for psychiatric detention to remain lawful for the purposes of Article 5 there must be objective medical evidence of unsoundness of mind of a kind or degree warranting confinement. The most disturbing aspect of the ruling in X v UK from the Home Office's point of view was the possibility that an offender who was given a hospital order with restrictions for a serious offence would be entitled to seek discharge before a Mental Health Review Tribunal after only six months in hospital and might be discharged after a comparatively short period of detention if the unsoundness of mind which originally justified the detention was no longer present. Offenders committing crimes meriting 10 or 15 years in prison might be found no longer to be mentally disordered to a degree warranting detention shortly after admission and might then be discharged after only a few months' detention.

In reality, a person is likely to spend longer in detention under a hospital order than they would if given a determinate prison sentence. Offenders committing crimes meriting two years imprisonment might well find themselves detained under the 1983 Act for a considerably longer period before they are judged well enough to leave. They may be detained as long as they continue to suffer from a mental disorder of a nature or degree warranting detention, regardless of the seriousness of the offence. From a risk-management point of view, therapeutic detention of offenders under the Mental Health Act has the advantage that it is potentially indefinite. It can extend until the offender is deemed well enough to leave hospital. The Mental Health Act offers the possibility of extending detention beyond the duration of whatever prison sentence is proportionate to the gravity of the offence. But after X v UK, detention under the Mental Health Act could not guarantee that the offender would spend a minimum period in detention.

Mental disorder has a very broad meaning under the 1983 Mental Health Act, including mental illness, psychopathic disorder, mental impairment and severe mental impairment. An offender who is mentally disordered may be detained in prison or in hospital. Which route they follow, therapeutic or penal, depends on whether they are identified, by psychiatrists willing to treat them, as being mentally disordered within the meaning of the 1983 Act. In the case of patients with mental impairment or psychopathic disorder, the doctors must consider that medical treatment is likely to alleviate or prevent a deterioration in their condition (in short that they are treatable). Section 37 of the 1983 Act allows for the detention of mentally disordered offenders in hospital under hospital orders. Section 37 also allows the community disposal of a guardianship order, placing the offender under the guardianship of the local authority. It is important to recognize that the system of hospital and guardianship orders requires no causal connection between the mental disorder and the offence. The only relevant considerations are the offender's mental condition at the time of sentencing. Detention or guardianship may be prolonged by the psychiatrist in charge of the patient's treatment, the responsible medical officer, who may furnish a report to the hospital managers 'renewing' the authority after six months and thereafter at annual intervals. Hospital order patients may be discharged to the community subject to 'supervised discharge' under Sections 25A–J of the Mental Health Act 1983.

If an offender is given a hospital order and the Crown Court feels it necessary to impose restrictions on discharge because of the need to protect the public from serious harm, they may impose a restriction order. Restrictions may be imposed for a prescribed period, or without limit of time. This has the effect of requiring the leave of the Home Secretary via the Home Office Mental Health Unit before the patient can be granted leave, transferred to another hospital, or discharged. At the end of 1995 there were 2482 mentally disordered offenders detained in hospital subject to Home Office restrictions on discharge, more than in any of the previous ten years.[15] Restriction order patients may be subject to conditional discharge, which means that they remain liable to recall to hospital at any time during the currency of the restriction order.

Local health and social services authorities are under a joint duty to provide after care on discharge for patients who have been detained under long term sections of the Mental Health Act or who have been transferred from prison to hospital. The duty applies for as long as the authorities jointly consider the patient to need the care.[16] Restricted patients may receive community care as a condition of their discharge and may be recalled by the Home Office if they remain mentally disordered and do not comply with treatment or show signs of relapse. Non-restricted patients may be subject to compulsory supervision under Sections 25A–J of the 1983 Act.[17] This range of legal mechanisms and services enables the Home Office to pursue a policy of 'graduated relaxation of security' whereby a person might progress from special hospital to a regional secure unit and thence to supervision in the community, possibly via a local non-secure hospital. But it is a difficult policy to operate efficiently. The rehabilitation of a mentally disordered offender is often a long drawn out affair, made even longer by the decision-making processes involved in moving patients from greater to lesser security. These may arise from lack of hospital or hostel places, from clinical disputes about treatability or suitability for less restrictive conditions, or from inability to find supervising psychiatrists or social workers.

---

[15] One difficulty in assessing the scale of the use of therapeutic disposals is that the Home Office issues statistics of mentally disordered offenders which are collected by calendar year and which cover mainly restricted patients. Meanwhile, the Department of Health collects statistics by financial year of all admissions to psychiatric hospitals, including those of the many offenders admitted without restrictions.

[16] Mental Health Act 1983, Section 117.

[17] As inserted by the Mental Health (Patients in the Community) Act 1995.

Prisoners

The legal status of prisoner means, for Convention purposes, that the person is detained following conviction for a criminal offence (Article 5(1)(a)), and in these cases it is possible to stipulate a minimum period to be served in detention which is proportionate to the gravity of the offence. In *Thynne Wilson and Gunnell v UK*[18] the European Court held that in the case of discretionary life prisoners it was allowable for a criminal court to impose a minimum tariff period of detention to reflect the gravity of the offence and the culpability of the offender, and for detention to be extended beyond that period if the prisoner remained dangerous. To comply with Article 5, the sentencing court must specify the amount of the sentence attributable to the gravity of the offence and the culpability of the offender (the tariff period). After this, the basis of detention is continued dangerousness, which is susceptible to change with the passage of time. Because of this, as soon as the offender enters the protective part of the sentence, Article 5(4) is engaged. This requires that the prisoner must have the right to seek review of the continuing need for his detention and to challenge the view that he remains dangerous before a court or tribunal with the power to order release.

Section 34 of the 1991 Criminal Justice Act was enacted to take into account the consequences of the *Thynne* ruling.[19] Certain offences carry a discretionary life sentence, where the dangerousness and instability of the offender are the determining factors. The 1991 Act entitles discretionary life prisoners to have their cases referred to the Parole Board once the tariff part of the sentence has been served. The Board can direct release if satisfied that the prisoner is not likely to be dangerous, regardless of the views of the Home Secretary.

Whilst a hospital patient has the right to seek review of detention after the first six months of detention, a life prisoner has to wait until the tariff period has expired before becoming entitled to review. The legal status of prisoner has always had advantages over that of patient if the goals of policy are to ensure that an offender will be detained for a minimum period commensurate with the gravity of the offence and the level of blameworthiness. Following *Thynne* it was clear that the convention represented no obstacle to extending detention beyond that tariff period on grounds of dangerousness, as long as there were opportunities for review. The possibility of indefinite detention on grounds of dangerousness, which used to be the advantage of patient status from the risk-management point of view, was now available in relation to prisoners.

However, an offender who is given a determinate sentence must be released when he has served that sentence, regardless of dangerousness. With violent or sexual offences the courts have the power under Section 2(2)(b) of the Criminal Justice Act 1991 to increase the duration of the prison sentence to such longer term as they consider

---

[18] Series A No. 190 Judgement of 25 October 1990.

[19] See now Crime Sentences Act 1997, Section 28.

necessary for the public protection.[20] A longer than normal sentence remains a determinate sentence, but offenders initially sent to prison may be transferred to psychiatric hospital with a restriction direction at any time during the sentence of imprisonment. If they recover from their mental disorder before the expiry of their sentence, the Home Secretary decides whether they should be discharged or returned to prison to serve out the sentence. Where the sentence of a transferred prisoner expires whilst he is in hospital, he may be kept in detention and his detention may be renewed by the doctor if the patient is mentally disordered and detention is necessary. This means that transfer to hospital can be and is used at the end of a sentence to extend a patient's detention if he or she is thought to be mentally disordered and to pose a risk. From time to time concerns have been raised about the fairness of transfers close to the end of sentence, in terms of proportionality between the time spent in detention and the gravity of the index offence.[21]

In recent years there have been significant developments in so-called 'protective sentencing'. Section 4 of the Criminal Justice Act 1991 introduced a requirement that, before imposing a custodial sentence on a person who is or who appears to be mentally disordered, a court must obtain and consider a medical report, and must consider the likely effect of a custodial sentence on the offender's condition and on any treatment which may be available for it. Failure to obtain such a report does not invalidate any sentence passed, but a court considering an appeal against sentence must obtain a report if none was furnished to the court of first instance, or consider afresh any report which was provided. Section 28(4) of the 1991 Act provides that nothing in the Act shall be taken as requiring a court to impose a custodial sentence on a mentally disordered offender or to restrict the powers under the 1983 Act to impose a therapeutic disposal. A mentally disordered offender may well receive a prison sentence, especially if mentally impaired or psychopathically disordered, and the reporting psychiatrists consider him or her to be untreatable. That sentence may well be determinate, in which case the prisoner will be released regardless of risk to the public, unless he is transferred to psychiatric hospital before the sentence ends. The other possibility is that the offender will receive a protective sentence or a discretionary life sentence where, once the penal element is served, parole will depend on the degree of risk.

There are three provisions in English law for protective sentencing: life imprisonment, protective sentencing under Sections 1(2)(b) and 2(2)(b) of the Criminal Justice Act 1991, and the new procedures for mandatory minimum sentences in the Crime (Sentences) Act 1997, whereby conviction of a second serious offence attracts an automatic life sentence.

----

[20] A second serious sexual offence or violent offence will put the offender at risk of a life sentence under the Crime Sentences Act 1997 'two strikes and you're out' principle.

[21] Grounds, A. (1990) Transfers of sentenced prisoners to hospital. *Criminal Law Review*, 544–55 and (1991) The transfer of sentenced prisoners to hospital 1960–1983: A study in one special hospital. *British Journal of Criminology*, **31**, 54–71.

Life imprisonment is the maximum sentence for crimes such as manslaughter, rape, robbery, wounding with intent and arson. A life sentence may only be imposed for these offences if three criteria (The 'Hodgson' criteria) are met: (1) the offence or offences are in themselves grave enough to require a very long sentence; (2) where it appears from the nature of the defendant's offences or from the defendant's history that he is a person of unstable character likely to commit such offences in future; and (3) where if such offences are committed the consequences to others may be specially injurious, as in the case of sexual offences or crimes of violence.[22] On the question of instability, it has been held that there need not be mental disorder within the terms of the 1983 Act but there must be some evidence of mental disturbance which goes beyond a mere reference to a personality disorder.[23] Medical reports are usually provided, most often giving evidence of untreatable personality disorder or learning disability, but in exceptional circumstances the court can find instability on the basis of the circumstances of the offence if it involves particularly savage or grotesque violence. The judge should specify the period to be served before the offender's case can be considered by the Parole Board. Counsel should be invited to address the court on the length of the tariff period, and reasons for the court's decision should be given.[24] Since account must be taken of the early release provisions in the 1991 Act, the tariff period is usually set at around two-thirds of the proportionate sentence. In very exceptional cases, that is the most serious cases, where the judge considers that detention for the offender's natural life is warranted by the seriousness of the offence, no period need be specified. After the expiry of the specified period, the offender is entitled to periodic review of his continued dangerousness before a Discretionary Life Sentence Panel of the Parole Board. This is to comply with the requirement of regular review in Article 5(4).

Section 1(2)(b) of the 1991 Criminal Justice Act permits a court to pass a sentence of imprisonment if it considers that 'only such a sentence would be adequate to protect the public from serious harm from him.' Section 2(2)(b) allows the Crown Court, when imposing imprisonment for a violent or sexual offence, to fix the term at such length, beyond what the gravity of the offence would merit but within the statutory maximum, as may be necessary to protect the public from serious harm.[25] 'Serious harm' is elaborated in Section 31(3) which provides that it refers to 'protecting the public from death or serious personal injury, whether physical or psychological'.

---

[22] *R v Hodgson* (1967) 52 Cr. App. Rep. 113. *R v Waller* (1995) 16 Cr. App. Rep. (S) 251.

[23] Ashworth, A. (1995) *Sentencing and Criminal Justice* (2nd edn), p. 179.

[24] *Practice direction (crime: life sentences)* (1993) 1 WLR 223.

[25] For a full discussion of the protective sentencing provisions in the 1991 act see Ashworth, A. (1995) *Sentencing and Criminal Justice* (2nd edn), pp. 172–182. London: Butterworths and Henham, R. (1996) Sentencing policy, appellate guidance and protective sentencing. *Journal of Criminal Law,* 424–446.

Although there is no requirement for a psychiatric or psychological report addressing the issue of risk, in *Fawcett* the Court of Appeal held that where the risk arises from a mental or personality problem the sentencing court should require a medical report before invoking Section 2(2)(b).[26] Henham has argued for mandatory psychiatric assessment in all Section 2(2)(b) cases. As Ashworth has noted, in most reported cases where a report has been requested, it has referred to a personality disorder which is not regarded as treatable, and therefore does not require treatment under the 1983 Act.[27] The courts have adopted the approach of stating what the proportionate sentence would be and then stating how much they are adding for public protection. The Court of Appeal has held that where there is insufficient evidence of instability to bring the offender within the second *Hodgson* criterion, a sentence under Section 2(2)(b) should be considered.[28]

So far there has been no successful challenge to the UK government's refusal to grant review hearings to Section 2(2) prisoners where the 'tariff' period has been served. In *Mansell v UK*[29] the European Commission on Human Rights held that there was no breach of the requirement of review in Article 5(4) where a Section 2(2)(b) prisoner sentenced to five years was not afforded a personal hearing before the Parole Board after the expiry of the tariff part of the sentence. The judge had stated that, had there been no need to protect the public, the appropriate sentence would have been two and a half years. The applicant argued that, following the expiry of that period, he should have had the same opportunities for a hearing as were available to a discretionary life prisoner, or the same parole entitlements and review procedures which applied to a normal punitive sentence. The Commission somewhat ducked the issue by holding that the five year sentence was 'essentially retributive and deterrent in character'. There was therefore no need for the controls and safeguards in Article 5(4), as these had been incorporated in the original conviction and sentence.

The protective sentencing provisions in relation to discretionary lifers and protective determinate sentencing are characterized by wide discretion and an absence of precise criteria in relation to instability or the need for protection. Henham has observed that 'the present protective provisions militate unfairly against mentally disordered offenders who are more likely to be adjudged dangerous because they are more likely to commit violent or sexual harm within the meaning of the Act.'[30] Be that as it may, the experience with protective sentencing shows that it is applied predominantly to one class of offenders, those with personality disorders who are viewed as unlikely to

---

[26] *R v Fawcett* (1995) Cr. App. Rep. (S)55.

[27] Ashworth, A. (1995) *Sentencing and Criminal Justice* (2nd edn), p. 174.

[28] *R v Spear* (1995) Cr. App. Rep. (S)242.

[29] (1997) EHRR 666.

[30] Henham, R. (1996) Sentencing policy, appellate guidance and protective sentencing. *Journal of Criminal Law*, 424–446.

respond to psychiatric intervention, so-called 'untreatable psychopaths.' An offender whose crime resulted from mental illness will probably benefit from a reduction of any determinate term of imprisonment imposed, but a personality disordered offender will probably have his mental disorder taken into account to increase his sentence. Only if the personality disorder is regarded as treatable will the offender be admitted to hospital.

The 1997 Crime (Sentences) Act introduced two protective sentencing provisions. Section 2 provides that a second serious offence[31] will attract a life sentence unless there are exceptional circumstances relating to either of the offences or to the offender. In *R v Newman*[32] it was held that a defendant's acute mental illness at the time of committing a second serious offence was not, of itself, an exceptional circumstance which justified the court in not passing a life sentence. The Court of Appeal noted that the rationale of Section 2 was based entirely on risk management, 'that those convicted of two qualifying serious offences presented such a serious and continuing threat to public safety as to require their liability to indefinite incarceration and, if released, to indefinite recall to prison.' That being the case, where such a danger was apparent, 'the court could hardly consider itself justified in imposing a lesser sentence.' Section 37(1) of the Mental Health Act was amended by the 1997 Act so as to preclude the making of a hospital order in any case where a mandatory life sentence is required by Section 2 of the Crime (Sentences) Act. Referring to this provision in *Newman*, the Lord Chief Justice said that it was a matter for concern that a defendant 'so obviously and acutely' mentally ill should be ordered to prison, not to hospital.

Even though in practical terms the difference between the two orders might lie less in the mode of treatment after sentence than in the procedure governing release and recall, the court regretted its inability to make what appeared on the medical evidence to be the more appropriate order.

Sections 3 and 4 of the 1997 act also provide for minimum sentences of seven years for a third Class A drug trafficking offence, and three years for a third domestic burglary, again unless there are exceptional circumstances relating to the offences or to the offender. A court is not precluded from passing a hospital order in Section 3 or 4 cases.[33]

The 1997 act represents a key step in the process of convergence between the penal and psychiatric legal regimes by providing for a 'hybrid order' whereby a mentally disordered offender may be given a sentence of imprisonment coupled with an immediate direction to hospital, resulting in the offender being returned to prison in the event

[31] The offences defined as serious include the following: (1) serious offences involving harm to the person (attempted murder soliciting murder, conspiracy or incitement to murder, manslaughter, wounding or causing grievous bodily harm with intent); (2) serious sexual offences (rape, attempted rape, intercourse with a girl under 13); and (3) offences involving firearms.

[32] *The Times* 3 February 2000.

[33] 1983 Mental Health Act, Section 37(1A).

of the mental disorder being successfully treated before the expiry of the prison sentence. Under this sentencing power, the mentally disordered offender is given a prison sentence which is calculated in accordance with normal sentencing principles, but is directed to hospital in the first instance. If he recovers prior to the expiry of the sentence, he will be remitted to prison to serve the remaining sentence. This avoids the problem of the Mental Health Review Tribunals discharging patients 'early', because if the offender is no longer mentally disordered, the Home Secretary has the ultimate say in whether he returns to prison.

From diversion[34] to risk management

The Home Office has issued two circulars specifically on mentally disordered offenders: Circulars 66/90 on diversion of mentally disordered offenders from custody and 12/95 on inter-agency working. Circular 66/90, issued in the wake of a spate of suicides in prison in the late 1980s and research surveys which suggested that up to 25% of the prison population suffered from problems of mental ill health, reaffirmed Government policy of diversion of mentally disordered offenders from custody into the mental health system. Circular 12/95 was issued following concerns about failures adequately to supervise discharged offender patients. It supplements Circular 66/90, giving guidance on inter-agency working with in- and out-patients and examples of good practice in diversion of mentally disordered offenders, and shifts the emphasis firmly towards protection of the public.

The key Department of Health policy documents are the 'Code of Practice on the Mental Health Act 1983' which gives guidance on the use of powers under the Act and the torrent of policy documents on community care of mentally disordered people issued since 1990 (see Chapter 11). In 1990, the inherently parlous nature of risk management in community settings was revealed by the inquiry into the killing of a social worker, Isabel Schwarz, by a psychiatric patient.[35] The inquiry's report led to the inauguration by the Department of Health of the 'care programme approach' for people with a mental illness referred to the specialist psychiatric services, requiring monitoring of the patient's progress by a 'key worker' with responsibility for ensuring that care is delivered.

Within two years came the Inquiry into the Care of Christopher Clunis,[36] a formerly detained patient who was supposedly receiving community care and supervision, who killed Jonathan Zito at random on a London Underground platform. Since 1993 the

---

[34] For an analysis of diversion in theory and practice see Laing, J. (1999) *Care or Custody: Mentally Disordered Offenders in the Criminal Justice System*. Oxford: Oxford University Press.

[35] Report of the Committee of Inquiry into the care and after-care of Miss Sharon Campbell (The Spokes Report) Cmd 440, 1988.

[36] Ritchie, J., Dick, D and Lingham, R. (1994) Report of the inquiry into the care of Christopher Clunis. HMSO.

prime focus of public concern has been on homicides by people who have been psychiatric in-patients, a focus maintained by the fact that Health Authorities are required to institute an inquiry chaired by an independent person every time such a homicide occurs.[37]

In 1994 new 'Guidance on discharge of mentally disordered people and their continued care in the community'[38] was published, and this laid unprecedented emphasis on risk assessment. Also in 1994, guidance was issued requiring purchasing health authorities to include terms in their contracts with provider bodies that providers would maintain a supervision register for patients felt to pose a risk to self or to others.[39] The 1995 Mental Health (Patients in the Community) Act introduced a further element of compulsion into community care in the form of supervised discharge. In 1996, following disquiet over continuing evidence of community care 'failures', the Conservative administration issued a new set of guidance emphasizing the need for effective risk-management through a 'spectrum of care' ranging from secure hospital beds through to community care.[40]

Community care and mentally disordered offenders

Mentally disordered offenders may be required to receive community care as part of their sentence in two ways. The first is by being sentenced to community care through a psychiatric probation order or a guardianship order. The second is by being required to accept community care as a condition of discharge from hospital following detention as an offender patient.

Community care sentences

Psychiatric probation

Probation orders with a condition of psychiatric treatment have been recommended by the Reed Committee as a valuable alternative to custody.[41] But in fact whilst the total number of probation commencements annually has been running at over 40 000 since 1987, the use of probation with a condition of psychiatric treatment has steadily declined and remains a tiny proportion of all probation work —with less than 500

---

[37] Department of Health (1995) *Building Bridges: A Guide to Inter-Agency Working for the Care and Protection of Severely Mentally Ill People*. Department of Health 5.1.18.

[38] HSG(94)27 LASSL(94)4.

[39] HSG(94) 5.

[40] *Spectrum of Care: Audit Pack for the Care Programme Approach.*

[41] *Review of Health and Social Services for Mentally Disordered Offenders and Others Requiring Similar Services* (Chairman Dr John Reed) (The Reed Report) Cm 2088 1992. Powers of the 1973 Criminal Courts Act, Section 3; see also Criminal Justice Act 1991, Schedule 1, Para. 5, which inserts a new Schedule 1A in the 1973 act and is in substantially the same terms as Section 3 of the 1973 act.

probation orders per annum with a condition of out-patient treatment and under 100 with a condition of in-patient treatment.[42]

The offender's mental condition must be 'such as requires and may be susceptible to treatment but is not such as to warrant his detention in hospital'.[43] The court must have received evidence that the criteria are met from a doctor with recognized psychiatric expertise. The court must have explained all the effects of the order to the offender and he must consent to it.[44]

The offender must attend hospital for psychiatric treatment, either as an in-patient or an out-patient, or must accept treatment from a specified medical practitioner. Psychiatric probation orders are generally encouraged by the courts for mentally disordered offenders, provided there is no significant risk of injury to the public as a result.[45] Probation is a criminal justice penalty. The offender must consent to the order to begin with. He may withdraw consent but if he does so risks being returned to court for breach. Section 6(7) provides that the offender cannot be dealt with for breach of the probation order for refusal to consent to surgical, electrical or other treatment, if the court decides that the refusal is reasonable in all the circumstances.[46]

Guardianship orders

The other community care sentence is a guardianship order under Section 37 which lasts for six months, renewable for a further six months and then for periods of one year at a time. The offender must be at least sixteen years of age and suffering from mental illness, psychopathic disorder, mental impairment or severe mental impairment of a nature or degree which warrants reception into guardianship. The court must be of the opinion, having regard to all the circumstances, including the nature of the offence and the character and antecedents of the offender and to other methods of dealing with him, that the most suitable method of disposing of the case is by means of a guardianship order. The effect of a guardianship order is that the local social services authority will be empowered to order the patient to live at a specified place and to attend specified places for training, education and treatment. They may also order that access to the patient be given to health and social services personnel. In an effort to

----

[42] Source: HM Inspectorate of Probation (1993) *Probation Orders with Requirements for Psychiatric Treatment: Report of a Thematic Inspection*, p. 9. Ashworth, A. (1995) *Sentencing and Criminal Justice* (2nd edn), pp. 325. London: Butterworths.

[43] Powers of the Criminal Courts Act 1973, Section 3(1); Criminal Justice Act 1991, Schedule 1, Para. 5(1)(a),(b).

[44] *Ibid.*, Section 2(6).

[45] *R v Ballester* (1971) Crim LR 111.

[46] Although the requirement of consent to the making of a probation has been largely abolished, it has been retained for psychiatric probation and for probation to treat drug or alcohol addiction. See Powers of the Criminal Courts Act 1973, Sched. 1A, para. 5(4) as inserted by the Crime (Sentences) Act 1997, Section 38(3).

encourage the use of guardianship orders, in 1991 courts considering making a guardianship order were empowered to request the local social services authority (or any other social services authority considered by the court to be appropriate): (1) to inform the court whether it or any person authorized by it is prepared to receive the patient into guardianship; and (2) if so, to give such information as it reasonably can about how it or the other person could be expected to exercise guardianship powers.[47] Although there are no precise figures on guardianship orders under Section 37 it is clear that the provision is little used. Guardianship is on the increase, from 337 patients in 1992 to 950 cases in force at the end of March 1999. It is not clear how many of these are in respect of offender patients, and the overall rate of guardianship is small compared with the 27 000 compulsory admissions to hospital during 1998–9.[48]

Compulsory community care following hospital detention

Local health and social services authorities have a duty under Section 117 of the 1983 Mental Health Act to provide aftercare for patients who leave hospital having been detained:

- after civil admission for treatment under Section 3 of the Act
- under a hospital order made by a criminal court (Section 37) or
- following a transfer direction from prison (Section 47 or 48).

This duty also applies in relation to restriction order and restriction direction patients. It applies whether or not the person leaves hospital immediately after ceasing to be liable to be detained, so authorities cannot escape it by taking the patient 'off section' before discharging him, and it also applies to a person who has been transferred back to prison prior to release. It continues until the authorities are jointly satisfied that the person no longer needs community care. In *R v Ealing District Health Authority ex parte Fox*, which concerned a restriction order patient, Otton J held that the proper interpretation of Section 117 was that it was a continuing duty in respect of any patient who may be discharged and who falls within its scope, although the duty is only triggered at the moment of discharge.[49]

Section 117 services are community care services for the purposes of the 1990 National Health Service and Community Care Act. This means that local social services authorities have a duty to prepare and publish an annual community care plan which will include provision to address the needs of mentally disordered offenders. They also have a duty under Section 47 of the 1990 act to assess people's needs for community care services. Where it appears to a local authority that any person for

---

[47] Mental Health Act 1983 section 39A.

[48] In-patients formally detained in hospitals under the Mental Health Act 1983 and other legislation, England: 1988–9 and 1994–5 to 1998–9. *DoH Statistical Bulletin* 1999/25.

[49] (1993) 3 All ER 170 at 181.

whom they may provide or arrange to provide community care services may be in need of any such services, the authority must carry out an assessment of his needs for those services and, having regard to the results of that assessment, must then decide whether his needs call for the provision by them of any such services. Responsibility for ensuring that the person's health care needs are met lies with the local authority, which may invite the relevant Health Authority (HA) to supply services to meet health needs. However the Act does not place a duty on the HA to co-operate, nor to provide services which the local authority decides are needed.[50]

The Department of Health takes the view that, unlike other community care services, Section 117 services cannot be charged for, so local social services authorities will have to foot the bill. This view has been upheld by the High Court in *R v Richmond London Borough ex parte Watson,* [51] which is subject to appeal at the time of writing. This is a disincentive to arrange services which may prove an expensive long-term commitment. The Reed Committee recognized this problem and recommended specific earmarked funding for community care for mentally disordered offenders.[52]

The care programme approach

In 1990 the Department of Health issued a circular to health and social services authorities promoting a care programme approach (CPA) for mentally ill people referred to specialist mental health services.[53] This requires needs assessments, a written care plan based on the needs assessment, a key worker whose task is to ensure that the services are delivered and received, and regular review. The CPA applies to all patients receiving care from specialist psychiatric services, whether or not they have been in hospital.[54] In 1993 the Home Office issued Circular 29/1993 drawing the attention of probation services to community care arrangements introduced following the 1990 Act, and pointing out that people in contact with the criminal justice system might require services as defendants on bail, whilst serving community sentences, or on release from custody.[55]

The 'audit pack' for monitoring the CPA, issued in 1996, identifies three tiers of CPA: 'minimal' for clients with no risk indicators who require the attention of only one key worker, 'complex' for clients who require attention from two or more mental health workers, and 'full multi-disciplinary CPA' for clients assessed as presenting

---

[50] National Health Service and Community Care Act 1990, Section 47(3).

[51] *The Times* 15 October 1999.

[52] The Reed Committee Report Cm 2088 1992, para. 11.263–11.269.

[53] HC(90)23/LASSL(90)11 Care programme approach for people with a mental illness referred to the specialist psychiatric services.

[54] *Spectrum of Care: Audit Pack for Monitoring the Care Programme Approach – Background and Explanatory Notes.* NHS Executive HSG 96(6).

[55] *Community Care Reforms and the Criminal Justice System.* Home Office Circular 29/1993.

considerable risk. In 1999 the Department of Health issued a 'policy booklet' entitled 'Effective care co-ordination in mental health services: modernizing the care programme approach'. This re-emphasizes the Government's commitment to the CPA but 'streamlines' it by replacing the elaborate system of tiers with a single distinction between 'standard' and 'enhanced' care programmes. Key workers will henceforth be known as care co-ordinators, and the 'mental health national service framework' sets a standard which requires that those on the CPA should be able to access services 24 hours a day, 365 days a year.

Chapter 27 of the Mental Health Act Code of Practice deals with aftercare for former in-patients, whether or not they have been detained. It states the function of aftercare as being to enable patients to cope with life outside hospital and function there successfully without danger to themselves or other people. Before the decision is taken to grant leave to or discharge a detained patient, it is the responsibility of the responsible medical officer (RMO) to ensure, in consultation with the other professionals concerned, that the patient's needs for health and social care are fully assessed and that the care plan addresses them. The RMO is responsible for ensuring that a proper risk assessment is carried out, that consideration is given to whether the patient meets the criteria for supervised discharge or guardianship, and that consideration is given to whether the patient ought to be placed on the supervision register (to be abolished when the 'modernized care programme approach' is introduced). The modernized CPA shows further the interweaving of the psychiatric and penal systems. It will apply not only to offenders coming out of hospital: 'It is as applicable to service users in residential set-tings (including prisons) as it is to those in the community.'[56] If service users have to reside in prison and they are known to have longer term and complex mental health needs, the responsible psychiatric team should maintain contact with the individual and make plans for care on the person's release in collaboration with prison and probation staff as appropriate.

If the patient is due to have a hospital managers' hearing or a Mental Health Review Tribunal to consider his fitness for discharge, a discussion of aftercare needs should take place beforehand so that a plan can be implemented if the patient is discharged.[57] The patient's wishes and needs are to be taken into account in the assessment, as are the views of any relevant relative, friend or supporter.[58] The patient is entitled to an assessment following the CPA or the Welsh Office Mental Illness Strategy.

There are two ways in which formerly detained patients may be compelled to accept community care services. Patients who have been detained under the civil power in Section 3 for treatment, or who have been subject to hospital orders or transfer directions without restrictions, may be placed under compulsory supervision in the

[56] Department of Health (1999) *Effective care co-ordination in mental health services: modernising the care programme approach: a policy booklet*, para. 23.

[57] *Spectrum of care: audit pack for monitoring the care programme approach – background and explanatory notes*. NHS Executive HSG 96(6), para. 27.5–6.

[58] *Ibid.*, para. 27.9.

community under Sections 25A–J of the 1983 Act. Patients subject to restriction orders or restriction directions may be discharged conditionally upon agreeing to accept treatment, to reside at a specified place, and to accept community care services.

Compulsory supervision in the community—supervised discharge

The Mental Health (Patients in the Community) Act 1995 added provisions (Sections 25A–J) to the 1983 Act to allow for supervised after-care of non-restricted patients subject to long-term detention. They came into force in April 1996, as part of a 'ten point plan to reinforce the care of mentally ill people in the community', announced in August 1993 by Virginia Bottomley, the Secretary of State for Health, following an internal review by the Department of Health. This followed two highly publicized incidents in December 1992 involving former psychiatric in-patients, Ben Silcock and Christopher Clunis. Silcock was a young schizophrenic who jumped into the lion's enclosure at London Zoo. Although badly mauled, he survived. The whole affair was captured on amateur video and appeared on network news. In December 1992 Jonathan Zito, a young musician barely three months married, was killed by Christopher Clunis, a paranoid schizophrenic with a long history of violence. Clunis had been released from hospital three months before the attack. An inquiry was instituted by the health authorities concerned and reported in February 1994. The inquiry identified a woeful catalogue of failure to provide adequate care for Clunis: there had been no Section 117 after-care plan and the authorities had failed to manage or oversee provision of health and social services for him.[59] Since then there have been many inquiries into incidents involving former in-patients, most notably 'The falling shadow: one patient's mental health care 1978–1993'[60] and 'The case of Jason Mitchell: report of the independent panel of inquiry'.[61]

Sections 25A–J introduced a new power of supervised discharge. An addition to the Mental Health Act Code of Practice was made, entitled 'Guidance on supervised discharge (after-care under supervision) and related provisions'.[62] The ten-point plan

[59] Ritchie, J. H., Dick, D. and Lingham, R. (1994) *The Report of the Inquiry into the Care and Treatment of Christopher Clunis*, p. 106. London: HMSO.

[60] Blom-Cooper, L., Hally, H. and Murphy, E. (1995) London: Duckworth.

[61] Blom-Cooper, L, Grounds, A., Guinan, P., Parker, A. and Taylor, M. (1996). London: Duckworth.

[62] In England Sections 25A–H should also be read in conjunction with Health Circulars HC(90)23/LASSL(90)1 (The care programme approach), HSG(94)27/LASSL(94)4 (Guidance on the discharge of mentally disordered people and their continuing care in the community) and HSG(94)5 (on supervision registers). In Wales the applicable guidance is WHC(95)40 (Guidance on the care of people in the community with a mental illness). See also Department of Health (1995) *Building bridges—a guide to arrangements for inter-agency working for the care and protection of severely mentally disordered people* (1995), LASSL(96(16) HSG(96)6 *The spectrum of care—a summary of comprehensive local services for people with mental health problems, 24 hours nursing beds for people with severe and enduring mental illness, An audit pack for the care programme approach and the patients' charter*, and NHS EL(97)1 *The patients' charter and mental health services: implementation guidelines*.

included a series of shorter-term measures to make greater use of existing powers. Amendments to the Mental Health Act Code of Practice were introduced in 1993 which encouraged early readmission of patients relapsing following cessation of medication. To prepare the way for supervised discharge, the Department of Health issued two further sets of guidance. The first introduced supervision registers, a form of 'at risk' register for mentally disordered adults.[63] The patient went on a register if a 'care programme review meeting' considered he was suffering from serious mental illness, and would be 'liable to be at risk of committing serious violence or suicide, or of serious self neglect.'[64] When the modernized CPA comes into force, supervision registers will be abolished. However, the policy makes it clear that supervision registers would be otiose given the 'information requirements' which it stipulates, and the guidance given on information sharing between health, social services and criminal justice agencies.

The information requirements are that local service providers are to 'ensure that a system is in place to collect data on all service users, including total numbers in contact with services and the numbers whose care is managed through enhanced and standard CPA'. The CPA is to be subject to local audit which 'should move away from a focus on simply numbers and more towards assessing the quality of CPA implementation, including the quality of care plans, the attainment of treatment goals and, particularly for those with multiple needs, the effectiveness of inter-agency working'.[65]

Paragraphs 45–49 are entitled 'The CPA, the criminal justice system and information sharing'. The following advice is offered where a service user is 'not in formal contact with the criminal justice system' but is assessed as being a potential risk to others.

> Careful liaison with the police to manage the risk is necessary. In this context it is important to note that the common law duty of confidence requires that, in the absence of a statutory requirement to share information provided in confidence, such information should only be shared with the informed consent of the individual. This duty is not absolute and can be overridden if the holder of the information can justify disclosure as being in the public interest (including a risk to public safety). Further guidance on the operation of the common law is included in the Department of Health publication *HSG (96)18 The Protection and Use of Patient Information*. Decisions to disclose information against the wishes of an individual should be fully documented and the public interest justification clearly stated.

The right of privacy under Article 8 of the European Convention allows for exceptions to the confidentiality of medical records if it is in accordance with law and necessary in a democratic society for the prevention of crime, for health, or for the protection of the rights of others. Those making decisions to share information without the consent of the subject should be aware of the need to restrict this to a need to know basis, and to bear in mind the principle of proportionality, that the method

---

[63] NHS Management Executive, Health Service Guidelines HSG(94)5 Supervision Registers.

[64] HSG (94)5, Annex A, para. 4.

[65] Department of Health (1999) *Effective care co-ordination in mental health services: modernising the care programme approach: a policy booklet*, para. 29–30.

chosen to achieve the protection of the public interest does not go beyond what is strictly necessary for that purpose.

The guidance states that 'information that is to be shared between different agencies should be governed by strict protocols to ensure that all parties concerned, including the service user, are aware of how information will be used, who will have access to it and how it will be safeguarded'. All National Health Service organizations are required, under 'Health Service Circular 1999/012', to have in place 'guardians of patient information' charged with overseeing information-sharing protocols and the policy booklet recommends that other agencies adopt this model.

The booklet concludes that 'Protocols enable information to be shared confidently and effectively between staff in agencies providing services within agreed and appropriate parameters'. The purpose of this passage is to bridge the information barriers between health and social services with their emphasis on individualistic health and social care values such as confidentiality, and the police, whose primary task is risk management. This necessarily entails the incorporation of the police into what previously were health and social care decisions, as is evidenced by the following passage from the new guidance.

> The framework that the CPA provides should be used by all agencies involved in the complex care arrangements necessary for an individual who has mental health problems. It should be supported by probation, police and housing colleagues who will need to be involved in ongoing risk assessment, risk management and review of care arrangements.[66]

With this level of information gathering and information sharing between police and health and social services, supervision registers become redundant.

A second set of guidance, issued in May 1994, relates to the discharge of mentally disordered people and their continuing care in the community.[67] The guidance particularly emphasizes that those taking individual decisions about discharge have 'a fundamental duty to consider both the safety of the patient and the protection of other people. No patient should be discharged from hospital unless and until those taking the decision are satisfied that he or she can live safely in the community, and that proper treatment, supervision, support and care are available':[68]

> In each case it must be demonstrable that decisions have been taken after full and proper consideration of any evidence about risk that the patient presents.[69]

Extensive information and advice are given in the guidance on the assessment of risk.[70]

The responsible medical officer of a patient detained under Section 3, 37, 47 or 48 has the power to consider supervised discharge if the patient is suffering from (1)

---

[66] Ibid., para. 48.

[67] NHS Management Executive, Health Service Guidelines HSG(94)27.

[68] NHS Management Executive, Health Service Guidelines HSG(94)27, para. 2.

[69] Ibid., para. 23.

[70] Ibid., para. 23–31.

mental illness; (2) severe mental impairment; (3) psychopathic disorder; or (4) mental impairment. There must be a substantial risk of serious harm to the health or safety of the patient or the safety of other persons, or of the patient being seriously exploited, if he were not to receive the after-care services to be provided for him under Section 117 after he leaves hospital. Finally, his being subject to aftercare under supervision must be likely to help to secure that he receives the after-care services to be so provided.[71]

Every patient has a 'community responsible medical officer', who is in charge of medical treatment in the community, and a supervisor.[72] The supervisor must maintain sufficiently close contact with the patient to be satisfied that he is receiving the agreed after-care services and is complying with the requirements, and must convene a meeting of the care team if care is not being received. He must be alive to signs of deterioration and other warning signs and must be accessible to people with whom the patient is living and listen to their concerns. He must ensure that the team reviews the care plan well before the date when it falls to be reviewed, and whenever any shortfall in the arrangements is identified.[73]

Once patients are subject to aftercare under supervision, the responsible after-care bodies[74] have power to impose requirements for the purpose of securing that they receive aftercare. These include: (1) that the patient reside at a specified place; (2) that he or she attend at specified places and times for the purpose of medical treatment, occupation, education or training; and (3) that access to the patient be given, at any place where he or she is residing, to the supervisor, any doctor or any approved social worker, or to any other person authorized by the supervisor.[75]

The conditions of supervision are modelled on the conditions of mental health guardianship. The major difference is that the act introduces a power to 'take and convey' to any place which the patient is required to attend for treatment, although once at that place there is no power to administer treatment forcibly unless there is an emergency requiring restraint under common law.[76] The Code emphasizes that the

---

[71] Mental Health Act 1983, Section 25A(4).

[72] 1983 Mental Health Act, Section 34(1A), as inserted by the 1995 Mental Health (Patients in the Community) Act, Schedule 1, para. 4(5).

[73] Amendment to the *Code of practice guidance on supervised discharge (after care under supervision) and related provisions*, para. 43, 46, 48.

[74] The bodies which have the joint duty under Section 117, see Section 25D(2).

[75] *Ibid.*, Section 25D(3).

[76] Paragraph 50 of the amendment to the code emphasizes that the power to take and convey, or the threat of using it should never be used to coerce a patient into accepting medication, and that where a patient has been conveyed, medical and other staff need to be satisfied that his or her consent to any subsequent treatment is genuine and not forced. 'A patient who has been conveyed to a clinic and then insists on leaving cannot be kept there or given treatment against his or her will (except in circumstances allowed by common law where it may be permissible to administer treatment to deal with the immediate emergency)'.

patient cannot be required to accept medical treatment and the power should only be used if the supervisor is satisfied that it is likely to lead to the patient co-operating with the services being provided. The supervisor should also consider whether the problem might be overcome by an adjustment to the care package, or whether it may point to a need to reassess the patient for compulsory admission.

In October 1998 the Government appointed an expert 'scoping group' to consider the reform of the 1983 Mental Health Act. Paul Boateng, then Under Secretary of State for Health, addressed the group on their appointment, emphasizing that individual patients had a responsibility to comply with their agreed programmes of care: 'Non-compliance can no longer be an option when appropriate care in appropriate settings is in place … [T]his is not negotiable'. The minister then went on to say:

> We are not talking about forcibly administering treatment over the individual's kitchen table. The new arrangements should only require treatment in an appropriate clinical setting and therefore may need powers for compulsory conveyance … Your delivery of this central object- ive will be critical to the whole process of reform.[77]

The Government has issued a Green Paper 'Reform of the Mental Health Act 1983: proposals for consultation'[78] which proposes a system of compulsory orders to be imposed by a Mental Disorder Tribunal which would determine whether the patient needs treatment in hospital or in the community. When applied in the community, the proposed order would be able to stipulate the patient's place of residence, define the proposed care and treatment plan and require the patient to allow access and be present for scheduled visits by case workers. It would impose a duty on the authorities to comply with the arrangements, and it would stipulate the consequences of non-compliance, which could include the power to enter premises, to convey the patient to the place specified for care and treatment, or to convey the patient to hospital.[79] The initial order could provide for readmission to hospital in the event of non-compliance and deterioration in the patient's mental health.[80] The Green Paper is silent on the question of whether there would be a power to treat forcibly once the patient has been conveyed to the clinical setting, but the Expert Committee recommended that the tri- bunal should be able to authorize the administration of compulsory medication in hospital out-patient settings. However they sounded the cautionary note that they were not satisfied that the necessary services are yet in place to render the forcible administration of medication in a non-hospital setting either safe or advisable.[81]

---

[77] Department of Health (1999) *Review of the Mental Health Act 1983: report of the Expert Committee* November, p. 142.

[78] *Reform of the Mental Health Act 1983: proposals for consultation.* Cm 4480, 1999.

[79] *Ibid.*, p. 38.

[80] Department of Health (1999) *Review of the Mental Health Act 1983: report of the Expert Committee* November, pp. 4–75.

[81] *Ibid.*

These proposals go further than the existing law in that they will authorize forcible medication in hospital out-patient clinics and will allow readmission subject to appeal to a tribunal. All proponents of compulsory community supervision are agreed that they do not want a power to treat forcibly in the patient's own home (concerns described by Geller as reflecting ideas of territorial propriety) and that any compulsory medication would take place not in 'their community', but in 'our institution'.[82] There are also concerns that a power to treat in the patient's own home would be a disproportionate protection of health and the rights of others and therefore risk contravention of the protection of privacy, home and family life guaranteed by Article 8.

Conditionally discharged restricted patients

In 1987 The Department of Health and the Home Office issued three sets of guidance in relation to the supervision and aftercare of conditionally discharged restricted patients. The first was to hospitals preparing for the discharge of such patients. The second was for the guidance of supervising psychiatrists, and the third was for social supervisors.[83] The 'Notes for psychiatrists' state the purpose of supervision as protecting the public from further serious harm by assisting the patient's reintegration into the community and by monitoring his mental health and risk. Conditional discharge enables a period of assessment before the patient is absolutely discharged. Absolute discharge means that the patient ceases to be subject to supervision and ceases to be liable to recall by the Home Secretary. Psychiatric and social supervisors must communicate effectively and report regularly to the Mental Health Unit at the Home Office which supervises restricted patients centrally.

The Home Secretary has a power under Section 42(3) of the 1983 Act at any time to recall a conditionally discharged patient to hospital, and this is not limited by any express statutory criteria. The 'Notes for guidance for psychiatrists' state that a report to the Home Office should always be made if:

- there appears to be a risk to the public
- contact with the patient is lost
- the patient is unwilling to co-operate with supervision
- the patient needs further in-patient treatment or
- the patient is charged with an offence.

---

[82] Geller, J. L. (1986) The quandaries of enforced community treatment and unenforceable outpatient commitment statutes. *Journal of Psychiatry and Law* **151,** 149–158.

[83] Home Office and Department of Health and Social Security (1987) *Mental Health Act 1983: The supervision and after-care of conditionally discharged restricted patients: notes for guidance of hospitals preparing for the conditional discharge of restricted patients, notes for the guidance of supervising psychiatrists,* and *notes for the guidance of social supervisors.*

Although there are no express statutory criteria governing the recall power, recall is a form of psychiatric detention subject to the requirements of Article 5 of the convention. One of the conditions of lawful detention under Article 5(1) is that, except in the case of an emergency detention, there must be objective evidence of mental disorder of a kind or degree warranting detention. In *James Kay v UK*[84] important limits were placed on this discretion, requiring that unless there is an emergency, recall to hospital must be based on objective evidence of mental disorder. Kay was a conditionally discharged restricted patient. He reoffended shortly after discharge and this time was given a prison sentence instead of a hospital order. At the end of his sentence the Home Secretary recalled him to Broadmoor Special Hospital without first obtaining medical reports. The Commission declared the application admissible, finding that when the recall decision was made, certain minimum conditions of lawfulness were not respected. In particular, there was no up-to-date objective medical expertise showing that he suffered from a true mental disorder, or that his previous psychopathic disorder persisted. The disorder was only confirmed a month after recall. In the absence of any emergency there were no circumstances to justify this omission and therefore the recall contravened Article 5(1)(e).

Between 1972 and 1994 2781 restricted patients were conditionally discharged, 530 of whom were recalled to hospital by the Home Secretary.[85] This is probably an underestimate of the numbers readmitted to hospital, since supervising psychiatrists often prefer to admit voluntarily or under the civil powers in Sections 2 and 3 of the 1983 Act (admission for assessment or treatment). This avoids involving the Home Office in the decision when to discharge, which can be time consuming. Psychiatrists justify this as serving the interests of a patient who needs a brief period as an in-patient to stabilize his condition or re-establish him on medication.

The lawfulness of using civil powers of detention as an alternative to recall was raised in *R v The Managers of the North West London Mental Health NHS Trust ex parte Stewart*.[86] In June 1995 Stewart, a conditionally discharged patient, was compulsorily admitted to hospital under Section 3 of the Act, after consultation with the relevant officer at the Home Office. His consultant psychiatrist felt that only a short admission was required. The doctor feared that if the patient were recalled by the Home Secretary under Section 42, the Home Secretary's consent to his rerelease would be necessary and this might prolong his stay in hospital which would not be in his best interests. He was released 14 days later. The patient challenged his admission under the civil powers and argued that the Home Office, the Department of Health 'Notes for the guidance of supervising psychiatrists' and the Department of Health 'Code of practice

---

[84] Application No. 17821/91 (Report of the Commission Adopted on 1 March 1994).

[85] Kershaw, C., Dowdeswell, P. and Goodman, J., *Restricted patients—reconvictions and recalls by the end of 1995: England and Wales*. Home Office Statistical Bulletin 1/97.

[86] (1997) 4 All ER 871.

on the Mental Health Act 1983' were erroneous in law because they advised that the powers of civil detention under Section 3 could be used as an alternative to the recall procedure. The High Court and the Court of Appeal upheld the legality of the guidance, notwithstanding the confusing legal position in which it places a patient. If a person is admitted under the civil powers to detain, they may appeal to the Mental Health Review Tribunal for discharge. If the Tribunal were to discharge them, it would be a discharge in relation to his liability to detention under Section 3 which would in no way affect the Secretary of State's power to recall him as a restricted patient under Section 42. The important aspect of this case is that it indicates the professional and the official preferred route of recall of restricted patients is by using the powers of civil admission in Part ll of the Act.

Recall is a sword of Damocles hanging over the head of every restricted patient. Doctors and patients wish to avoid the involvement of the Home Office if the admission will only be brief, and this ruling endorses the flexible approach of the 'Home Office guidance' and the 'Code of Practice'. But the flexibility brings disadvantages in terms of a patient's ability to know his legal position with certainty. The Home Office can recall a patient at any time in an emergency. If there is no emergency there must objective evidence that he suffers from mental disorder of a nature or degree warranting detention.[87] The power of recall may be exercised whether or not the patient is already in hospital under civil detention at the time of recall.[88]

On average 120 restricted patients are conditionally discharged each year. Of the 2871 restricted patients conditionally discharged between 1972 and 1995, 586 persons are known to have been reconvicted of a standard list offence by the end of 1995, and 177 were convicted of a grave offence. Reconviction rates of a standard list offence within two years have gone down in the period since 1987 when they averaged 5%, as opposed to 17 % between 1972 and 1986. The Home Office considers that this may be due to more effective supervision for conditionally discharged restricted patients. [89]

Over the same period (1972–1994), 1691 life prisoners were released on licence. Of these, 362 had been convicted of a standard list offence and 66 of a grave offence by the end of 1995. 307 licensees had been recalled during the period, and 28 given a further life sentence.[90] The reconviction rates for restricted patients and life licensees compare favourably with other prisoners where the reconviction rates for standard list offences within two years approach 50%. This may be explained by any of a number of factors.

---

[87] *James Kay v UK* Application No. 17821/91. Admissibility Decision 7 July 1993. Decision on the merits 1 March 1994, para. 50 and 63–65.

[88] *Dlodlo v Mental Health Review Tribunal for the South Thames Region and Others* (1996) 36 BMLR 145.

[89] Kershaw, C., Dowdeswell, P. and Goodman, J., *Restricted patients— reconvictions and recalls by the end of 1995: England and Wales.* Home Office Statistical Bulletin 1/97.

[90] Kershaw, C., Dowdeswell, P. and Goodman, J., *Life licensees—reconvictions and recalls by the end of 1995: England and Wales.* Home Office Statistical Bulletin 2/97.

For example, it may be due to the close supervision exercised by the Home Office, probation and community care agencies over these two groups of offenders, to their age, or to the fact that mentally disordered offenders may be convicted of offences, such as homicide, with low recidivism rates.

The Government's Green Paper on Reform of the 1983 Act concludes that the offender patient provisions of the 1983 Act are fundamentally sound, and that the restriction order plays an indispensable function in the safe management of those offenders who pose a risk of serious harm to others. The Government proposes that there should be a single power to remand to hospital for a period of assessment with or without treatment, and a restriction order would not be able to be imposed unless there had been a full risk assessment. As for conditional discharge, the Government's view is that it is one of the most effective safeguards for the public in the management of dangerous offender patients:

> The Committee recognizes that the structure provided by the community treatment order for improved treatment and supervision in the community might not suffice in the case of the most dangerous offenders. We agree.[91]

Indeed there is very little disturbance proposed to the existing provisions of Part lll. Transfers from prison to hospital will remain the mechanism to effect compulsory treatment of sentenced prisoners. Once their sentence ends, however, they would be able to be detained as non-offender patients only, instead of the position at present, where they are detained as if they had been sentenced to a hospital order made by a criminal court.

Offender patients will continue to have rights to appeal to the Mental Health Review Tribunal, which will continue to have the power to discharge as required by Article 5(4) of the European Convention on Human Rights. Although the Convention is described as a 'living instrument' and represents 'a floor not a ceiling', it is a creature of its time, designed to protect against totalitarian interference with basic freedoms. The main provisions relevant to the situation of mentally disordered offenders are Article 3, the protection against inhuman and degrading treatment, Article 5 which protects against arbitrary detention and gives patients a right to periodic review of the continued need for their detention, and Article 8 which protects the right of privacy and family life. The Human Rights Act 1998 came into force in October 2000 requiring the courts to take into account the case law of the Strasbourg Court of Human Rights and where possible to interpret statutes so as to give effect to Convention rights. This raises the question of the extent to which the Convention offers rights to community care provision.

---

[91] *Reform of the Mental Health Act 1983: proposals for consultation.* Cm 4480, 1999, 52.

Community care rights

The 1997 judgement of the European Court of Human Rights in *Stanley Johnson v UK*[92] has potentially serious implications for the rights of offender patients to community care services. Johnson complained of breaches of Article 5(1), that he had been detained without objective evidence of unsoundness of mind, and of Article 5(4), which requires the right to seek review of the lawfulness of detention before a court which must have the power to order discharge. Johnson had been found not to be suffering from mental disorder by a Mental Health Review Tribunal which had given him a conditional discharge, deferred until suitable arrangements could be made for his reception into a hostel. Patients are entitled to seek review of their detention before a tribunal once in every 12 months. Where a tribunal defers conditional discharge until suitable arrangements can be made, if no arrangements are made before the case next comes before a tribunal, the order for conditional discharge lapses. Johnson was found by three tribunals (1989, 1990 and 1991) not to be suffering from mental disorder, but his conditional discharge was deferred until a suitable hostel could be found, and none ever was. He was finally released following a tribunal hearing in 1993. He complained that his detention contravened Articles 5(1) and 5(4) because the unsoundness of mind, which formed the necessary basis of his continued detention, was no longer present.

The Court rejected the argument that a finding by an expert authority that a person is no longer suffering from the form of mental illness which led to his confinement must inevitably lead to his immediate and unconditional release into the community. This would be an unfortunate curtailment of the expert authority's discretion to assess, part of the 'margin of appreciation' left to the national authorities. Nevertheless, the Court held that there had been a breach of Article 5(1) as discharge must not be unreasonably delayed and there must be safeguards, including judicial review, to prevent this. The tribunal had to have the powers to ensure that a placement could be secured within a reasonable period of time. This will necessitate tribunals being given powers to ensure that discharge arrangements will not be unduly delayed and to investigate in cases where this happens. The fact that given adequate community care support a person would not require detention could be used as an argument based on Article 5. Failure to provide, and failure to fund, that care could be breaches of Article 5 because they are consigning a person to detention which they would not otherwise need. By failure to provide community care services, the patient's rights against arbitrary detention may be infringed.

Personality disorder: treatment or preventive detention

All the recent major legal developments in relation to mentally disordered offenders result from the conundrum posed by personality disordered offenders. The concern of

---

[92] European Commission on Human Rights decision on admissibility 18 May 1995 32520/93. Judgement of the European Court of Human Rights 24 October 1997.

the Home Office is that the protective sentencing powers outlined above are being insufficiently used by the judiciary, and that offenders who pose a high risk on account of personality disorder will receive determinate sentences. This means that the offender will have to be released at the end of sentence, regardless of the risk to the public, unless he is transferred to hospital before it expires. He can only be transferred on grounds of psychopathic disorder if that disorder is deemed treatable. The consultation document on severe personality disorder summarizes the difficulty from a risk-management point of view in these terms:

> All offenders on whom the courts have passed fixed term prison sentences have to be released from custody at some point. The vast majority serving one or more years in prison are subject to some form of supervision following release. But once the compulsory period of supervision in the community ends there is no mandatory provision to continue supervision even though the individual may continue to present a risk. Probation officers may refer clients about whom they have continuing concerns to other agencies but there is no certainty that this will result in the risk being reduced.[93]

These worries underlie the proposals of the Fallon Committee for reviewable sentences for dangerous personality disordered offenders[94] and have led to the Government's proposals for management of this group by allowing for their indefinite detention on grounds of risk. In *E v Norway* the European Court of Human Rights held that it is lawful under the convention to extend the period of detention on grounds of dangerousness, as long as the extension is necessary and is carried out in accordance with a procedure prescribed by law.[95] In that case the patient was detained under a Norwegian law allowing for preventive detention if the offender had an impaired mental capacity and posed a serious risk. E satisfied both criteria. His preventive detention was lawful under Article 5(1)(e) (unsoundness of mind), but Article 5(4) required that he be given access to periodic review of his continued impaired capacity and dangerousness before a court with power of discharge. The proposals for personality disorder raise contentious ethical issues about the boundary between therapy and preventive detention. Whilst there is consensus among psychiatrists that drug therapy and ECT are effective in treating mental illness, no such consensus exists about the treatment of personality disorder, or even what severe personality disorder is.

Although advances in the treatment of personality disorder have been pioneered in the special hospital and secure unit sectors of the hospital system, many personality-disordered offenders have been 'treated' in the prison system. The most disruptive are

---

[93] The Home Office and Department of Health Discussion Document—Managing dangerous people with a severe personality disorder: proposals for policy development, July 1999, para.[18].

[94] Department of Health, Report of the Committee of Inquiry into the personality disorder unit, Ashworth Special Hospital (1999 HMSO) Cm 4194.

[95] *E v Norway* Series A, Vol. 181, 1990

detained in 'close supervision centres'. Some are in vulnerable prisoner units or on prerelease sex offender treatment programmes. Some are benefiting from therapeutic communities in prisons, and others are in Grendon Underwood Prison, which is run on therapeutic community lines. Nevertheless, the Government's conclusion is that most dangerous offenders with severe personality disorders receive little consistent or long-term help with their disorders either while they are in prison or on release.[96]

Even though mental illness and personality disorder are often the result of an abusive upbringing, and both in different ways often cause pain to the sufferer, there is undoubtedly a moral hierarchy of mental disorder. In crude terms, the mentally ill are seen as the 'afflicted mad or the deserving mad', whilst people with personality disorder are seen as the 'bad mad or the undeserving mad'. The principal reason is the disruptive and often highly manipulative behaviour exhibited by people with personality disorders. The concept of psychopathic disorder was introduced in the 1959 Mental Health Act, an act which is said to reflect therapeutic optimism about the treatment of personality disorder.[97] But it was an optimism tempered with a degree of realism. Psychopathy was defined as 'a persistent disorder or disability of mind which results in abnormally aggressive or seriously irresponsible conduct on the part of the patient and requires or is susceptible to hospital treatment'. So there was a 'treatability' test in the 1959 Act, albeit less elaborate than the current 'medical treatment for mental disorder is likely to alleviate or prevent deterioration in the patient's condition'. Both reflect hesitancy in authorizing detention on a purely medical condition whose precise boundaries are unknown and where there was little science about effective therapies. Under the 1959 Act there was also an age limit, reflecting contemporary perception that it was necessary to tackle psychopathy while the patient was still young to have any prospect of success. A person classified as psychopathically disordered could not be compulsorily admitted under the power to admit for treatment if they were over the age of 21.[98] If they were admitted before the age of 21, their detention could be renewed until they were 25, but no further unless they were either dangerous to themselves or to others[99] or they had committed a criminal offence.

The contributions of the psychiatrist and medical Members of Parliament who spoke in the debates express reservations which might be expressed differently today,

[96] The Home Office and Department of Health Discussion Document, Managing dangerous people with a severe personality disorder: proposals for policy development, July 1999, para.[17]

[97] The Home Office and Department of Health Discussion Document, Managing dangerous people with a severe personality disorder: proposals for policy development, July 1999, refers to the 'enthusiasm and optimism dating from the 1940s and 1950s for treating people with personality disorder having given way over the past 15 years to greater realism as it has become apparent that outcomes relating to reduction in risk, improvements in quality of life, and social integration remain uncertain.

[98] Mental Health Act 1959, Section 26.

[99] Mental Health Act 1959, Section 44.

but which persist within contemporary psychiatry.[100] Dr Bennett MP referred to the requirement in the definition of psychopath that the patient's condition must be susceptible to treatment and remarked that so far as he could make out the treatment was 'custodial'. 'Perhaps', he continued, 'the treatment intended for the psychopath is simply ageing in custody, in which case it seems unnecessary to commit him to hospital'.[101] Dr Bennett also referred to the disruptive influence of psychopaths in hospitals. 'No hospital can stand more than one or two psychopaths in the whole hospital, let alone in one ward. The whole place becomes a bear garden. They put the other chaps up to tricks and they are frightfully clever at finding out bright ideas for perhaps the duller members of the community or the more disturbed ones'.[102] Indeed many who spoke advocated the development of separate specialist units for psychopaths on these very grounds.[103] The 1983 Act abolished the age limits and introduced a new treatability test, that medical treatment must be likely to alleviate or prevent deterioration in the patient's condition. Hence the question became one of pure clinical judgement for psychiatrists.

One of the hopes expressed during the debates on the 1959 Act was that the introduction of psychopathy into the legislation would enable this group to be identified and worked with and medical science to develop effective treatment interventions. Kenneth Robinson MP welcomed the fact that 'at last the nettle had been grasped':

> The Bill makes a great stride forward, in that it enables patients to be placed for the first time in a category. Hitherto we have been thinking and talking of psychopaths as a kind of spectrum of behaviour disorders, a word meaning different things to different psychiatrists. Now at any rate we have a definition of a certain kind which will enable a certain amount of isolation and categorisation to take place. That will facilitate, and for the first time make possible social and clinical research into these cases.[104]

This hope has not been realized, and 40 years later the same nettle fails to be grasped. The Government's proposals for dangerous people with severe personality disorders (DSPD) express the view that 'psychiatrists are poorly equipped by training' to deal with this group, and 'most psychiatrists are reluctant to recommend that dangerous people with severe personality disorder should be admitted to hospital unless they also suffer from mental illness'. The current Government proposals are based on the same

---

[100] Cope, R. (1993) A survey of forensic psychiatrists' views on psychopathic disorder. *Journal of Forensic Psychiatry*, **4**, 227–229; Lewis, A. (1974) Psychopathic personality: a most elusive category. *Psychological Medicine*, **4**, 133–40; Collins, P. (1991) The treatability of psychopaths. *Journal of Forensic Psychiatry*, **2**, 103–110.

[101] Hansard HC Debs Series 5, Vol. 598, col. 783–784, 26 January 1959.

[102] *Ibid.*

[103] Dr Bennett MP argued for the establishment of some special sort of accommodation and Mr Iremonger MP advocated the establishment of small pilot units for the treatment of the intelligent psychopath. Hansard HC Debs Series 5, Vol. 605, 6 May 1959 col. 423 and 432.

[104] Hansard HC Debs Series 5, Vol. 605, 6 May 1959 col. 434.

premise as their forbears, namely that a prerequisite of the development of 'robust' national assessment criteria and effective treatment interventions is the introduction of powers to detain this group.

The Government's proposals in relation to people with DSPD are basically designed to provide authority for their detention on the basis of the risk they present and, if necessary, for that detention to be indefinite.[105] In order to ensure that these changes comply with the European Convention on Human Rights, detention would be based on evidence from an intensive, specialist assessment and would be subject to a process of appeal and regular review. If a DSPD individual is before the courts on remand or following conviction the court will be able to refer him or her for specialist assessment where there is evidence of mental disorder from preliminary psychiatric reports and evidence from the police or probation service of risk to the public.

In the case of individuals not currently before the courts, prisoners, offenders under statutory supervision and others, referral for specialist assessment will be made in what the Government calls 'civil proceedings' and will be subject to appeal. The main target group is probably prisoners who are due to come out of prison after a determinate sentence and who present a significant risk. Referral will be on the basis of prior psychiatric reports together with evidence of probable risk. Evidence of risk will be presented to a Mental Disorder Tribunal through reports from the police, probation or prison service. In time such evidence is likely to come from the local multi-agency public protection panels and risk panels that are being set up around the country as part of the overall management of risky populations.

The Government puts forward two options. Both rely on the development of 'new, more rigorous, procedures for assessing risk associated with presence of severe personality disorder'. Under each option the specific aim is to ensure that the arrangements for detention and management focus on reducing these risks. Both options involve closing off the possibility of the hospital order for a DSPD offender. Hospital orders will be reserved for mentally ill and mentally impaired people. This will avoid the problem that Mental Health Review Tribunals are obliged to discharge psychopathically disordered patients if they consider that medical treatment for their disorder is unlikely to alleviate or prevent deterioration in the patient's condition.

In terms of powers for the criminal courts, Option A would encourage greater use of the discretionary life sentence by improving the quality of information available to the courts and extending its availability to a wider range of offences, and providing new powers for remand and specialist assessment. Legislation would be 'strengthened' to ensure that prisoners identified as DSPD would not be released at the end of their sentence.

For non-offender patients the 'treatability' requirement for detention and renewal of

---

[105] The Home Office and Department of Health Discussion Document, Managing dangerous people with a severe personality disorder: proposals for policy development, July 1999, p. 13.

detention would be removed and new powers would be introduced for compulsory supervision and recall of DSPD individuals following discharge from detention.

In terms of service provision, services would be provided within the prison and hospital systems, including the creation of better specialist facilities and better procedures for assessment and court reporting. Specialist facilities would be established within the prison and health services (potentially including independent sector providers) and drawn closer together, for example by ring fencing funding and setting up one central agency to commission services for DSPD individuals in both the prison service and the health service.

The general tenor of the document leads to the conclusion that Option B is the preferred course. This involves the creation of new institutions, neither hospital nor prison, 'a third way.' A new specialist service would be set up, separate from, but with close links to, the prison service. These specialist units would contain 50 beds with 8–12 to a ward. Option B involves powers for the indeterminate detention of dangerous severely personality disordered people in both criminal and civil proceedings. Those detained under the new orders would be managed in facilities run separately from prison and health service provision. The location for detention would be based on the risk that the person presented and their therapeutic needs, rather than whether they had been convicted of an offence.

If there was evidence that an offender was suffering from a severe personality disorder and as a consequence presented a serious risk to the public, the offender could be remanded for assessment in a specialist facility. The disposal would be subject to appeal and periodic review. A DSPD direction could be attached to any sentence passed by the higher courts, except mandatory life sentences which are fixed by law (analogous to the existing procedures for making a hospital direction under Section 45A of the 1983 Mental Health Act). The effect of a DSPD direction would be that the offender would be detained in a specialist facility until such time as they were no longer considered to present a serious risk on the grounds of their disorder. At that point they would be released into the community or returned to prison to serve the remainder of their sentence. Release to the community would be subject to formal supervision and, as necessary, compliance with specified conditions. A person who had been detained on a DSPD direction would be liable to recall for further assessment. Sentenced prisoners, including those subject to mandatory life sentences, could be referred for consideration of making a DSPD order at any time during their term of imprisonment. Such an order would be made under the non-offender procedures and would result in the transfer of the individual from prison to specialist facilities.

In these cases, the DSPD order would be made by the Mental Disorder Tribunal under the non-offender provisions of the legislation. It would be subject to appeal and periodic review. The order would be available on the basis of evidence that the individual was suffering from a severe personality disorder and as a consequence of the disorder presented a serious risk to the public. A DSPD order could only be made following a period of compulsory assessment in a specialist facility. The effect of an order would be that the individual would be detained in a specialist facility until such time as they were no longer considered to present a serious risk on grounds of their disorder and could (subject to any necessary supervision) be released safely into the community; but there would be provision for transfer elsewhere for treatment of other mental disorders if necessary. A person who had been detained on a DSPD order would remain liable to recall into detention for further assessment.

These proposals effectively replace treatment with risk management. The treatability test will disappear for personality disorder to be replaced by risk assessment and risk management. The references to rigorous, robust etc. methods of assessment and management are necessary to achieve 'Convention compliance' because the only ground on which people who have not committed any offence, or who are coming out of prison after a determinate sentence, will be detained is 'unsoundness of mind' (Article 5(1)(e)). This means there must be objective evidence of unsoundness of mind which goes beyond mere deviance from society's norms. The international diagnostic manuals of mental disorder are replete with categories of personality disorder, so this requirement will be satisfied.

In 1998 in *Aerts v Belgium*[106] the European Court of Human Rights held that, where the sole basis of detention is unsoundness of mind (Article 5(1)(e)), an anti-therapeutic environment may contravene Article 5(1), even if it is not severe enough to amount to inhuman and degrading treatment. Mr Aerts was arrested in November 1992 after attacking his ex-wife with a hammer. In January 1993 a Belgian Court ordered his detention in an institution to be designated by the relevant mental health board and specified that, pending the Board's decision, he was to be provisionally held in the psychiatric wing at Lantin Prison. He remained in prison until October 1993, even though a clinic had been designated in March.

Aerts complained of breaches of Article 3 and Article 5(1). The prison psychiatric wing where he was had been criticized in 1994 by the European Committee for the Prevention of Torture and Inhuman and Degrading Treatment as unsuitable for the care of people with mental health problems, since there was neither regular medical attention nor a therapeutic environment. Nevertheless, the Court followed the line adopted in previous case law on Article 3, adopting a very strict view of the level of severity required to bring ill treatment under the umbrella of inhuman and degrading treatment. The Committee for the Prevention of Torture had found the standard of care at the prison fell below the minimum acceptable from an ethical and humanitarian point of view and that prolonging patients' detention there for lengthy periods carried an undeniable risk of deterioration in their mental health. However, the Court held that there was no proof of deterioration in the applicant's mental health. The living conditions in the prison did not seem to have had such serious effects on his mental

---

[106] Judgement of European Court of Human Rights 30 July 1998.

health as to bring them within Article 3. They did not reach the level of severity necessary to amount to inhuman or degrading treatment.

The most interesting feature of the Court's ruling from the point of view of advancing the idea of the right to therapy came in relation to the Article 5(1) complaint regarding his detention in the psychiatric wing of the prison after the March 1993 decision to detain him in the clinic. The Court upheld this complaint because the proper relationship between the aim of the detention and the conditions in which it took place had been deficient. As he had not been convicted of any offence, his detention could not be justified under Article 5(1)(a). The only permissible justification left was Article 5(1)(e)—detention on grounds of unsoundness of mind. The Court held that there had to be some relationship between the ground of permitted deprivation of liberty relied on and the place and conditions of detention. In principle, the detention of a person as a mental health patient would only be lawful for the purposes of Article 5(1)(e) if effected in a hospital, clinic or other appropriate institution. In Aerts' case the Belgian Mental Health Board had expressed the view that the situation was harmful to him, as he was not receiving the treatment required by the condition giving rise to detention. Obviously, standards and conditions will have to fall very low indeed for the therapeutic purpose to be destroyed. However, it seems now that where the detention is based on Article 5(1)(e) alone, complaints about conditions and the absence of basic therapeutic standards in the place of detention are better brought under Article 5 than Article 3.

The question with the 'third way' institutions is whether they are genuinely offering therapy which has some prospect of reducing the risk to a level where the DSPD person can be released, or whether the primary purpose is to achieve a form of indefinite preventive detention. Undoubtedly, if there were a humane environment and if some scientific therapeutic efforts were being made there would be no risk of the Aerts ruling applying, although we should remember that the convention rights are a floor, not a ceiling. This is what makes the development of the necessary science to offer effective therapy a pressing imperative.

Conclusion

The proposed arrangements for DSPD individuals represent the apotheosis of the cross fertilization of risk management and therapeutic strategies between the penal and the psychiatric systems which we have described as a convergence. They would allow the indefinite detention usually associated with the psychiatric system but without the tiresome requirement of treatability. The need for risk management is enough. The proposals would also ensure that the psychiatric system would effectively be closed off to these people, yet they would be receiving treatment for their riskiness in 'third way' institutions. Dangerous people with severe personality disorder would also be liable to recall into detention indefinitely.

The convergence of the penal and the psychiatric systems continues apace, and the ethical dilemma for psychiatrists is where they draw the boundary between therapy and preventive detention or 'growing old in custody'. We conclude by offering some observations on the development of a model of community care along the lines of Jeremy Bentham's Panopticon, the model upon which both the penitentiary and the asylum system were based, where a large number of inmates could be supervised with relative ease from a central point. The new system into which we are moving is increasingly characterized by controls exercised from an institutional base where patients can be detained if necessary and where they can be brought by force by specialist teams of paramedics for compulsory treatment. Those posing a risk will be tracked in the community. Supervisors in the community will assume responsibility for ensuring that patients receive community care.

What are the likely consequences of the convergence we have described in terms of the relationship between therapist and patient? Increasingly, psychiatrists are becoming involved in decision making about risk in the penal system, whether sitting as medical members of the various panels of the Parole Board or giving expert evidence on risk before those panels. The modernized CPA suggests a significant role for the police in what has traditionally been health and social care decision making about risk management and community care. Confidentiality has always been open to exceptions, both at national law and under the European Convention. The ethics of health care are based around the primacy of therapy (primum non nocere) and key notions such as respect for autonomy, informed consent and confidentiality. The ethics of criminal justice and risk management afford primacy to deterrence, retributivism, social protection, information sharing, selective incapacitation and recognition of the rights of victims. The erosion of the boundaries between the medical world with its values and the criminal justice system with its own very different concerns results in the concept of confidentiality being redefined to accommodate the information sharing requirements of effective risk management.

There can be no more vivid illustration of the primacy of risk management than the personality disorder proposals. What makes them so interesting is that therapy is so far behind risk management that it is almost out of sight. Frantic efforts are under way to agree what DSPD is, with debates about how many different DSM-1V categories of personality disorder have to be present to merit the appellation 'severe'. What about the dangerous person without a personality disorder, or is it to be taken as given that all really nasty and risky people have a disordered personality?

The proposal to remove the treatability criterion from the conditions for renewable detention of DSPD individuals comes at a time when the treatability criterion is legally at its widest following the *Reid* decision. The Government's worry appears to be that, however broad the concept may be legally, clinicians cannot be relied upon to certify that the 'risky' are even personality disordered, let alone treatable. Their proposals purport to be offering treatment, but do not require treatability. National protocols are being developed for the identification and treatment of severe personality disorder. The proposed 'third way' institutions offer the certainty of risk management, but only the possibility of therapy. The 'third way' institutions are based on ideas of incapacitating or 'taking out'. The primary goal is to achieve the possibility of indeterminate detention of the risky and the secondary goal of therapy, as evidenced by the 'detain now, develop the science on the hoof' approach adopted by the Government. A cynic might say that the main product of all this will be the indeterminate detention of significant numbers of people with personality disorders, a more sophisticated taxonomy of the untreatable, but little by way of significant therapeutic advances.

The personality disorder debate has rekindled the age-old controversy about the relationship between psychiatry and the state. English law describes the psychiatrist in charge of a detained patient's treatment as the RMO. The RMO has the power to renew detention. If the family seek to discharge the patient from detention, the RMO has the power to block discharge on grounds of the patient's likely dangerousness to self or others. The RMO's role, even for a 'civilly' detained patient, involves the exercise of state authority, the power to detain. Effective psychiatric therapy of people who require detention involves a strong element of risk management, because of the nature and consequences of mental disorder. The kaleidoscopic mix between risk management requirements and therapeutic values is constantly changing. As one moves across the spectrum from those whose primary risk is to themselves to those who pose a severe risk of danger to others, the balance between therapeutic values and risk management imperatives alters in subtle ways. These tensions are inherent in psychiatry. Psychiatrists, insofar as they are RMOs, exercise public functions in relation to the renewal of detention. Therefore they will be public authorities for the purposes of the 1988 Human Rights Act. Therefore they will be required to act compatibly with Convention rights.

Lurking not far from the surface of every psychiatrist/patient relationship is a potential tension between psychiatrists' therapeutic duty, essentially individual patient-centred, and their more public, collectively oriented, role as risk manager in protecting society. Often the circle is easily squared by the argument that it cannot be in the therapeutic interests of a patient if he or she is prematurely released and commits criminal offences. But often it will involve more complex calculations such as whether the level of assessed risk justifies a breach of medical confidence. The contours of the doctor–patient relationship are being steadily altered to accommodate the demands of state penal policy. The legal and policy developments described above reveal one pre-eminent master. Risk management dominates every aspect of community care policy towards mentally disordered people in general, and mentally disordered offenders in particular.

Index